Contents

List of Boxes

List of Figures

List of Tables

Preface

THE WORLD BANK IS ACTIVELY ENGAGED in supporting pension policymakers worldwide. As part of this ongoing effort, in 1994 the Bank published *Averting the Old Age Crisis,* a book that reflected a massive research effort on the economics and political economy of pension reform. Recently, the Bank launched the "Pension Primer" to help governments design and implement reforms. The Bank's Pension Reform Options Simulation Toolkit (PROST), which is used in more than 50 countries, has become a standard actuarial software for quantitative analysis.

Given the impact of the multipillar approach proposed in *Averting the Old Age Crisis*—and the diversity of its implementation—the fifth anniversary of the book seemed a particularly auspicious moment to reexamine both the evidence and the thinking on pensions and retirement security. When the Bank convened the New Ideas about Old Age Security conference in September 1999, its purpose was to summarize developments in pension reform that had taken place in the late 1990s so that they could be incorporated into the second-generation reforms many countries were contemplating. The selected and revised conference papers comprising this book represent a sample of the most recent thinking in the global debate over pension reform.

Acknowledgments

MANY PEOPLE INSIDE AND OUTSIDE the World Bank supported the conference preparation and the revision and editing of the papers. We would like to thank in particular Louise Fox, Estelle James and Peter Orszag for their conceptual inputs and editorial support; David Ellerman and Joanne Lee for their help in organizing the conference; the participants in the conference for their comments on the papers presented; and Ian Mac Arthur for organizing and handling the revisions and editing of the conference volume in such a superb manner.

List of Contributors

Max Alier works for the Western Hemisphere Department of the International Monetary Fund. At the time his paper was written he was with the Fiscal Affairs Department. His work has focused mainly on fiscal policy issues, including social security arrangements and fiscal policy sustainability.

Axel Börsch-Supan is professor of economics at the University of Mannheim, Germany, and member of the scientific advisory board of the German ministry of economy. He has published widely on German and international pension reform issues.

Sarah Brooks is a graduate student in political science at Duke University. Her research in international and comparative political economy centers on the politics of institutional reform in developing countries. Her dissertation examines the political economy of pension reform in Latin America.

Paulette Castel has been working for the World Bank since 1994 in the area of poverty reduction and economic management in transition economies. She holds a doctorate in economics from the Sorbonne, Paris. Ms. Castel advised the government of Kyrgyz on the reform of its pension system. She is currently working on the evaluation of fiscal, macro, and micro aspects of pension reforms in several countries in the Eastern Europe and Central Asia region.

Jose Cuesta is an economist at the Oxford University conducting research on the impact of social transfers—education and health—on income distribution and labor supply in Chile. He has worked in the economics department of Universidad de Chile and the United Nations Economic Commission for Latin America and the Caribbean in Santiago. He is currently working for the United Nations Development Program in Honduras.

Peter Diamond, professor at the Massachusetts Institute of Technology, is a key figure in international and U.S. pension reform discussion. He has been a member of many research and policy panels and has written extensively on the economic foundation of social security issues.

Kshama Fernandes, of Goa University, has worked on the issues of index fund management, performance comparisons between active and passive management, and VAR estimation in equity and currency markets.

Louise Fox is one of the World Bank's senior specialists in social sector economics. She has provided policy advice to governments and led teams involved in policy analysis and preparation of investment projects supporting social sector reform. Her research has examined poverty, income distribution, and adjustment in Brazil; female-headed households and child welfare; and social sector reforms in transition economies.

Joaquin Gutierrez is currently manager of the Latin American Group of the Bank of Spain, in charge of supervising the overall activities of large Spanish conglomerates in Latin America. From 1989 to 1998 he was a financial advisor in the World Bank and worked on financial sector programs and operations in Latin America, Central Europe, and Africa. His responsibilities included bank restructuring, development of legal and regulatory frameworks for banking and banking supervision, and the creation of training programs for country supervisors. From 1976 to 1989 he was bank examiner in the Bank of Spain, which involved all core supervisory functions: off-site surveillance unit (team leader), examination (inspector chief), and policy research leading to regulatory development.

Richard Hinz is the Director of the Office of Policy and Research of the Pension and Welfare Benefits Administration (PWBA) of the U.S. Department of Labor. He manages a program of policy and legislative analysis on issues related to the development, regulation, and supervision of the private employee benefits system in the United States. His organization supports the Department of Labor's policy and legislative initiatives on pension and health care issues, publishes statistics on employer-sponsored benefits, conducts economic analysis of proposed regulatory actions, and provides economic research on a range of private employee benefits issues.

Robert Holzmann is director of the Social Protection unit of the Human Development Network of the World Bank, a unit that, among other things, is in charge of conceptual and strategic thinking in the area of social risk management, including pensions. He has published widely on pension issues and has been involved in pension reforms in many countries. While working for the Organization for Economic Cooperation and Development, he wrote a comprehensive report on pension reform, and while working for the International Monetary Fund he was involved in fiscal and pension reform issues in Eastern Europe. He is on leave of absence from the University of Saarland (Germany) where he is professor of economics and director of the European Institute. His research includes public finance, international economics, European integration, and economics of transition.

Augusto Iglesias is the director of PrimAmérica Consultores, based in Santiago, Chile. He has written extensively on pension reform in Chile and in the last decade has worked on pension reforms in Egypt, Romania, Macedonia, and many Latin American countries.

Estelle James is currently director of the Flagship Course on Pension Reform at the World Bank Institute. She was previously lead economist in the Policy Research Department at the World Bank. Ms. James is principal author of *Averting the Old Age Crisis: Policies to Protect the Old and Promote Growth*, a World Bank study providing the first global analysis of economic problems associated with population aging. Since the publication of this book, she has given numerous presentations on public pension plans at scholarly meetings, conferences for government officials, think tanks, and financial institutions. Her recent research has focused on social security reform, including the political economy of the reform process, administrative costs of individual account systems, and the impact of population aging on health care systems. Before joining the World Bank in 1991, she was professor of economics at the State University of New York, Stony Brook, where she also served as chair of the Economics Department and provost, Social and Behavioral Sciences.

Mamta Murthi is research fellow in economics at Clare Hall, Cambridge University. Her work is supported by the John D. and Catherine T. MacArthur Foundation's Network on Inequality and Poverty in Broader Perspectives. She was formerly an economist at the World Bank.

J. Michael Orszag is lecturer in economics at Birkbeck College, University of London. His research focuses on pensions, personnel economics, and social insurance.

Peter R. Orszag is president of Sebago Associates, Inc., an economics and public policy consulting firm, and a lecturer in macroeconomics at the University of California, Berkeley. Before founding Sebago Associates, Mr. Orszag served as special assistant to the president for economic policy at the White House. He has also served as an economic adviser to the government of Russia, and as senior economist and senior adviser on the President's Council of Economic Advisers.

Robert J. Palacios is senior pension economist at the World Bank. A member of the team that produced *Averting the Old Age Crisis: Policies to Protect the Old and Promote Growth* in 1994, Mr. Palacios has written extensively on topics in pension reform. He has also been involved in pension reform operations in many countries, having worked for several years with the Hungarian government on their pathbreaking pension reform in 1997. He is currently working in Korea and India and manages a working paper series called the Pension Reform Primer. The Primer papers and notes can be found at www.worldbank.org/pensions.

Edward Palmer heads the Division for Research and Evaluation at the Swedish National Social Insurance Board and serves as professor of social insurance economics at Uppsala University. He received a doctorate in economics from Stockholm University. Mr. Palmer has written extensively on a variety of topics in the fields of household consumption and saving, social insurance, and income distribution. He has worked as an adviser on pension reform in countries such as Sweden, Latvia, Poland, and Russia.

Truman Packard is an economist working with the Social Protection unit in the Latin America and Caribbean Regional Office of the World Bank. Truman was trained at the University of Oxford and has worked on social security and pension reform projects in Argentina, Uruguay, Mexico and Brazil. He is conducting research, initiated with the Social Risk Management Survey (PRIESO) in Santiago, Chile, focused on coverage of social insurance, household saving and investment, and labor market efficiency in countries that have established individual retirement savings accounts.

Roberto Rocha, a Brazilian citizen, finished his graduate studies at the Vargas Foundation in Brazil and at the Massachusetts Institute of Technology. He has taught at the Vargas Foundation and served as a financial consultant for Brazilian banks. Mr. Rocha has worked at the International Monetary Fund, and since 1985 has worked for the World Bank primarily on issues of macroeconomic and financial sector reforms in transition countries, writing numerous articles pertaining to these areas. In 1993 he moved to the World Bank's regional office in Central Europe, located in Budapest, as a lead economist. Since then, Mr. Rocha has led the World Bank's work in the areas of financial sector reform and pension reform in several Central European countries.

Ajay Shah, of the Indira Gandhi Institute for Development Research, works in the areas of index construction, index funds, risk measurement, market microstructure, policy issues in securities markets, and pension reform. He has worked on several real-world efforts in developing stock market indexes, launching index funds and exchange-traded stock index derivatives, and creating reference rates from dealer markets. Apart from academic research, he has been closely associated with policy formulation in the financial sector in India, and has done consulting work for numerous brokerage firms and money managers in several countries.

James Smalhout is a visiting fellow at the Hudson Institute and the author of *The Uncertain Retirement: Securing Pension Promises in a World of Risk*. He has worked as a financial analyst at the Pension Benefit Guaranty Corporation and as an economist at the Federal Reserve Board of Governors. His previous research focused on private pensions, financial guarantees, and the economics of individual retirement accounts. Mr. Smalhout is a contributing editor of *Euromoney Magazine* and writes often for the business and financial press.

Joseph E. Stiglitz currently works at the Brookings Institution. He was formerly senior vice president of development economics and chief economist at the World Bank. From June 1995 until he joined the World Bank, Mr. Stiglitz was chairman of the President's Council of Economic Advisers and, from 1993, a member of the Council. He is presently on leave from Stanford University, where he is the Joan Kenney Professor of Economics. Previously, Mr. Stiglitz was a professor of economics at Princeton and Yale universities and All Souls College, Oxford University. He is a fellow of the National Academy of Sciences, the American Academy of Arts and Sciences, and the American Philosophical Society, as well as a corresponding fellow of the British Academy.

Salvador Valdés-Prieto is professor of economics at the Catholic University of Santiago de Chile and one of the Latin American key researchers on pension issues. He has written extensively about the Chilean pension reform, published "The Economics of Pensions" in 1997, and served as an advisor on pension reforms in Latin American and East Asian countries.

Dimitri Vittas works with the Research Development Group of the World Bank. He specializes in financial sector issues, especially the promotion and regulation of pension funds, insurance companies, and mutual funds. Mr. Vittas served as a member of the team that produced the 1989 *World Development Report* on "Financial Systems and Development" and the 1994 World Bank report *Averting the Old Age Crisis: Policies to Protect the Old and Promote Growth*.

Jan Walliser is an economist in the Fiscal Affairs Department of the International Monetary Fund. Between 1996 and 1998, he was a fiscal policy analyst at the U.S. Congressional Budget Office. Mr. Walliser received a doctorate in economics from Boston University in 1998 and a Diplom-Volkswirt degree from Kiel University, Germany, in 1993. He has been an author and coauthor of several articles on intergenerational redistribution through fiscal policy, tax reform, macroeconomic aspects of pension reform, and annuitization of retirement income.

Introduction

Robert Holzmann and Joseph E. Stiglitz

POLICYMAKERS ACROSS THE GLOBE are struggling to adapt their pension systems to the reality of aging populations, globalization, and tightening budgets. The World Bank is actively engaged in supporting these policymakers, from helping them to identify the economic and demographic challenges facing their countries to highlighting potential policy responses and providing implementation support.

Averting the Old Age Crisis, published in 1994, advocated a multipillar approach to pension reform. The multipillar system includes an unfunded mandatory pillar, a funded mandatory pillar, and a voluntary private pillar. The book was influential in focusing the minds of policymakers worldwide and in providing support to politicians who have thought independently in the same direction. This led to a spread of multipillar pension systems, which many countries throughout the world have adopted, including Argentina, Bolivia, Columbia, Hungary, Kazakhstan, Latvia, Poland, Sweden, and Uruguay.

As it emerged, the World Bank's multipillar pension reform approach became a benchmark rather than a blueprint, and the World Bank has supported different approaches in different countries despite the perception that it favors a specific approach (Holzmann 2000). For example, in Lithuania, the World Bank helped the government fashion and implement a relatively modest pay-as-you-go scheme with a redistributional formula; continues to work with the government in developing the regulatory framework for voluntary supplementary schemes; and has left to the future the decision of a mandatory funded pillar. The Bank suggests a similar route for the old Bulgarian, the young Korean, and the nascent Thai unfunded schemes. In Latvia the reform has taken the path of a notional defined contribution system, with a very modest funded add-on under preparation. In

1

Hungary and Poland, the mandatory funded component will deliver about one-third to one-half of the total replacement rate. In Kazakhstan the reform completely replaced the pay-as-you-go scheme with a funded scheme, and Bolivia, Mexico, and Peru are adopting a similar approach. The reforms in Argentina and Costa Rica favor a two-pillar approach.

Given the impact of the proposed multipillar approach and the diversity in its implementation, the fifth anniversary of *Averting the Old Age Crisis* seemed a particularly auspicious moment to reexamine the evidence and thinking on pensions and retirement security. While helping countries to design and implement pension reforms, Bank staff encountered many issues that required looking anew at basic old questions and addressing many new ones. The 1999 conference, New Ideas about Old Age Security, and this resulting volume examine global issues on pension reform that help put in perspective three major sets of pension reform questions.

A first set of questions deals with generic issues that concern policymakers worldwide, almost independently of approaches to reform. Perhaps most prominent but also least understood are the economic policy questions regarding the economic circumstances that are most conducive to the initiation of a reform and to its eventual success. Equally important are questions relating to the coverage of the labor force under a reformed system. While it was expected that a reformed system would induce workers in the informal sector to join the formal sector (since distortions were presumably reduced), these expectations have not been realized in most instances. Other questions concern the distributive effects of reformed systems with respect to generation, income group, and gender.

A second set of questions is linked with a move toward funded provisions under a multipillar approach. The high administrative costs of privately managed, defined contribution accounts (also referred to as *individual accounts*) in many countries figure prominently in the academic and political discussion. A related set of concerns involves the cost of annuitizing accumulated assets upon retirement. In addition, the recent global financial crisis has focused attention on the problems of income security under individual account systems, especially when funds are invested in high-volatility markets. As a result of such volatility, the replacement rate (during retirement) for a given contribution rate (during a working career) may differ substantially among individuals contributing and retiring at different times.

A third set of questions concerns the multipillar reform approach itself. A wide consensus has emerged inside and outside the World Bank about the multipillar framework, and it now includes the International Labor Office, which in the past has been rather cautious on the topic (Gillion 2000). But that consensus does not extend to several key issues regarding how the framework should be implemented in practice. The first issue relates to the size of the second pillar and, indeed, whether a mandated, second, funded and privately managed pillar is needed at all. Can a reformed first, unfunded pillar and a third pillar with funded but voluntary (and, perhaps, tax-preferred provisions) achieve the objectives of a sustainable and equitable pension system? Another issue involves the nature of the second pillar. While it has widely been assumed that the second prefunded pillar should be privately managed, the large transaction costs, difficulties of regulating private providers, lack of sophisticated financial education even in advanced countries, and existence of efficient public trust funds (for example, in Denmark and the United States) have led some observers to urge consideration of a publicly managed second pillar. Other observers note the far-from-stellar performance of publicly managed funds in most other countries that have them. There are also questions about the first pillar: most importantly, how can pension systems create a sustainable unfunded pillar? Several countries are undertaking experiments with notional defined contribution schemes, in which workers have individual "accounts" within a pay-as-you-go system.

In many of these areas, a key question is whether we should examine average experience or best practices. Can developing countries learn from those that have had the most successful experiences in managing public trust funds or in reducing administrative costs on individual accounts? Or are the problems associated with public malfeasance on the one hand, or administrative costs on the other, inherent in public or private approaches respectively? What is inherent and what is avoidable?

This introduction provides a short summary for each of the chapters in the volume and concludes with a discussion of policy issues—the main areas of agreement and disagreement—and on areas requiring further research.

The Costs and Benefits of a Privately Managed Second Pillar

The first chapter, written by Peter Orszag and Joseph Stiglitz, provides an overall perspective on pension reform issues and delineates a series of myths that the authors claim have been used to advocate one specific approach to multipillar reform. The authors argue that policymakers have too often interpreted the multipillar system as requiring that the second, funded pillar entail private management and defined contributions (an "individual account" approach). In contrast, Orszag and Stiglitz defend a more expansive view of the second pillar, involving public (as well as private) management and defined benefit (as well as defined contribution) funded plans.

Orszag and Stiglitz emphasize four distinct aspects of pension reform that are often combined in privately managed, defined contribution pension systems: (i) *privatization*, in which a privately managed pension system replaces a publicly run one; (ii) *prefunding*, which entails the accumulation of assets against future pension payments;[1] (iii) *diversification*, which involves allowing investments in a variety of assets, rather than government bonds alone; and (iv) *defined benefit versus defined contribution plans*, which concerns the assignment of accrual risk to the sponsor or individual worker, respectively. The key point, according to Orszag and Stiglitz, is that any combination of these four elements is possible, and that individual account proposals typically wrap them all together rather than allowing a choice on each component separately.

The authors also highlight the importance of clarifying which elements of any pension system are inherent to that specific system and which elements are merely common in how that system has been implemented in practice. Comparing an idealized version of individual accounts to an as-implemented version of public, defined benefit plans is not likely to prove insightful, yet many discussions of individual accounts do just that. It would be better to determine which elements of public, defined benefit systems are inherent and which reflect less-than-optimal implementation and then factor out the latter before undertaking the comparison to a similarly "optimized" privately managed, defined contribution system.

The chapter by Orszag and Stiglitz emphasizes that in evaluating the effect of pension reform, initial conditions are important. In particular, one must be careful not to confuse the issue of whether a shift to individual accounts would be socially beneficial with the separate issue of whether, in a tabula rasa sense, an individual account system would have been preferable to a public, defined benefit system in the first place. For many countries, initial choices have largely been made, and it makes little sense to ignore those decisions in analyzing pension reforms.

The chapter then discusses 10 of the myths that Orszag and Stiglitz believe are present in many discussions of individual accounts. Underlying their analysis of these myths is the role of incentives and behavior at the individual and macro levels. For instance, the relationship between what an individual contributes (whether under an individual account or under a standard public program) and the benefit received primarily determines work incentives. It is this relationship, not whether the system is funded or not, publicly run or not, that matters most for labor market incentives. To be sure, under many public, unfunded programs, the relationship between contributions and benefits distorts incentives.

Despite this disadvantage, public programs typically incorporate important elements of insurance, which, while they may deleteriously affect incentives, have generally had markedly positive welfare benefits in and of themselves. If markets worked well (and insurance markets are notoriously imperfect), individuals might actually choose to purchase the insurance provided by public plans, which would affect their behavior just as the publicly provided "insurance" does. For example, individuals may not know when they will be unable to work effectively—not so disabled that they qualify for public disability, but with a declined productivity that diminishes the pleasure they receive from the work, which then affects their choice between leisure and work. Many workers may want to purchase insurance against this risk. But currently, while social insurance provides some insurance of this type, most private markets do not. Removing some of the insurance provided under public plans may increase labor supply, but the objective of public policy is to maximize social welfare, not to maximize work. Eliminating insurance components that limit labor supply may not necessarily enhance welfare, particularly when broader distributional concerns enter the analysis. A careful delineation of the underlying reasons for government programs—including an analysis of the underlying market failures—is therefore not only essential in designing pension reforms, but may also suggest complementary reforms (such as in capital markets and their regulation or in the government provision of insurance, for example, through indexed bonds or disability insurance).

The authors conclude that the debate over pension reform would benefit substantially from a more expansive view of the optimal second pillar, which should incorporate well-designed, funded, public, defined benefit plans. Such a perspective would allow policymakers to weigh appropriately all the trade-offs they face, including private versus public systems; prefunding versus not prefunding; diversification versus nondiversification; and defined contribution versus defined benefit pension plans.

The commentators on the Orszag-Stiglitz chapter hold markedly different positions. Peter Diamond of the Massachusetts Institute of Technology agrees with all 10 myths in the chapter; he writes that the "the economic and political advantages of defined contribution individual accounts have been exaggerated." He goes on to add an 11th myth, that defined contribution schemes are often claimed to be more "transparent" than defined benefit schemes.

Robert Holzmann of the World Bank, in contrast, argues that the myths were misleading because of the way in which they were formulated and because many of the issues have been long recognized within and outside the Bank. He points out that since the publication of *Averting the Old Age Crisis*, countries and the World Bank have progressed in their thinking and pension reform implementation, which already reflect the differentiation and sophistication that Orszag and Stiglitz claim should exist in the field.

Estelle James of the World Bank starts by emphasizing the substantial shift toward consensus on many points, including the desirability of some

degree of prefunding, the recognition that prefunding is a different concept
than privatization, and that we should look at systems in practice, not only
systems in theory. She then notes several points of disagreement with the
Orszag-Stiglitz chapter, particularly with regard to the political economy
judgements that underlie some of the so-called myths. In effect, she agrees
with Orszag and Stiglitz that the World Bank indeed has a specific perspective on how to undertake pension reforms but stresses that sufficient
evidence exists to support that position.

Axel Börsch-Supan from the University of Mannheim argues that the
core question is whether prefunding should be done publicly or privately. The fundamental disagreement in the debate, according to Börsch-
Supan, involves the decisions regarding which choices to leave to the people and which choices the government should undertake on their behalf.

Salvador Valdés-Prieto from the Catholic University of Santiago de
Chile focuses on the differences between pension reform in the advanced,
industrialized economies and developing economies. For the latter, he
argues that the standard interpretation of *Averting the Old Age Crisis*—that
the second pillar should include a privately managed, defined contribution
scheme—is still valid.

New Approaches to Multipillar Pension Systems

The chapter by Louise Fox and Edward Palmer begins with a brief survey
of pension reform developments since the publication of *Averting the Old
Age Crisis* and concludes that the late 1990s was a period of blossoming
innovation. The largely unfunded debt of pay-as-you-go systems is challenging countries with very diverse historical backgrounds to find solutions
to financing income support for their aging populations in the coming
decades. They are retooling single-pillar, defined benefit schemes to meet
these challenges.

The chapter identifies three major emerging trends in pension reform in
the 1990s. First, countries are modifying pay-as-you-go systems to strength-
en the links between contributions and benefits, increase full-benefit pension ages, and phase out seniority arrangements and special privileges. The
notional defined contribution system is the newest tool to achieve this
goal, and countries in Western Europe (Italy and Sweden) and those with
economies in transition (China, the Kyrgyz Republic, Latvia, Mongolia, and
Poland) have adopted this approach. Second, privately managed individual
account systems are growing. Third, countries with large pension debts are
finding it difficult to finance a transition to more funding. These countries
are not aspiring to full funding but instead are retaining pay-as-you-go

systems indefinitely. Emerging reform issues identified in the chapter include (i) how to hold down the administrative costs of privately managed financial account systems, (ii) how to assign risks ex ante, and (iii) what low-income countries should do.

The Political Economy of Structural Pension Reform

The chapter by Estelle James and Sarah Brooks examines the political economy of shifting from a publicly managed, pay-as-you-go, defined benefit system to a system that includes defined contribution, funded, privately managed pillars. In particular, the chapter examines the connection between preexisting conditions in a country and the probability of adopting such a multipillar system.

The chapter addresses three central questions: (i) How have political and economic forces influenced the probability of adopting a multipillar system with individual accounts? (ii) How have these various factors influenced the nature of reform, especially its public-private mix? (iii) How have reforming countries overcome resistance from powerful interest groups? The authors use quantitative analysis to answer the first two questions, and they use qualitative case studies of a smaller number of reforming countries in Latin America and the transitional economies to address the third question.

The authors conclude that factors such as cultural, linguistic, and geographic proximity to countries that have already reformed their pension systems play a key role in explaining how multipillar reform ideas diffuse across countries; that the existence of private financial organizations (such as funded voluntary pension plans) signals institutional interests that speed the adoption of a funded, mandatory, private pillar; and that a large implicit pension debt raises the prominence of pension reform on the political agenda but also reduces the probability of adopting a multipillar system with individual accounts.

The Regulatory Framework for Pension Funds

The increasing role of private, funded systems in the provision of retirement income has led to an increasing interest in the analysis of regulatory and supervisory frameworks in the pension industry. The chapter by Roberto Rocha, Richard Hinz, and Joaquin Gutierrez reviews the regulatory framework for pensions across countries and examines whether there is scope for improvements in regulation and supervision.

In carrying out its analysis, the chapter also briefly examines the regulatory framework for banks and whether lessons from bank regulation can apply to pension regulation. Banks and pension funds are different in many ways, but the authors argue that such an analysis is still insightful—especially because the regulatory framework for the banking system has evolved in response to episodes of crisis and by regulators' efforts to avoid future crisis. Given the increasing role of private pensions and the need to ensure the safety of the industry, it is natural to ask whether there are aspects of banking regulation and supervision that could be applicable to pensions. Rocha, Hinz, and Gutierrez conclude that there are possible lessons from banking regulation in the area of guarantees, portfolio diversification, and the structure and techniques of supervision.

The chapter also notes that bank supervision has been shifting from a basic inspection of compliance with quantitative regulations to a more general assessment of the quality of risk management in banks. Pension regulators could learn from this experience.

Managing Public Pension Reserves:
Evidence from the International Experience

The chapter by Augusto Iglesias and Robert Palacios investigates an important issue of the international pension reform discussion, namely the success or failure of public management of public pension reserves. Many pension schemes mandated by governments have accumulated large reserves, reaching more than 50 percent of gross domestic product in a few countries. The management of these funds has a direct effect on financial sustainability and potential benefit levels, since high returns allow for a lower contribution rate. It also has important indirect effects on the overall economy when the funds are large (for example, on the functioning of financial markets and corporate governance). While substantial consensus exists about the advantages of some prefunding of public pension benefits, there is major disagreement about its management—public or private.

Iglesias and Palacios survey some of the available cross-country evidence on publicly managed pension reserves, covering more than 20 countries in the industrial and developing world. They find that publicly managed pension funds (i) are often used to achieve objectives other than providing pensions, (ii) are difficult to insulate from political interference, and (iii) tend to earn poor rates of return compared to relevant indices. These findings are consistent across countries of all types, but returns are especially dismal in countries with poor governance. The authors conclude that the experience to date suggests that the public management of pension reserves has seriously undermined the rationale for prefunding. In consequence, they suggest that countries with serious governance problems should probably avoid funding altogether.

Administrative Costs and the Organization of Individual Account Systems: A Comparative Perspective

One of the biggest criticisms associated with defined contribution individual accounts is that they are too expensive. The chapter by Estelle James, James Smalhout, and Dmitri Vittas investigates the cost-effectiveness of two alternative methods for constructing funded social security pillars: individual accounts invested in the retail market with relatively open choice, and individual accounts invested in the institutional market with constrained choice among investment companies. The authors also examine the most cost-effective way to organize a mandatory system of individual accounts.

For the retail market, the authors use data from mandatory pension funds in Chile and other Latin American countries and from voluntary mutual funds in the United States. For the institutional market, they use data from individual accounts systems in Bolivia and Sweden and from large pension plans as well as the federal Thrift Saving Plan in the United States. These institutional approaches aggregate numerous small accounts into large blocks of money and negotiate fees on a centralized basis. Some choice by workers remains. But fees and costs are kept low by constraining choice to investment portfolios that are inexpensive to manage, reducing incentives for marketing and avoiding excess capacity at the start of the new system. In the retail Chilean Administradoras de Fondos de Pensiones industry and the U.S. mutual fund industry, the authors conclude that average annualized fees range between 0.8 and 1.5 percent of assets. They find that use of the institutional market in individual account systems has reduced annualized fees to less than 0.5 percent per year, and in some cases to less than 0.2 percent.

The authors conclude that the biggest potential fee cuts stem from constrained portfolio choice, especially from a concentration on passive investment in index funds. This option is most readily available in countries with well-developed financial markets—that is, the more advanced industrial countries. The biggest cost saving for a given portfolio is due to reduced marketing activities, which is the main option available to countries with weak financial markets. The authors suggest that such constrained approaches to individual accounts are worthy of serious consideration, especially for systems with small contribution and asset bases and in the start-up phase of a new multipillar system.

Administrative Costs under a Decentralized Approach to Individual Accounts: Lessons from the United Kingdom

Since 1988 workers in the United Kingdom have been allowed to opt out of the nation's social security system and into individual accounts. Mamta Murthi, Michael Orszag, and Peter Orszag link together existing sources on U.K. personal pension costs to form a comprehensive database on firm-level administrative and other costs within the U.K. system. Their analysis of that data finds significant administrative costs.

Murthi, Orszag, and Orszag show that the administrative costs associated with any system of individual accounts can be broken down into three components. The *accumulation ratio* captures fund management and administrative costs for a worker contributing funds to a single financial provider throughout his or her career. As the study finds, and as previous studies also have documented, this factor reduces the value of an account in the United Kingdom by an average of 25 percent over an individual's working years. The *alteration ratio* measures the additional costs of failing to contribute consistently to a single financial provider over an entire career. It includes any costs from switching from one financial provider to another or from stopping contributions altogether. In the United Kingdom, this factor reduces an account's value by at least 15 percent over a career, on average. The *annuitization ratio* reflects the costs of converting an account to a lifetime annuity upon retirement. This factor reduces the value of an account in the United Kingdom at retirement by approximately 10 percent, on average. Taking into account interaction effects, these estimates indicate that, on average, various fees and costs consume between 40 and 45 percent of the value of individual accounts in the United Kingdom.

Murthi, Orszag, and Orszag note that costs depend on the structure of individual accounts. They agree with James, Smalhout, and Vittas that lower costs result from individual accounts that take aggressive advantage of potential economies of scale through centralized provision and that limit investment options. However, they conclude that the U.K. experience suggests that a decentralized, unconstrained approach to individual accounts may involve significant administrative costs. The cost ratio is likely to be even larger in developing countries with smaller accounts and less developed capital markets.

The Relevance of Index Funds for Pension Investment in Equities

Ajay Shah and Kshama Fernandes examine the role of index funds in facilitating pension investments in equities. They note that the rise of index

funds has been one of the most remarkable phenomena in the fund industry over the last 25 years. The traditional rationale for the success of index
funds is based on market efficiency, net of transaction costs. In addition,
Shah and Fernandes argue, the agency conflicts between active fund managers and investors, and the low power of statistical tests of performance,
could play an important role in encouraging the growth of index funds.

Most of the empirical evidence about the superiority of index funds
comes from the United States. Shah and Fernandes discuss the use of index
funds in developing countries and the policy issues in the financial sector
that affect the market infrastructure for index funds. They conclude that in
developing countries there are avenues through which policymakers can
improve the viability of index funds in pension investments. The main
issues faced are primarily those of market mechanisms used on the equity market and the construction of the market index. Possible improvements in these will benefit market efficiency at large and the viability of
index funds in particular.

Regulation of Withdrawals in Individual Account Systems

Another challenge for individual account systems is transforming the
accumulated account into a retirement benefit. During the accumulation
phase of an individual account system, workers invest a percentage of their
income in approved investment products. Following retirement, workers
withdraw the accumulated assets to finance consumption in old age. Quite
naturally, much of the initial interest in designing the new pension systems
has focused on the accumulation phase. With the maturation of some individual account systems, Jan Walliser notes that policy questions surrounding the design of the withdrawal phase will require more attention.

Standard pay-as-you-go systems in industrial economies generally offer
an inflation-indexed pension for the duration of a worker's life. Can private insurance markets replicate such a pension—a real life annuity—at reasonable cost? What flexibility should retirees have in choosing insurance
products that convert their retirement account balance into retirement
income? What form of government oversight and regulation would strike
a reasonable balance between the interests of retirees and taxpayers who
finance income protection programs? These are among the core questions
that policymakers face in reform countries.

Walliser concludes that government regulation of withdrawals from
individual accounts should mandate the purchase of inflation-indexed life
annuities exceeding income available from government welfare programs
for the retiree and potential survivors. However, he argues, proper functioning of insurance markets does not require annuitizing the entire account

balance. Instead, more flexibility for the choice of withdrawals could be permitted for any remaining funds, helping to tailor income streams to individual needs and living arrangements.

Personal Pension Plans and Stockmarket Volatility

In addition to administrative costs, one of the strongest objections against personal pension plans is that they transfer investment risk to individual workers, who are then exposed to the vagaries of equity and bond markets. Max Alier and Dmitri Vittas examine this issue using historical data from the United States. In particular, they investigate the impact of investment return volatility on replacement rates in the context of personal pension plans and also explore simple financial strategies to cope with this problem.

The "coping" strategies examined by Alier and Vittas include portfolio diversification, a late gradual shift to bonds, gradual purchase of annuities, and the purchase of variable annuities. They conclude that the latter strategy seems to be the most promising to reduce the dispersion of replacement rates across generations. But they also note that substantial risk continues to reside with the worker regardless of the strategy adopted, especially in terms of persistent deviations of investment returns from long-term trends.

Gender in Pension Reform in the Former Soviet Union

Restructuring the pension system in the former Soviet Union has been an important part of the challenge of the transition. The inherited system, designed to alleviate old age poverty, embodied a set of gender norms, which included encouraging women to leave the labor force early. Reforms in many countries have sought to change these norms by linking benefits much more closely with work histories, to encourage a long working life. While the new norms may on the surface appear gender neutral, they have important gender dimensions that are often undetected at the time the reforms were formulated.

Paulette Castel and Louise Fox analyze the gender implications of pension reform in Kazakhstan, the Kyrgyz Republic, Latvia, and Moldova. The authors observe that in all cases the new systems deliberately penalize early retirement and reward longer careers, so that with no change in behavior or policy, women's pensions will be, on average, less than men's. The implicit financial returns for women, however, remain on average higher than for men, because of women's longer life expectancy and because of redistributory minimum pensions. Overall, the net change in wealth from the reforms is higher on average for men than for women because they will work longer and get a higher pension. Women's longer life expectancy means that women can expect to spend their last years of life alone. If their pensions are too low owing to their work histories, an increase in elderly poverty may result.

Pension Coverage under Multipillar Systems

In many countries that have adopted multipillar systems, coverage rates have remained low—many workers remain outside the pension system. Robert Holzmann, Truman Packard, and Jose Cuesta examine the causes of low coverage rates, with special emphasis on two Latin American countries. They present and analyze a set of preliminary hypotheses and use econometric testing to explain low rates of participation.

The authors hypothesize specifically that it is the working poor and self-employed who, in particular, have a specific and strong rationale for avoiding participation in any pension system, including a multipillar one, and that transaction costs, system design issues, and problems of credibility negatively influence the decision of members of the labor force to participate. The authors subject these hypotheses to exploratory econometric tests using available household survey data for Chile and Argentina. The results support the conjecture that socioeconomic characteristics matter for nonparticipation and that the poor, the uneducated, and the self-employed pose a special challenge to the extension of pension coverage. Holzmann, Packard, and Cuesta propose further research to confirm the results presented in their chapter.

Conclusions and Areas for Future Research

The chapters in this volume explore a wide variety of pension reform issues. On many elements of pension reform, the participants in the conference and the contributors to this volume appear to agree. For example, all observers seem to concur that the government must play some role in pension provision, that a well-designed pension system has multiple pillars, and that the design of the pillars (as well as their relative importance) will ultimately differ across countries.

Despite these areas of agreement, however, various areas of disagreement remain. Three factors underlie much of that disagreement: (i) judgments about whether countries can learn from past mistakes to redesign programs in ways that reflect best practices and whether average past performance (for example, of public programs) provides the best evidence of likely future performance; (ii) judgments about the significance of market failures and limitations of the market more generally (transaction costs, volatility, lack of investor information, and missing insurance markets)— their magnitude, their implications, and the speed with which they will be reduced; and (iii) judgments about the significance of political failure (over-commitment, mismanagement of reserve funds, ad hoc benefit system changes and credibility, reform incapacity) and the effectiveness of potential means to keep the political risk in check through private management or self-binding mechanisms, such as long-term actuarial projections of unfunded schemes by an independent body and generational accounting. Differences in the judgments about political economy are most visible in the discussion about whether prefunding of pension commitments should be publicly or privately managed.

The results of the chapters and the remaining differences clearly dictate further research on multiple fronts. First, what are the best ways to isolate publicly managed prefunding arrangements from political risk or to prevent government bailouts of privately managed arrangements? While the limited best practice in highly industrialized economies such as Denmark and Canada may provide some guidance on a public approach, and the limited best practice in other industrial countries may provide some guidance on a private approach, caution may be required in the implementation in the World Bank's typical client environment. As seasoned World Bankers like to say, if our clients could implement best practices, they would not be developing economies. How can we best overcome these restrictions?

Second, the level of high transaction costs in funded systems needs continued attention. Are there changes in policy design and implementation that can substantially reduce costs? Current suggestions include the restriction of choice in individually selected funds and products to produce lower fees. Others, however, see the solution in stronger competition among alternative providers with a level playing field. More research is needed to guide design decisions and implementation.

Third, the analysis of the political economy of pension reform is still in its infancy. The available results provide some guidance for policymakers and the World Bank, but they cannot really answer the two main questions: What starts a pension reform, and what makes it successful? While the rising number of pension reforms undertaken worldwide enhance the information pool and the possibility to discriminate better among competing hypotheses, more data and more research are clearly required.

Fourth, while there are potential large benefits from prefunding, the mechanism through which they emerge and the distribution of the benefits between and within generations has not been sufficiently studied. Many of the benefits from prefunding arise from increases in national saving in the economy, but what is the best way to effect such higher saving?

In developing countries, pension reform may help to develop financial markets, and this in turn may have positive effects on economic growth. The evidence of such linkages, however, remains limited, and the conditions under which such benefits arise—and the kinds of reforms that are most likely to produce them—are still being debated and need further research.

Finally, despite the benefits of prefunding, pay-as-you-go systems are clearly here to stay in many countries over extended periods of time. It is therefore crucially important to explore ways of improving such pay-as-you-go systems, by modifying incentives (which includes avoiding disincentives for work among the elderly) and ensuring their long-term financial viability.

But there is also a second set of research issues on old age income support that goes beyond formal pension systems (and making them more equitable, less distortionary, and financially more sustainable), and these issues must be urgently addressed. This research is important to strengthening the poverty agenda of the World Bank.

First, we have to provide better guidance to policymakers regarding how to help the elderly poor, particularly those who have never been able to join a formal pension system and have never had sufficient resources to prepare for their old age. Research should provide insights about equitable and financially sustainable noncontributory schemes, about community-based systems, and about the possibilities to induce families to provide support for their elderly members.

Second, we have to investigate the instruments for informal sector workers to prepare for their old age. Many of these informal workers—self-employed and workers in rural and urban areas—are the current nonpoor but risk becoming the future poor when old because they often have little or no means to save in a safe and cost-efficient manner. Since they need access to savings during their working years to cope with other risks, they have little incentive to join a formal system that makes their contributions illiquid until retirement. Research is needed to explore the appropriate instruments and institutions that can serve both as a means for development as well as the prevention of poverty in old age.

Last but not least we need a better understanding of how to reform civil service pensions, including those for the military. In many client countries, these expenditures consume an important share of budgetary resources to the detriment of poverty-oriented public expenditure. But their reform is intimately linked to the overall compensation package for civil servants.

Both researchers and policymakers will continue to debate the best way to address the economic and demographic challenges of pension systems. Many pension plans are clearly unsustainable, and difficult reforms will be necessary. And we will have to go beyond formal pension systems if we want to ensure that the elderly are not left in poverty. We hope that this volume helps to enlighten researchers and policymakers around the globe on the costs and benefits of different approaches to pension reform.

Notes

1 The authors distinguish between broad and narrow prefunding and emphasize that only broad prefunding—an increase in national saving—affects the economy.

References

Gillion, C. 2000. "The Development and Reform of Social Security Pensions: The Approach of the International Labor Office." *International Social Security Review* 53(1): 35-63.

Holzmann, R. 2000. "The World Bank Approach to Pension Reform." *International Social Security Review* 53(1): 11-34.

World Bank. 2000. Pension Reform Primer. Washington, D.C. (*www.world-bank.org/pensions*).

1

Rethinking Pension Reform: Ten Myths about Social Security Systems

Peter R. Orszag and Joseph E. Stiglitz

Averting the Old Age Crisis, the World Bank's (1994) pathbreaking publication on pensions, trenchantly notes that "myths abound in discussions of old age security." This chapter examines 10 such "myths" in a deliberately provocative manner.

It is testimony to the power of *Averting the Old Age Crisis* that many of today's myths at least partially emanate from that report's unmasking of yesterday's myths. Yet the rejection of one extreme is not the affirmation of the other, and the pendulum seems to have swung far, perhaps too far, in the other direction. The complexity of optimal pension policy should caution us against believing that a similar set of recommendations would be appropriate in countries ranging from Argentina to Azerbaijan, from China to Costa Rica, and from Sierra Leone to Sweden. We are reminded of the joke about the professor who kept the same questions each year but changed the answers. Ironically, that joke may offer us some sound guidance. We should be wary of offering a single answer across the globe in response to the question, "What should we do about our pension system?"

The answer to this question is also unlikely to be "nothing." The problems that have motivated pension reform across the globe are real. In many developing countries, soaring deficits—gaps between pension fund obligations and revenues—not only threaten economic stability but also crowd out necessary investments in education, health, and infrastructure. Too often, the benefits of pension programs have accrued to those already privileged; forcing poor farmers to finance the largesse of the urban elite is hardly equitable. Furthermore, the structure of the pension programs in many cases has weakened the functioning of labor markets and distorted resource allocations. In other words, reforms have been and are needed. And while countries may be able to muddle through in the short run, averting a crisis in the long run will not be so simple.

17

The necessity of serious reforms in many countries tells us nothing about which specific reforms should be undertaken in which countries. Unfortunately, a set of myths that have dominated public discussions and derailed rational decision-making have too often clouded evaluations of such reform options. The purpose of this chapter is to dispel those myths— or, at the very least, to raise questions concerning their universal validity.

In principle, the "three pillars" delineated in *Averting the Old Age Crisis* are expansive enough to reflect any potential combination of policy measures—especially if the second (funded) pillar incorporates both privately and publicly managed systems.[1] But in practice, the book has often been interpreted as advocating one specific constellation of the pillars: a publicly managed, unfunded, defined benefit pillar; a privately managed, funded, defined contribution pillar (with no redistribution); and a voluntary private pillar. For example, Weaver (1998) writes that *Averting the Old Age Crisis* advocated "a three-tier model in which the role of public pensions would focus on a minimal poverty reduction role, complemented by a fully-funded, mandatory defined-contribution savings second tier . . . and a third tier of voluntary savings." That interpretation—especially the inclusion of a *privately managed, defined contribution* component—is common among policymakers and pension analysts, regardless of whether it fully reflects the nuances of *Averting the Old Age Crisis* itself.[2] And it is precisely the private, defined contribution pillar of that "best practice" model that we wish to explore.

Over the past decade, following the seminal reforms in Chile in the early 1980s, and with support from the World Bank, many nations have moved away from a public defined benefit pension system and toward a private defined contribution one. Important reforms in this direction have occurred in, among other places, Argentina, Bolivia, Columbia, Hungary, Kazakhstan, Latvia, Peru, Poland, Sweden, and Uruguay.[3] The focus throughout the chapter will therefore be on whether this type of shift—to a private defined contribution (individual account) pension system—is as *universally* beneficial as many of its proponents claim.

Many of today's myths emanate from a failure to distinguish several aspects of a pension system. As Geanakoplos, Mitchell, and Zeldes (1998, 1999) and others have emphasized, the failure to clearly distinguish the different aspects of individual account proposals has obscured many underlying realities. In particular, most discussions of individual account systems conflate privatization, prefunding, diversification, and the distinction between defined benefit and defined contribution pensions:

- *Privatization.* Privatization is the replacing of a publicly run pension system with a privately managed one.

- *Prefunding.* Prefunding means accumulating assets against future pension payments. As discussed below, prefunding can be used in a broad or narrow sense.
- *Diversification.* Diversification involves allowing investments in a variety of assets, rather than government bonds alone.
- *Defined benefit versus defined contribution.* Defined benefit plans assign accrual risk to the sponsor; conditional upon a worker's earnings history, retirement benefits are supposedly deterministic, although they may depend on nonaccrual factors affecting the earnings history, such as productivity increases. Defined contribution plans, on the other hand, assign accrual risk to the individual worker; even conditional upon an earnings history, retirement benefits depend on the efficacy with which contributions were financially managed.

Any combination of these four elements is possible. Indeed, *in practice, all of these elements contain spectra of choices—making it particularly important to examine specific institutional details. An idealized model is likely never to be realized in practice, and choices are inevitably characterized by degrees of gray rather than being black or white.* For example, a public system is one that is organized and administered primarily by the government; a private system is one that is organized and administered primarily outside the government. Yet a public system may involve some private firms; for example, a private firm may be chosen as the money manager for a public trust fund. Similarly, a private system likely involves some public role, at the very least in enforcing its rules (Heclo 1998).[4] Prefunding and diversification are also matters of degree: pensions can be partially prefunded, and degrees of diversification are possible. Finally, the distinction between defined benefit and defined contribution plans is not as pure as it may initially appear. Indeed, a defined benefit plan could be thought of as a defined contribution plan combined with an appropriate mix of options to eliminate the residual risk to the worker.[5]

Before examining the myths, four further background points are worth highlighting to inform our subsequent analysis of individual accounts:

- *Inherent features versus imperfect implementation.* A key issue surrounding both public defined benefit systems and individual accounts is which elements are inherent to the system and which elements are merely common in how that system has been implemented in practice. That is to say, we observe that system Z is not working properly. Should we propose a switch to system Y, or instead work on improving system Z? Surely, comparing an idealized version of Y to an as-implemented version of Z is not likely to prove insightful. A first step may therefore be to compare the idealized features of Y and Z and then examine whether political economy constraints differentially affect the two models (in terms of their idealized versus *expected* implementation features).[6] Many of the myths arise from mixing comparisons between idealized and as-implemented features. Our initial focus is on inherent features, for it is these inherent features that would tend to make one system or the other universally applicable. Statements about historic tendencies regarding implementation must be treated with much more caution than inherent features, especially since the historic tendencies in one nation are not necessarily reflective of those in another one.

- *Tabula rasa choices versus transformation choices.* In evaluating the effect of pension reform, initial conditions are important. One must be particularly careful not to confuse the issue of whether a *shift* to individual accounts would be socially beneficial with the separate issue of whether, in a tabula rasa sense, an individual account system would have been preferable to a public defined benefit system in the first place. In other words, the social effects of transforming a mature pension system into a system of individual accounts may be substantially different than the social effects of the *initial* choice between a public defined benefit system and individual accounts, and the differences between a transformation and an introduction must be taken into account. Very few nations face that initial choice in a pure sense; almost all have some form of old age insurance program. Out of the 172 countries included in the 1997 edition of *Social Security Programs Throughout the World*, only six (Bangladesh, Botswana, Malawi, Myanmar, Sierra Leone, and Somalia) lack an old age, disability, and survivors program (Social Security Administration 1997).[7] It should be emphasized that many of the extant programs have relatively low coverage; even then, however, the cost of including them in any reform or the consequences of not including them must be taken into account.

- *Intergenerational analysis.* Politicians are known for focusing exclusively on the short run, ignoring the long-run costs (or even viability) of public programs. In analyzing transitions and reforms, however, we have to be careful not to make the opposite mistake of focusing exclusively on the long run and ignoring short-run costs. Consider, for example, a reform that leads to higher steady-state output and consumption but only at the cost of reduced welfare for intervening generations. When some generations are made worse off, and some better off, we face a complex welfare calculus—how to weigh the gains of one generation against the losses of another.[8]

- *Ultimate focus on welfare.* In a similar vein, we need to keep in mind our ultimate objective. Savings and growth are not ends in themselves but means to an end: the increase in well-being of members of the society. Thus we could perhaps induce people to save more by exposing them to more risk (for example, increasing variance in the real return of their pension plan).[9] The increased risk, however, would make them unambiguously worse off. Even the future generations that benefit from the higher wages associated with a larger capital stock may be worse off.

With these background points in mind, we now turn our attention to the myths. To help delineate the issues, we divide our 10 myths into three broad areas relating to macroeconomic effects, microeconomic efficiency, and political economy.

Macroeconomic Myths

We begin with myths in the macroeconomic arena, for these are perhaps the most vigorously propagated and also the ones for which a broad array of economists agree that popular slogans are misleading.

Myth 1: Private Defined Contribution Plans Raise National Savings

It is common to assert that moving toward a system of "prefunded" individual accounts would raise national saving (James 1995; Feldstein 1997). To analyze the validity of this claim, we must introduce another distinction in addition to the ones delineated in the introduction: "prefunding" can be used in a narrow or broad sense. In its narrow sense, prefunding means that the pension system is accumulating assets against future projected payments. In a broader sense, however, prefunding means increasing national saving.[10]

Prefunding in the narrow sense need not imply prefunding in the broader sense. For example, consider a system of individual accounts that is prefunded in the narrow sense. If individuals offset any contributions to the individual accounts through reduced saving in other forms, then total private saving is unaffected by the accounts. In other words, in the absence of the individual account system, individuals would have saved an equivalent amount in some other form. If public saving is also unaffected, then national saving is not changed by the narrowly prefunded set of individual accounts—and so no prefunding in the broad sense occurs.[11] Similarly, consider a "partially prefunded" public system with a trust fund. If the presence of that trust fund causes offsetting reductions in nonpension taxes and/or increases in nonpension benefits, and if private behavior is unaffected by the public pension system, then the public system would not affect public saving or national saving, and thus would not be prefunded in a broad sense (even though it is prefunded in the narrow sense). In summary, narrow prefunding can be a misleading guide to broad prefunding. Furthermore, narrow prefunding has no macroeconomic implications; only broad prefunding offers potential macroeconomic benefits.

Privatization and broad prefunding are distinct concepts, and privatization is neither necessary nor sufficient for broad prefunding. To see why, consider a pay-as-you-go system in which each individual's benefits are directly tied to contributions. Each individual has an account with the social security administrator, showing contributions at each date. These contributions are then translated into benefits using actuarial tables. Now assume the government decides to prefund these accounts in the narrow sense, transferring to each the full value of the cumulative contributions. The social security system thus becomes completely prefunded in the narrow sense. But to finance the contributions, the government borrows from the public. National saving is therefore constant; all that has happened is that the government has altered the form of the debt.[12] Such a switch should not have any real effects on the macroeconomy. To be sure, the implicit debt under the old system has become explicit. But in and of itself, that has no economic ramifications. *A debt-financed privatization does not involve any macroeconomic consequences— it does not engender broad prefunding—assuming the new explicit debt follows the same time path as the old implicit debt.*[13] The key is what is happening to the sum of implicit and explicit debt; transforming one into the other does not effect broad prefunding.[14]

Conversely, broad prefunding can be accomplished without privatization. In particular, the government can accumulate assets in anticipation of future benefit payments due under the public defined benefit plan. Such prefunding does not have to take the form of private market investments. Interestingly, those who argue that a public system cannot prefund have often pointed to the United States as their example of a country that has failed to do so. And yet over the past year, despite the lack of agreement on almost everything else, policymakers in the United States have largely agreed to protect Social Security surpluses from the demands of the rest of the budget—in other words, to ensure broad prefunding. Similarly, one study found that Malaysia's Employees Provident Fund contributed significantly to national saving—accounting for between 20 and 25 percent of national saving in the 1980s (Bateman and Piggott 1997).

Note that this myth highlights the tabula rasa point above. A large academic literature exists on whether the introduction of a pay-as-you-go social security system reduces national saving.[15] But that is a fundamentally different issue from whether shifting an *existing* pay-as-you-go system to one of individual accounts would raise national saving. Even if the introduction of a pay-as-you-go system reduces national saving (as some studies suggest), shifting to individual accounts in a manner that accomplishes only narrow prefunding would not raise national saving.

The fundamental issue involved in broad prefunding is, given the inherited level of implicit and explicit debt, the optimal policy of paying it off. This optimization problem does not depend on how or why the debt was acquired, and it is not affected by the introduction of narrowly prefunded individual accounts.[16]

The conclusion is that the trade-offs involved in *how* to prefund—for example, through a public or private approach—are distinct from the trade-offs involved in *whether* to prefund.[17] Indeed, broad prefunding— done either way—may not increase social welfare. In any case, some analysts argue that a prefunded, public, defined benefit system may be preferable to a prefunded, private, defined contribution system (Heller 1998; Modigliani, Ceprini, and Muralidhar 1999). Automatically linking privatization and broad prefunding, rather than examining each choice separately, fails to reflect the full range of policy options.

Myth 2: Rates of Return Are Higher under Individual Accounts

A second myth is that rates of return would be higher under individual accounts than under a pay-as-you-go system. For example, the *Financial Times* last spring reported that the "rate of return [on individual accounts] would be higher—perhaps 6 to 8 per cent on past stock market performance, against the roughly 2 per cent the social security system will produce."[18] Similarly, Palacios and Whitehouse (1998) argue that the higher rate of return under a private scheme "is an important reason for reform."[19] As in Myth 1, this myth conflates privatization with prefunding. In addition, most simple rate-of-return comparisons conflate privatization with diversification.

As Paul Samuelson showed more than 40 years ago, the real rate of return in a mature pay-as-you-go system is equal to the sum of the rate of growth in the labor force and the rate of growth in productivity (Samuelson 1958). In the decades ahead, fertility rates are expected to remain relatively low, and the world's population is expected to age. World population growth is expected to slow from 1.7 percent per year in the 1980s and about 1.3 percent per year currently to 0.8 percent per year, on average, between 2010 and 2050.[20] As a result, global labor force growth is also expected to slow, putting downward pressure on the rate of return under mature pay-as-you-go systems. Assuming productivity growth of 2 percent per year, the long-run real rate of return on a hypothetical, global, mature pay-as-you-go system would be about 3 percent per year.

In a dynamically efficient economy without risky assets, the real interest rate must exceed the growth rate.[21] Therefore, in a dynamically efficient economy, individual accounts—even without diversification—will *always* appear to offer a higher rate of return than a pay-as-you-go system. Appearances can be deceiving, however. The simple rate-of-return comparison, even without the diversification issues discussed below, is fundamentally misleading for two reasons: administrative costs and transition costs.

- *Administrative costs.* The simple rate-of-return comparison usually compares gross rates of return, even though administrative costs may differ even under idealized versions of the two systems and, ceteris paribus, higher administrative costs reduce the net rate of return an individual receives. Myth 7 addresses administrative costs in more detail. As that section explains (admittedly on an as-implemented basis), administrative costs are likely to consume a nontrivial share of the account balance under individual accounts—especially for small accounts. Such administrative costs imply that on a risk-adjusted basis, once the costs of financing the unfunded liability under the old system are incorporated (see below), the rate of return on a decentralized private system is likely to be lower than under the public system.
- *Transition costs.* Since individual accounts are financed from revenue currently devoted to the public social security system, computations of the rate of return under individual accounts need to include the cost of continuing to pay the benefits promised to retirees and older workers under the extant system. Assuming that society is unwilling to renege on its promises to such retirees and older workers, the costs remain even if the social security system is eliminated for new workers and replaced entirely by individual accounts. Since the payments to current beneficiaries are not avoided by setting up individual accounts, the returns on individual accounts should not be artificially inflated by excluding their cost.

The fundamental point is a simple one. If the economy is dynamically efficient, one cannot improve the welfare of later generations without making intervening generations worse off. Reform of pension systems must thus address equity issues both within and across generations.[22] The comparison of rates of return is thus misguided because *higher returns in the long run can be obtained only at the expense of reduced consumption and returns for intervening generations.*

An example may be helpful in making this point more explicitly.[23] Imagine a simple pay-as-you-go system, under which one generation pays $1 while it is young and receives $1 while old. Generation A is old in period 1 and therefore receives $1. That $1 is paid for by Generation B, which is young in period 1. Then in period 2, Generation B is old and receives $1, paid for by Generation C, which is young in period 2, and so on. Table 1.1 presents the operation of the system. Assume further that the market interest rate is 10 percent per period. Now consider the system from the perspective of Generation C during period 2:

- Under the pay-as-you-go system, Generation C pays $1 during period 2 and receives $1 back during period 3. The pay-as-you-go system's rate of return is zero (which also follows from the assumption of zero productivity growth and zero population growth).
- Under an individual accounts system, Generation C would invest the $1 contribution and receive $1.10 in period 3. The rate of return would appear to be 10 percent.

It would therefore appear that a switch from the pay-as-you-go system to individual accounts would produce substantially higher returns for Generation C—10 percent rather than 0 percent. But if Generation C put $1 into individual accounts during period 2, that $1 could not be used to finance the benefits for Generation B. Yet Generation B's benefits must be paid for somehow, unless society is willing to allow Generation B to go without benefits.

Assume that Generation B's benefits are financed through borrowing and that the interest costs are paid for by the older generation in each period. With an interest rate of 10 percent, the interest payments would cost 10 cents per period. The net benefit to Generation C during period 3, therefore, would be $1 ($1.10 from its individual accounts minus 10 cents in interest costs). Thus Generation C would earn a zero rate of return just as under the pay-as-you-go system, once the interest costs are included. Indeed, for Generation C and each generation thereafter, *the extra return from the individual account is more apparent than real: it is exactly offset by the cost of the debt that financed Generation B's benefits.*

Rate-of-return comparisons for *specific individuals* may also reflect the redistribution component of different systems. To be sure, current systems

Table 1.1. The Simplified Pay-as-You-Go System

| Period | Generation | | | |
	A	B	C	D
1	+$1	-$1		
2		+$1	-$1	
3			+$1	-$1
4				+$1

Source: Authors' data.

entail considerable redistribution, a result of which is that some individuals (those who are "paying" for the redistribution) receive a lower rate of return than they would in a system that does not involve such redistribution, even if the aggregate returns are the same under the two systems. We may or may not believe that such redistributions are desirable or deserved. If the redistributions are not desirable, they—and not necessarily the public system that currently embodies them—should be abolished.[24] In other words, as emphasized in the introduction, the fact that the public systems *as implemented* have been less than ideal means that they should be changed, not necessarily dramatically scaled back. With respect to pension programs in Europe, Boldrin, Dolado, Jimeno, and Peracchi (1999) write, "Their use as camouflaged redistributional devices, motivated by rent-seeking and political purposes, has turned into an abuse, and, in about three decades, almost lead to their financial bankruptcy. We insist on the fact that, in the justifiable and commendable process of getting rid of such redistributional distortions, one does not want to 'throw away the baby with the dirty water.' PAYG public pension systems do serve a useful purpose, which should be salvaged and enhanced by a deeper reform of the European Welfare State."[25]

Risk issues raise further complications for the simple rate-of-return comparison. Most simple rate-of-return comparisons conflate privatization and diversification (out of government bonds). The two need not go together; one can imagine private accounts that are restricted to risk-free financial assets, and public systems that invest in risky assets.

Diversification should produce higher average financial returns over long periods of time. But individuals generally dislike risk; a much riskier asset with a slightly higher rate of return is not necessarily preferable to a much safer asset with a slightly lower rate of return—so some adjustment to observed rates of return is necessary. And if capital markets are perfect, the higher mean return from diversification should merely compensate for additional risk (assuming that the portfolio holds a sufficient number of different risky assets). In other words, in efficient markets, returns are commensurate with risk, and if individuals wish more or less risk than associated with the government program, they can engineer such changes at minimum cost.[26]

For example, by many common measures, stocks are relatively risky—at least over the short run. Standard & Poor's (S&P) 500 index in the United States has declined (in nominal terms) by more than 10 percent in eight of the past 70 years.[27] (In inflation-adjusted terms, the number of years of substantial decline is larger.) Moreover, individual stocks are considerably riskier than broad portfolios such as the S&P 500; many stocks decline even in years when the market rises overall. And the recent turmoil in developing countries' financial markets provides more than ample evidence of short-term variance: Relative to the end of 1996, for example, stock market capitalization fell by 40 percent in Indonesia, 55–60 percent in Malaysia and Thailand, and 35–40 percent in South Korea and Singapore by early 1998.[28] Stock returns also tend to be risky in the sense of being high when the marginal utility of consumption is low and vice versa.

Analysis conducted by Gary Burtless of the Brookings Institution highlights the risks embodied in stocks. Burtless studied the replacement rates that workers would have achieved (that is, the percentage of their previous wages that their retirement incomes would equal) if they had invested 2 percent of their earnings in stock index funds each year over a 40-year work career and converted the accumulated balance to a retirement annuity upon reaching age 62. Workers reaching age 62 in 1968 would have enjoyed a 39 percent replacement rate from those investments (that is, the monthly benefit from their retirement annuity would equal 39 percent of prior wages). By contrast, the replacement rate for workers retiring in 1974—only six years later—would have been only 17 percent, or less than half as much (Burtless 1998). While the precise estimates can be criticized, the central point that emerges from them cannot be: stock returns embody substantial variation from year to year.

If we are willing to assume that markets are fully efficient, we do not need to bother with risk adjustments—we can merely assume that all properly risk-adjusted returns on sufficiently diversified portfolios are equal. If we are *not* willing to assume that markets are fully efficient, however, we must undertake complicated risk adjustments. For example, it is difficult to determine the precise degree of risk aversion in individuals. "Risk" also may depend on a wide variety of factors. For example, over long enough periods, stocks may not be particularly risky relative to nominal bonds (Siegel 1998). Another critical question is whether the observed equity premium merely reflects risk, or whether it includes a component of supernormal returns on stocks even on a risk-adjusted basis (Mehra and Prescott 1985). A related question is how to make projections of the risk premium.

Other complicating factors exist for risk adjustments to public versus private systems. In purely financial terms (abstracting from any potential differences in political risk), diversification undertaken through a public defined benefit system involves less risk for any given individual than diversification undertaken through a private defined contribution system. The reason is that a public defined benefit system can spread risk across generations in a way that is not possible under a private defined contribution program. In other words, while the public program can attain any profile of risk (and diversification) that the private program can, the converse is not true. To be sure, government guarantees on returns under a private defined contribution system (see Myth 9) facilitate some degree of intergenerational risk sharing. But note that they do so only by transforming the pure private defined contribution system into a mixed private defined contribution-public defined benefit system.

Full risk analysis of a public defined benefit system relative to individual accounts would entail evaluations of not just diversification, but also a wide variety of other risks inherent in the typical as-implemented forms of the two systems. For example, defined benefit systems are usually progressive and therefore provide a form of lifetime earnings insurance.[29] If lifetime earnings are lower than expected, the replacement rate is higher than expected, at least partially cushioning the blow in retirement of the lower-than-expected earnings. Furthermore, even under a nonprogressive defined benefit plan, pensioners do not face accrual risk, although many systems often included under the "defined benefit" heading still contain residual risks of various kinds (for example, real risks arising from imperfect indexation or demographic risks from the adjustment of benefits depending on the status of public finances).[30] Finally, once we depart from an idealized comparison and examine the political economy of the two systems, a variety of political risk issues arise with respect to public systems that may or may not be less extreme under private systems (see further discussion in Myth 9 and Myth 10). In any case, the simple rate-of-return comparison ignores these complicated risk issues.

Myth 3: Declining Rates of Return on Pay-As-You-Go Systems Reflect Fundamental Problems with Those Systems

Another myth surrounding reform of public pay-as-you-go systems is that observed declines in rates of return on pay-as-you-go systems are indicative of some fundamental flaw in those systems. Instead, that decline reflects the natural convergence of a pay-as-you-go system to its mature steady-state.

The Samuelson formula gives the rate of return on a *mature* pay-as-you-go system. In the early years of such a system, however, beneficiaries receive a substantially higher rate of return than the formula would suggest. Consider Generation A from the example above. That first generation in the pay-as-you-go system received $1 in benefits but had not contributed anything to the system. Generation A's rate of return thus was infinite.

In a similar vein, early beneficiaries under the Social Security system in the United States received extremely high rates of return because they received benefits disproportionate to their contributions (table 1.2). They contributed for only a limited number of years, since much of their working lives had passed before Social Security payroll contributions began to be collected. The earliest beneficiaries under Social Security—those born in the 1870s—enjoyed real rates of return approaching 40 percent.

This decline in rates of return from the earliest groups of beneficiaries is a feature of any pay-as-you-go system, under which the early beneficiaries receive very high rates of return because they contributed little during

Table 1.2. Average Real Annual Rate of Return on U.S. Social Security by Cohort

Year of birth	Average annual real rate of return
1876	36.5 percent
1900	11.9 percent
1925	4.8 percent
1950	2.2 percent

Source: Leimer 1995, table 3.

their working years. The rate of return for subsequent beneficiaries necessarily declines. As the system matures, that decline in rates of return may be attenuated or exacerbated by changes in productivity and labor force growth rates.

Two other points are worth noting. First, the decision to provide benefits at the beginning of the program to those who did not contribute over their entire lives—to make the system a pay-as-you-go one rather than a funded one—may be understandable in terms of political exigencies but may or may not make much sense in terms of intergenerational welfare policy. But unless we are now willing to let existing retirees or older workers suffer because earlier generations received a supernormal rate of return, we are forced to bear the consequences of that decision regardless of whether the pension system is privatized. Second, and relatedly, the supernormal rates of return enjoyed by early beneficiaries are the mirror reflection of the submarket rate of return on the mature system. As Geanakoplos, Mitchell, and Zeldes (1998) emphasize, the net present value of the pay-as-you-go system across all generations is zero. If some generations receive super-market rates of return, all other generations must therefore receive submarket rates of return. Again, the introduction of individual accounts does not change that conclusion.

Myth 4: Investment of Public Trust Funds in Equities Has No Macroeconomic Effects or Welfare Implications

Many analysts of pension reform believe that investing a public trust fund in equities rather than government bonds would have no macroeconomic or social welfare effects. The argument is simply that such diversification is merely an asset shift, and does not change national saving. It therefore may alter asset prices or rates of return but not the macroeconomy. As Alan Greenspan (1996) has stated:

> If the social security trust funds achieved a higher rate of return investing in equities than in lower yielding U.S. Treasuries, private sector incomes generated by their asset portfolios, including

retirement funds, would fall by the same amount, potentially jeopardizing their financial condition. This zero-sum result occurs because of the assumption that no new productive saving and investment has been induced by this portfolio reallocation process.

Note that this argument is not really one about whether public trust funds should be invested in equities. Rather, it is about whether social security funds should be shifted into equities through any mechanism—either through public trust funds or private accounts. In other words, the issue is purely one of whether *diversification* per se is beneficial. Interestingly, proponents of private accounts often hail the diversification potential of such accounts as a substantial social benefit, yet simultaneously claim that diversification undertaken through a public trust fund would yield no benefits. From a strictly economic perspective, that dichotomy does not seem to make much sense. To be sure, *how* to best accomplish diversification involves numerous issues, including both administrative costs and political economy issues, that are addressed below (see Myths 7 and 10).[31] For now, we focus on the effects of diversification absent such administrative cost or political economy concerns. For convenience, we therefore examine diversification undertaken through a public trust fund.

Underlying our examination of this myth is a fundamental theory—the public sector analogue to the Modigliani-Miller theorem—that provides conditions under which public sector financial structure makes no difference. The conditions were developed in a series of papers by Joseph Stiglitz (Stiglitz 1974, 1983, 1988). Given perfect capital markets and the ability of individuals to reverse the actions of government financial policies, such policies have no real effects.

Given imperfections in the financial markets, however, Stiglitz also shows that government financial policy—including its approach to investing its trust funds—could have important real effects. More recently, economists have highlighted imperfections or nonconvexities such as learning costs, minimum investment thresholds, or other factors. In the presence of such imperfections and assuming that pensioners assume some of the accrual risk from the government's financial policies (which means that the pension system is not a pure defined benefit plan), diversification can produce real welfare gains and possibly macroeconomic effects. The key insight is that, given the imperfections, many individuals do not hold equities—and government diversification can therefore produce a welfare gain.[32]

For example, Diamond and Geanakoplos examine a model in which there are two types of consumers: savers and nonsavers. The nonsavers participate in a social security program, and the government therefore "invests" on their behalf. Transferring some of the social security trust fund into equities—in other words, diversification—produces a welfare gain for these nonsavers. "Our major finding is that trust fund portfolio diversification into equities has substantial real effects, including the potential for significant welfare improvements. Diversification raises the sum total of utility in the economy if household utilities are weighted so that the marginal utility of a dollar today is the same for every household. The potential welfare gains come from the presence of workers who do not invest their savings on their own." (Diamond and Geanakoplos 1999).

Similarly, if a nontrivial share of households lacks access to capital markets, diversification (either through a trust fund or individual accounts) could raise welfare for these households. One study concludes that $1 of equity may be worth $1.59 to such constrained households (Geanakoplos, Mitchell, and Zeldes 1999). The myth of neutral diversification thus arises from the implicit assumption that all households are at interior solutions in terms of their financial portfolios; the papers explore the ramifications of having at least some households at corner solutions. In a somewhat different approach that nonetheless reaches similar conclusions about the non-neutrality of diversification, Abel (1999) finds that diversification could raise the growth rate of the capital stock in a defined benefit system.

Finally, it is also interesting to note that from a risk perspective the socially optimal system may be a diversified, *partially* funded one. Several papers have shown that combining an unfunded component (with a rate of return tied to earnings growth) with a diversified, funded component (with a rate of return tied to a market index) may reduce risk relative to a completely funded system (Merton 1983; Merton, Bodie, and Marcus 1987; and Dutta, Kapur, and Orszag 1999). The intuition is simply that partial funding provides access to an asset—the human capital of the young—that is not normally tradable on the financial markets, thereby providing further diversification relative to the set of assets available on financial markets. The historical correlations among annual GDP growth, earnings growth, bond returns, and stock returns in the United States, Germany, United Kingdom, France, Italy, and Japan are substantially less than 1, and often negative, leading one study to conclude that "diversification of risk provides an additional reason to invest in both human and physical capital." (Boldrin, Dolado, Jimeno, and Peracchi 1999).

Microeconomic Myths

Myth 5: Labor Market Incentives Are Better under Private Defined Contribution Plans

A common claim regarding individual accounts is that they provide better labor market incentives than traditional (defined benefit) social security systems. For example, Estelle James (1998) has written, "The close linkage between benefits and contributions, in a defined-contribution plan, is designed to reduce labor market distortions, such as evasion by escape to the informal sector, since people are less likely to regard their contribution as a tax." Similarly, in analyzing Social Security in the United States, Martin Feldstein (1998) has written that "the extra deadweight loss that results from these very unequal links between incremental taxes and incremental benefits would automatically be eliminated in a privatized funded system with individual retirement accounts."

Any differential labor market incentives of individual accounts result from differences in both risk and redistribution. It is therefore important to note:

- We are ultimately interested in welfare, not labor supply. It is possible to design structures that accentuate labor market incentives but reduce welfare. To do so would be to confuse means with ends. For example, if individuals were very risk averse, imposing a large random lump sum tax on individuals in the latter part of their lives may induce both more savings and more labor supply, since individuals would work harder as a precaution against this adverse contingency. Yet such a tax could have large adverse effects on welfare (Stiglitz 1982). A particular example of this point is the changes in risk associated with a movement from defined benefit to a defined contribution system. A mean-preserving increase in risk could lead to greater labor supply but would be undesirable from a welfare perspective (Rothschild and Stiglitz 1970, 1971).
- A key trade-off exists between redistribution and incentives. It is usually possible to provide more redistribution only at the cost of weakened incentives. Redistribution typically creates labor market distortions.[33] As Peter Diamond argues, "economists have raised the issue of the extent to which the payroll tax distorts the labor market. Suggestions that switching to a defined-contribution system will produce large efficiency gains are overblown. . . . Any redistribution will create some labor market distortion, whether the redistribution is located in the benefit formula or in another portion of the retirement income system." (Diamond 1998a).
- More generally, given other distortions in the labor market (for example, a progressive tax system), assessing how specific provisions of a pension program affect the efficiency of the labor market is a complicated matter (Diamond 1998b). As one example, the redistributive aspects of the Social Security program in the United States increase the return to work among the poor who, given the phaseouts associated with various other welfare programs, often face very high marginal tax rates (Stiglitz 1998; Lyon 1995).
- The distortion imposed by the payroll tax is not measured by the payroll tax itself, but rather by any difference between the net present

value of marginal benefits and the marginal tax (Feldstein and Samwick 1992). Similarly, the labor supply of those who do not fully value mandatory retirement savings—those who would not on their own have saved as much—will generally be affected by such a program, but it is wrong to infer that the mandatory savings program necessarily reduces labor supply. The key issue is what happens to the mean *marginal* utility of consumption, which could either increase or decrease (Stiglitz 1998).

- One of the most difficult questions in assessing any program is the appropriate counterfactual against which to judge it. For example, assume that workers who did not save for retirement—or who invested their contributions poorly—knew that they would be bailed out by the government. Funds for the bailouts would have to be raised through distortionary taxes, which would then affect labor supply. Savings, investment, and labor supply behavior would all be affected by the (potential) bailout and associated taxes. Whether they would be more or less affected than under an alternative social insurance program is an empirical question. Similarly, consider a program of privatization without prefunding. The additional taxes necessary to finance the debt generated by privatization without prefunding could distort labor market incentives. Indeed, in simulations reported by Corsetti and Schmidt-Hebbel (1997), a debt-financed transition to individual accounts *reduces* output by between 1 and 4 percent in the long run because of the distortions from higher income taxes necessary to finance the debt.
- Most of the discussion of the labor market effects of social insurance has focused on supply-side effects in competitive markets. Particularly in developing countries, the assumption of a perfectly competitive labor market seems inappropriate—suggesting that an exclusive focus on the supply side may be misplaced. Stiglitz has begun the exploration of labor market effects in a broader context (Stiglitz 1998).[34] More recently, Orszag, Orszag, Snower, and Stiglitz (1999) explore these issues in a model that incorporates interactions between the characteristics of the labor market and the pension system, while it is also capable of studying interactions between the pension system and the unemployment insurance system. They conclude that there is no simple dominance of one system over another in terms of labor market incentives.

Myth 6: Defined Benefit Plans Necessarily Provide More of an Incentive to Retire Early

The seminal work edited by Gruber and Wise (1999) shows that public defined benefit plans in the industrialized economies incorporate substantial taxes on work among the elderly, and that the provisions of those plans are often an important factor in early retirement. Some proponents of individual accounts have therefore suggested moving to a system of individual accounts as a way of avoiding this blandishment for early retirement.

This myth is thus related to Myth 5, but focuses specifically on older workers. This issue provides a vivid illustration of the "inherent vs. implemented" point we noted in the introduction. A public defined benefit plan need not necessarily impose an additional tax on elderly work. (An interesting question in evaluating the importance of such taxes is the degree to which we should be concerned about early retirement per se.)[35]

The net effect of a pension system on the incentive to retire comprises three components: the marginal accrual rate for additional work (additional benefits relative to additional taxes or contributions, for any given age of initial benefit receipt), the actuarial adjustment for delaying the initial receipt of benefits (regardless of whether work continues), and the rules for whether benefits are reduced because of earnings. In all three components, defined benefit plans need not provide more of a disincentive against work in favor of claiming benefits than a defined contribution plan. For example, benefit accrual rates are *higher* under many forms of defined benefit plans (some forms of final salary plans, for example) than under defined contribution plans—potentially providing a stronger incentive for continued work at older ages. The actuarial adjustment within a defined benefit plan is a policy parameter. And the presence or absence of an earnings test need not depend on the form of the pension system.

This comparison between a defined benefit and defined contribution approach therefore shows that the latter need not provide better incentives in theory. But what about the as-implemented comparison? Here, too, the situation is complicated. Many industrialized countries are reducing the incentives for early retirement within their defined benefit structures (Kalish and Aman 1997). In the United States, for example, Diamond and Gruber (1999) find small subsidies at age 62 and small net tax rates until age 65, with substantial tax rates from ages 65 to 69. Those large tax rates above age 65, however, will fall over time—under current law, the delayed retirement credit, which provides increased benefits to those who delay claiming benefits past 65, has been increasing, and is scheduled to reach 8 percent for each year of delayed claiming by 2005.[36] (That level is viewed as being approximately actuarially fair.)[37] Increasing the delayed retirement credit has a particularly strong effect on encouraging work among the elderly (Coile and Gruber 1999). Similarly, the economies in transition have generally increased the retirement ages within their traditional defined benefit programs over the past decade (Cangiano, Cottarelli, and Cubeddu 1998).

It is also worth noting that Sweden recently introduced a new pension system, including a "notional defined contribution" approach to the pay-as-you-go component,[38] that reflects concerns about the return to work among the elderly (Sundén 1998). A similar system was earlier implemented in Latvia and Poland (Fox 1997).

The key point is that the encouragement of early retirement is not a necessary element of a public defined benefit plan, and the Gruber-Wise findings do not necessarily provide a rationale for moving to individual accounts.

Myth 7: Competition Ensures Low Administrative Costs under Private Defined Contribution Plans

Another myth is that competition among financial providers will necessarily reduce administrative costs on individual accounts. For example, the *Economist* (1999) has stated that in creating individual accounts countries should "let many kinds of firms (banks, insurance companies, mutual funds) compete for the business. Fierce competition in sophisticated markets has driven down costs in these businesses. There is no reason why the same should not be true for pensions, although the need for adequate prudential and saver-protection regulation will clearly remain."

Competition, however, only precludes excess rents; it does not ensure low costs.[39] Instead, the *structure* of the accounts determines the level of costs. Furthermore, centralized approaches—under which choices are constrained and economies of scale are captured—appear to have substantially lower costs than decentralized approaches.

One approach to individual accounts would be to have centralized management with restricted investment options. In the United States, the Advisory Council on Social Security estimated that administrative costs under such a system would amount to roughly 10 basis points per year. Such costs, accumulated over 40 years of work, would reduce the ultimate value of an individual account by about 2 percent relative to its level without such transactions costs.[40]

An alternative approach would be a decentralized system of individual accounts, in which workers held their accounts with various financial firms and were allowed a broad array of investment options. Under such an approach, costs tend to be significantly higher because of advertising expenses, the loss of economies of scale, competitive returns on financial company capital, and various other additional costs. Administrative costs under such a system could easily amount to 100 basis points or more per year. Such costs would, over a 40-year work career, consume about 20 percent of the value of the account accumulated over the career.

Experience from both Chile and the United Kingdom is consistent with these predictions and indicates that a decentralized system of individual accounts involves significant administrative expenses (NASI 1999; Diamond 1999a; James, Ferrier, Smalhout, and Vittas 1998; Mitchell 1998). Both Chile and the United Kingdom have decentralized, privately managed accounts, and administrative costs in both countries have also proven to be surprisingly high (Diamond 1998a; Congressional Budget Office 1999).

Murthi, Orszag, and Orszag (1999a) present an accounting structure for administrative costs and then show that the administrative costs for individual accounts in the United Kingdom are substantial. The administrative costs associated with any system of individual accounts can be broken down into three components:

- The *accumulation ratio* captures fund management and administrative costs for a worker contributing funds to a single financial provider throughout his or her career.
- The *alteration ratio* measures the additional costs of failing to contribute consistently to a single financial provider over an entire career. It includes any costs from switching from one financial provider to another or from stopping contributions altogether (because of a withdrawal from the labor force, for instance). Many analyses have ignored the costs of transferring funds or stopping contributions.[41]
- The *annuitization ratio* reflects the costs of converting an account to a lifetime annuity upon retirement. These costs include mortality cost effects, since those purchasing an annuity in the United Kingdom (or elsewhere) tend to have longer average life expectancies than the general population. In a competitive market, such longer life expectancies will be reflected in higher annuity prices. Consequently, if someone with a typical life expectancy wishes to purchase an annuity, he or she must pay these prices, which means such a person will pay a higher price than the actuarially fair price for people with average life expectancies.[42]

Given interaction effects, various fees and costs consume between 40 and 45 percent of the value of an individual account for the typical worker in the United Kingdom. Furthermore, given the fixed costs associated with individual accounts, costs for smaller accounts (for example, in developing economies with lower levels of GDP per capita) would be even higher relative to the account size if the U.K. experience were replicated in such countries.

Charges can be high either because profits or underlying costs are high. The competitiveness of the individual account market in the United Kingdom and the departure of some providers from the market suggest the market is not excessively profitable. It is thus likely that charges primarily reflect underlying costs rather than unusually high profits for providers. Examples of the underlying costs include sales and marketing costs, fund management charges, regulatory and compliance costs, record-keeping, and adverse selection effects.[43]

The bottom line is that both the U.K. and Chilean experiences indicate that a decentralized approach to individual accounts is expensive—and the administrative costs would be even higher (relative to the account balances) if the accounts were smaller. A centralized approach to individual accounts could offer substantially reduced administrative costs. It is also worth noting that a centralized system could incorporate *some* competition, sufficient to obtain most of the benefits without the costs associated with a fully decentralized system.

Political Economy Myths

Myth 8: Inefficient Governments Provide a Rationale for Private Defined Contribution Plans

Some proponents of individual accounts argue that corrupt and inefficient governments provide a strong motivation for moving away from public systems toward private ones. To be true to our idealized versus as-implemented distinction, we should emphasize that this myth is very much in the as-implemented world: in an idealized world, democratic governments are not inefficient or corrupt, since political competition forces efficiency in the provision of public services, just as market competition does for private goods and services.[44]

On an as-implemented basis, however, the issue is more complicated than it may initially appear. Even under a private system, as Estelle James (1997) emphasizes, "considerable government regulation is essential to avoid investments that are overly risky and managers who are fraudulent. Some minimum reliability is required from the civil service for regulation to be effective." It is difficult to know why a government that is inefficient and corrupt in administering a public benefit system would be efficient and honest in regulating a private one.

To be sure, the likelihood of government malfeasance under different public programs—regulatory versus direct government management—may differ markedly, and we are only just beginning to understand the causes of any such differences. Among the relevant factors are undoubtedly transparency and complexity and, more generally, control systems within the public sector, as well as the magnitude of private incentives for abuses.[45]

Kazakhstan, which lacks a well-developed set of financial markets and has little of the infrastructure and regulatory prerequisites for the proper functioning of individual accounts, offers a good example of the risks. Even in industrialized economies with relatively efficient governments and well-developed financial markets, the scale of the regulatory challenge should not be underestimated. For example, according to Arthur Levitt (1998), chairman of the Securities and Exchange Commission in the United States, more than half of all Americans do not know the difference between a stock and a bond; only 12 percent know the difference between a load and noload mutual fund; only 16 percent say they have a clear understanding of the Individual Retirement Account; and only 8 percent say they completely understand the expenses that their mutual funds charge. The investor education and investor protection measures required to ensure that an individual account system operates well despite these knowledge gaps seem substantial, especially in developing countries.

The bottom line is that *public* malfeasance or incompetence can be just as dangerous under individual accounts as under public defined benefit systems. The key questions are the difficulties of constructing open, transparent systems under alternative regimes, and the capacities of individuals and organizations to monitor the public sector. In some cases, government failures may be so substantial that any form of prefunding—either through a public trust fund or through private accounts—would not be advisable.

Myth 9: Bailout Politics Are Worse under Public Defined Benefit Plans Than under Private Defined Contribution Plans

Another political economy myth is that bailout politics are more severe under public defined benefit plans than under private defined contribution plans. In other words, the assertion is that the government will experience greater pressure for social protection under a public defined benefit system than a private defined contribution one.

This myth, like the previous one, is largely based on comparing systems as they are implemented. After all, in an idealized world, programs would be designed with the "efficient" bail-out provisions. But even on an as-implemented basis, the distinction in this myth is overdrawn: it is simply not politically realistic to claim that governments will fail to come to the rescue in some way if financial disaster (say, a stock market crash) looms for a nontrivial share of the population.

In a sense, this myth is related to the previous one. If the government fails to do an effective job in regulating the private sector, and if individuals are allowed to invest in risky securities, those whose investment decisions turn out to be poor will likely turn to the government for assistance. In many countries, the guarantee is more than implicit: Governments often provide some sort of guarantee on the returns earned under the individual account approach.[46] As Rocha, Hinz, and Gutierrez stated in chapter 5, in most countries with a mandatory second pillar, some form of guarantee on returns exists. Such guarantees ultimately involve some type of explicit government backstop.[47]

Diamond and Valdés-Prieto (1994) examine the government guarantees inhering in the Chilean system at that time. They note that the government guaranteed 100 percent of an annuity up to the minimum pension, plus 75 percent of its value above the minimum pension; the minimum Administradoras de Fondos de Pensiones (AFP) relative return if the guarantee bonds posted by the AFPs are temporarily exhausted; and, finally, the minimum pension, so that the government shared in accrual risk (and longevity risk, if a phased withdrawal is chosen rather than an annuity). They further argue that "implicit government guarantees may exist because of the mandatory nature of contributions." (Diamond and Valdés-Prieto 1994).

Some analysts may argue that the government does not have to issue guarantees in the second pillar of a pension system if the first pillar were optimally constructed. Yet such an approach seems unlikely to be a political equilibrium. Dynamic inconsistency concerns are likely to loom large. Governments that regulate privatized systems—and surely some government regulation of the second pillar is necessary—are inevitably blamed for any failures in that system.[48] The comfort provided by the first pillar is unlikely to be sufficient to calm the political unrest resulting from any significant financial losses suffered by the middle and upper classes.

A more fundamental question is, if the first pillar were indeed so well designed that bailout pressures in a private second pillar were low, why bailout politics in a *public* second pillar would be so strong. The differences between a private, defined contribution system relative to a public, defined benefit one is difficult to assess ex ante. The outcome depends on a complicated political dynamic, which undoubtedly differs from country to country. To what extent does any increased risk under a defined contribution approach—and the related inability to spread risk across generations—increase the likelihood of a bailout? To what extent does the "privatized" nature of a private defined contribution system insulate the government from pressure for bailouts? These are important questions, and worthy of further study. We submit that the answers are far from clear at this point.

Concerns about potential bailouts following adverse financial performances are particularly germane to developing countries, since such economies typically experience substantially higher volatility than developed ones (Easterly, Islam, and Stiglitz 1999).[49]

Finally, the likelihood of a bailout of individual accounts may be heightened in postsocialist economies that had engaged in voucher privatizations.[50] In such voucher privatizations, shares in large and medium-sized companies were sold in exchange for vouchers. Since the normal fiduciary rules to be listed on a public stock exchange were bypassed by many firms undergoing privatization, shares in these firms are illiquid. Voucher investment funds, which were organized as intermediaries for the voucher privatizations, hold most of the illiquid shares.[51] Pension reform schemes in these countries may have the effect of transferring illiquid shares from the voucher funds to pension funds. Such a transfer may benefit the voucher funds but could also necessitate a government bailout of the pension funds should the illiquid shares prove to be worth less than their current "market price."[52] To be sure, the pension reforms are often touted as "deepening the stock market." Yet they may ultimately merely reallocate losses from one set of funds to another—and in a potentially regressive fashion.[53]

Myth 10: Investment of Public Trust Funds Is Always Squandered and Mismanaged

Another myth is that public trust funds are always squandered or mismanaged. Estelle James (1998) has written that "data gathered for the 1980s indicate that publicly managed pension reserves fared poorly and in many cases lost money—largely because public managers were required to invest in government securities or loans to failing state enterprises, at low nominal interest rates that became negative real rates during inflationary periods."

Several points are worth noting here. The first concerns the nature of the capital market. If capital markets were perfect, then it would simply not be possible (apart from corruption or a failure to diversify the portfolio across a sufficient number of assets) for funds to be badly invested. *Efficient markets ensure that returns are commensurate with risk*, as long as the investment portfolio is sufficiently diversified. Given efficient markets, those that accuse the government of investing poorly therefore must be accusing the government either of corruption or of choosing a portfolio that does not correspond to the risk preferences of pensioners. With respect to the latter, little evidence is typically presented. Furthermore, if individuals can undo the public fund portfolio by adjusting their own portfolio risk, public financial policy—including how the government invests its trust funds—is irrelevant (Stiglitz 1974, 1983, 1988). The assumption of perfect capital markets is not entirely convincing, especially in many developing countries. But then the opportunities for uninformed investors to make mistakes or to be exploited are increased.

Averting the Old Age Crisis noted that real rates of return on many public trust funds were negative during the 1980s. But that information alone does not tell us much: we would like to know how the real rate of return on the trust fund compared to other investments, after controlling for risk. Figure 3.7 in *Averting the Old Age Crisis* only offers one such comparison: between the U.S. Old-Age and Survivors Insurance trust fund and returns earned by U.S. occupational pension funds, and it does not control for risk. The risk adjustment is essential, since we should not be particularly concerned about funds that earn equal risk-adjusted rates of return but differ in their portfolios. Table 1.3 includes the other countries in *Averting the Old Age Crisis*, along with ex post real market interest rates between 1980 and 1990 computed from the International Monetary Fund's (IMF) *International Financial Statistics*. As it shows, a comparison with market interest rates indicates that the returns earned on public pension funds during the 1980s were indeed lower than risk-free market interest rates in most cases. But the degree of shortfall is much less pronounced than column (A) by itself

Table 1.3. Ex-Post Real Returns

	Real return on public fund, as published in Averting the Old Age Crisis[a] (A)	Average real ex-post discount rate, 1980–90, geometric mean[b] (B)	Difference (A)-(B)
Peru	–37.4	n.a.	n.a.
Turkey	–23.8	–4.4	–19.4
Zambia[c]	–23.4	–12.4	–11.0
Venezuela	–15.3	–6.4	–8.9
Egypt	–11.7	–4.1	–7.6
Ecuador	–10.0	–10.2	0.2
Kenya	–3.8	1.8	–5.6
India	0.3	0.8	–0.5
Singapore	3.0	4.3	–1.3
Malaysia	4.6	1.1	3.5

n.a. Not applicable.
a. Note that the time period in column (A) covers different subperiods of the 1980s for different countries, so the comparisons with columns (B) and (C) are not precise. Nonetheless, the qualitative results are similar regardless of the subperiod.
b. The real ex-post discount rate in any year is computed as

$$r = 100 \left\{ \frac{1+n}{1+\pi} - 1 \right\}$$

where r is the real interest rate, n is the nominal discount rate (line 60 in the International Financial Statistics), and π is the consumer price inflation rate (the percentage change in line 64 in the International Financial Statistics). The figure shown is then the geometric mean of the cumulative real return across 1980–90.
c. The real market rate is for 1980–88 because of data limitations.

would suggest. According to Iglesias and Palacios (see chapter 6), more recent research suggests that even after undertaking some risk adjustment, public trust funds tend to underperform private. But data problems plague the analysis, and undertaking an accurate risk adjustment is difficult.

In the United States, where the data are somewhat better than in many other countries, the debate over public pension investment performance has been particularly heated. On the basis of earlier research undertaken by Olivia Mitchell and others, Alan Greenspan has noted that state and local pension funds tend to underperform market rates of return (Mitchell and Carr 1996; Mitchell and Hsin 1997; Greenspan 1999). On closer analysis, however, the data do not seem to support this conclusion: Munnell and Sundén (1999) reexamined the evidence on state and local pension funds, and concluded that "public plans appear to be performing as well as private plans."

Finally, it is important to emphasize that countries are experimenting with institutional arrangements—such as independent boards, clear legislative mandates to avoid political investing, and restrictions on investments to broad market indexes—to protect trust funds from political pressures. For example, Canada has recently changed the regulations governing its Canada Pension Plan to allow that system to invest a portion of its reserves in private securities. Another interesting model, which is already fully operational, is the State Petroleum Fund (SPF) in Norway. The SPF, which, admittedly, is not formally a pension fund but still a public trust fund that may ultimately be used to pay pensions, held assets of about 15 percent of GDP at the end of 1998. It invests primarily in foreign bonds; its equity investments—which are mostly in managed and index funds—are externally managed by several foreign companies. The fund is managed at very low cost, and tracking errors relative to the benchmark have been relatively low (IMF 1999).

The impact of a trust fund's institutional structure deserves closer attention—funds with independent boards and sources of financing, a clear legal mandate to pursue competitive returns, and a focus on broad market index funds may fare better than other funds. (Active private fund managers do not tend to outperform index funds, so it is hard to argue—at least when the public trust fund would be a relatively small share of the market—that private funds would outperform a public fund that is invested solely in broad indexes.) Given the critical importance of prefunding in many countries, further scrutiny of whether public trust fund structures can be designed to avoid malfeasance and underperformance (even on a risk-adjusted basis) is crucial to a full evaluation of policy choices, particularly between public and private approaches to prefunding.

Conclusion

Underfunded public pension systems represent a potential threat to the fiscal soundness—and, more broadly, economic stability—of many developing countries. *Averting the Old Age Crisis* provided an invaluable service in drawing attention to this problem and in discussing specific policy changes to address the issue. Unfortunately, as often happens, the suggestions have come to be viewed narrowly—focusing on a second pillar limited to a private, nonredistributive, defined contribution approach. Most of the arguments in favor of this particular reform are based on a set of myths that are often not substantiated in either theory or practice.

The goals of pension policy—promoting old age security, developing a robust capital market, and encouraging domestic investment—often come into conflict, especially in developing countries. Private funds *may* help deepen domestic capital markets, but they may also expose the elderly to greater risks and dissipate more resources in administrative costs. Allowing investment of pension funds abroad, which is not politically popular in most countries, may reduce risk but could undermine the objective of deepening domestic capital markets. It may be possible to design arrangements that reduce risk without such adverse consequences—for example, swaps across countries—but these arrangements may be easier to undertake with public rather than private pension funds. Clearly, trade-offs exist, especially since developing country capital markets are imperfect and are likely to remain so for some time.

A move toward privately managed defined contribution pensions may or may not have an adverse effect on savings, welfare, labor supply, or the fiscal balance. We have identified a number of factors that affect the outcome in any specific country. In developing economies, there is not, we would argue, any presumption in favor of the conventional wisdom—a privately managed, defined contribution system. Less developed countries usually have less developed capital markets, with less informed investors and less regulatory capacity, making the scope for potential abuse all the greater. Moreover, the presence of greater volatility and the absence of many types of financial markets make many kinds of insurance provided by traditional defined benefit programs all the more valuable.

The debate over pension reform would benefit substantially from a more expansive view of the optimal second pillar, which should incorporate well-designed public defined benefit plans. A privately managed second pillar is not always optimal. A more expansive perspective would allow policymakers to appropriately weigh all the trade-offs they face, including private versus public systems; prefunding versus not prefunding; diversifying versus not diversifying; and defined contribution versus defined benefit pension plans.

Notes

1. Another crucial issue is whether the second pillar is redistributive. In general, the optimal system of redistribution involves taxes and subsidies in each "pillar," rather than confining the redistribution role to a single pillar.

2. The popular interpretation may be understandable, since many of the Bank's leading pension scholars could easily be misinterpreted as advocating it. For example, Estelle James writes that the second pillar should be "a mandatory, privately managed scheme....[The scheme] should be privately and competitively managed (through personal retirement savings accounts or employer-sponsored pension plans) to produce the best allocation of

capital and the best return on savings." See Estelle James, "Outreach #17: Policy Views from the World Bank Policy Research Complex," August 1995, pp. 2–3.

3. In Hong Kong, Croatia, and Venezuela, multipillar systems are scheduled to begin in 2000.

4 In addition, a private system may involve some public guarantees, such as those that ensure pensioners are protected when pension funds declare bankruptcy.

5. The cash balance plans becoming more prevalent in the United States are one example. It is also interesting that many analysts assume that retirees under a defined benefit pay-as-you-go system would partially share in any positive long-term productivity shocks. Such an assumption changes the nature of the system from a pure defined benefit one to an amalgam of defined benefit and defined contribution systems, with the accrual risk arising from productivity and demographic variables rather than financial markets.

6. An inherent feature of a program is one which would be true for *all* feasible implementation strategies and institutions.

7. Botswana is apparently in the process of implementing a pension scheme.

8. Precisely to avoid having to make trade-offs across these generations, economists typically look for Pareto improvements—reforms that make *everyone* better off while making no one worse off. Almost all proposed reforms, however, fail to meet this test. The situation therefore becomes much more complicated.

9. The conditions under which this effect occurs are complicated. The earlier literature analyzing the impact of (mean-preserving) increases in risk discussed them widely. See, for example, Diamond and Stiglitz (1974), and Rothschild and Stiglitz (1971).

10. The distinction between narrow and broad prefunding is similar to the distinction between "apparently funded" and "ultimately funded" pensions highlighted by Valdés-Prieto (1997).

11. The evidence from Chile on the impact of pension reform on national saving is somewhat mixed. The national saving rate rose substantially from the early 1980s to the mid-1990s, but it is unclear precisely how much of that increase should be attributed to the pension reform (Kay 1997).

12. Another issue that carries national saving implications—admittedly in the "as-implemented" category—is whether early (preretirement) withdrawals are allowed from individual accounts. In many cases, substantial political pressure may be applied to allow such early withdrawals. Yet succumbing to such pressures could reduce both narrow and broad prefunding. In the United States, for example, Samwick and Skinner (1997) show that nearly US$50 billion in pension assets were distributed prior to

age 59-1/2 in 1990, and that roughly half of those early distributions were spent rather than rolled over into other retirement accounts.

13. Holzmann notes that "a redistribution of total debt between implicit and explicit liabilities should have little effect on the pure interest rate. It affects the capital stock and national saving only marginally." (Holzmann 1997).

14. Note that we are assuming that from a macroeconomic perspective, implicit and explicit debt are equivalent. For further discussion of whether implicit unfunded liabilities are equivalent to explicit public debt, see Hemming (1998), pp. 15–16. Note that in asserting that *changes* in the sum of implicit and explicit debt do affect national saving, we are assuming that the conditions required for neo-Ricardian equivalence fail.

15. For references to the existing literature on pay-as-you-go systems internationally, see Mackenzie, Gerson, and Cuevas (1997). For references to the existing literature on the United States, see Feldstein (1998).

16. This proposition can be put somewhat more formally. For any program of gradual conversion of a public pay-as-you-go system to a narrowly prefunded individual account system, a set of taxes exists that would convert the public pay-as-you-go system to a narrowly prefunded public system and that would leave aggregate consumption and output at each date (in each state of nature) unaffected relative to the individual account system.

17. More generally, Samuelson's original paper on the consumption loan model illustrates this point quite vividly. Broad prefunding involves intergenerational trade-offs of the type discussed in the introduction.

18. Nicholas Timmins. "The Biggest Question in Town: America Faces Critical Choices Over the Future of Its Most Popular Spending Programme." *Financial Times*, March 20, 1998, p. 23.

19. Palacios and Whitehouse (1998), p. 5.

20. These projections are taken from the U.S. Bureau of the Census. See *Statistical Abstract of the United States 1998*, table 1340.

21. Dynamic efficiency requires that no generation can be made better off without making other generations worse off (for a fuller articulation, see Cass 1965). An economy that is dynamically inefficient could "dissave" and reduce its capital stock, increasing consumption for the current generation and every subsequent generation. While the conditions for dynamic efficiency have been widely discussed in hypothetical economies with no land, the issue typically is not even germane in the "real world" with land. Consider, for example, an economy with zero growth. Dynamic inefficiency would then require a negative real interest rate, which would produce the absurd result of land with infinite value! Also note that the conditions for dynamic efficiency in a stochastic setting are complicated (see, for example, Abel, Mankiw, Summers, and Zeckhauser 1989).

22. Ironically, there are cases in which a switch to a pay-as-you-go system can increase the welfare of earlier generations without making later

generations worse off. Indeed, that was Samuelson's fundamental insight in his consumption loan paper: In the reversal, from a pay-as-you-go system to a fully funded one, it is possible that every generation could be worse off. To be sure, our concerns about existing systems are somewhat different—Samuelson focused on Ponzi schemes that were viable in the long run, but most real-world systems do not seem to share that property. Some type of reform is inevitable.

23. This simplified example and much of its discussion is taken from Orszag (1999), which is itself based on Geanakoplos, Mitchell, and Zeldes (1998, 1999).

24. Some may argue that the only feasible way to abolish the redistribution would be to convert the program from a public one to a private one. Even if that were true, the choices involved would then become substantially more complicated than a simple rate-of-return comparison would suggest.

25. Boldrin, Dolado, Jimeno, and Peracchi (1999), p. 27.

26. This is an example of the more general theorem showing that public financial policy is irrelevant with efficient markets (Stiglitz 1983).

27. Council of Economic Advisers (1997), p. 113.

28. Heller (1998), p. 11.

29. It is often asserted that differential mortality rates by income imply that on a lifetime basis seemingly progressive systems are not actually progressive. In the United States, at least, that statement is somewhat misleading. See Steuerle and Bakija (1994); Garrett (1995); and Duggan, Gillingham, and Greenlees (1995).

30. As noted above, a defined benefit program could be thought of as a defined contribution program combined with appropriate financial options. In principle, the government could issue the options independently of the pension system, allowing individuals to create synthetically a defined benefit pension out of an otherwise defined contribution system. Yet there may be benefits—for example, in terms of bailouts—to bundling the options solely with the pension system.

31. A related concern is that government ownership of private equity would distort investment allocations. Restricting public investment to broad market indexes may attenuate such concerns.

32. Another implication of the failure of the public sector analogue to the Modigliani-Miller theorem is that a movement of government trust funds out of bonds and into stocks could increase interest rates on the government bonds. The higher interest costs to the government could then at least temporarily worsen the government's cash flow (e.g., if most of the short-run returns from holding equities are in the form of unrealized capital gains rather than dividends). The deterioration in cash flow could then require additional reliance on distortionary taxation, which could then affect labor supply. In effect, one could think of an investment restriction in which the

public trust fund holds only government bonds as a tax imposed on the pension system. Lifting the investment restriction then shifts the tax to a different base (all taxpayers).

33. Whether redistribution should be undertaken through the pension system or other means (such as the income tax system) is a serious question. If the redistribution is better undertaken through alternative mechanisms, then a complete analysis of defined benefit versus defined contribution pension systems must also take into account the distortions engendered by the alternative redistribution mechanism.

34. Consider, for example, an efficiency wage model in an environment in which an urban job entitles one to participate in a public social insurance program. The subsidies associated with such a system increase the rents of those who obtain jobs in the urban sector (one of the most often stated criticisms of such public systems), but the increased public subsidy shifts the no-shirking constraint (for example, in a Shapiro-Stiglitz model of efficiency wages) down, so that equilibrium wages are reduced and equilibrium employment increased. Whether social welfare increases from such a wage subsidy is thus a complicated matter.

35. Some social insurance programs implicitly provide "obsolescence" insurance against technological shocks that affect the value of human capital. Experience normally increases an individual's human capital, but rapid technological change may diminish its value, so that older workers face diminishing productivity and wages. Some workers may want to obtain insurance against this risk, in the form of an "option" to retire early. Carefully defined retirement insurance programs could provide an element of such insurance by providing early retirees some increment in the present value of benefits over contributions. To be sure, like most insurance, moral hazard concerns arise with such insurance: The provision of the insurance at the margin induces some individuals whose productivity has not fallen to retire earlier than they otherwise would have. Optimal insurance balances the risk reduction and moral hazard effects. It is a valid criticism to say that balancing has not been undertaken properly; it is not a valid criticism to say that some adverse incentive effect exists. In a related spirit, Diamond and Mirlees prove the optimality of taxing work for insurance purposes in an ex ante identical workers model (Diamond and Mirlees 1978, 1986, and forthcoming).

36. The delayed retirement credit applies to delays past the normal retirement age (currently 65). For claiming before the normal retirement age, the actuarial adjustments are 6.67 percent of the worker's Primary Insurance Amount per year. That is also approximately actuarially fair.

37. A difficult issue involved in actuarial "fairness" is which population's mortality projections to use in evaluating such fairness. For example, many of those retiring early are less healthy than average. In evaluating actuarial

fairness for early retirement, should the mortality experience of those actually choosing to retire early be used, or the mortality experience of the population as a whole? Similarly, a program that is actuarially fair for the population as a whole will generally not be actuarially fair for specific subsets of that population. See, for example, the discussion in Gruber and Orszag (1999).

38 A notional defined contribution system is a pay-as-you-go pension system in which the worker's benefit is accrued in a notional account, which is then uprated each year by wage growth (in Sweden's case, wage growth per capita). The "account" thus provides a real rate of return equal to real wage growth (per capita), which is why the system is referred to as a "notional defined contribution" system. Upon retirement, the value of pension rights is divided by remaining life expectancy. Therefore, the later benefits begin, the higher annual benefits will be, since the downward adjustment to reflect remaining life expectancy will be smaller. (Benefits can be claimed as early as age 61.)

39. Moreover, in a world with monopolistic competition (which, given imperfect information, is often a better description of markets than perfect competition), competition leads to zero profits but not necessarily economic efficiency.

40. More recent estimates suggest that costs may be somewhat higher under this approach (Diamond 1999a). Diamond also notes that the administrative costs for a decentralized approach may be 100 to 150 basis points, slightly higher than the 100-basis-point estimate applied to the Personal Security Account proposal in the Advisory Council report.

41. Murthi, Orszag, and Orszag (1999a) discuss these alteration costs in much more detail. The high level of alteration costs in the United Kingdom seems to reflect a particularly inefficient approach to implementation of individual accounts.

42. This point is related to one made in a footnote above: It is always important to ask "actuarially fair for whom?" It is also important to note that mortality selection effects are a cost to the typical individual but do not necessarily measure the profit to the provider, the loss of utility to the consumer, or the resource cost to society from the selection effect in the annuity market. Rather, they represent a financial loss for the typical person, if he or she decided to purchase an annuity, relative to an annuity that accurately reflected his or her life expectancy. For further discussion of the annuities market in the United Kingdom and the impact of selection effects, see Murthi, Orszag, and Orszag (1999b). For further discussion of the various selection effects in annuities markets—not all of which necessarily represent market failures—see James and Vittas (1999).

43. It is important to note that most studies examine the costs of individual accounts to consumers, not the resource costs to society. In many

situations, the two concepts may not be identical. For example, selection effects are of a somewhat different nature than many of the other costs listed above: most of the accumulation costs, for example, likely represent direct resource costs to society, whereas selection effects represent indirect costs (by discouraging individuals from participating in the insurance market). Similarly, such studies do not necessarily measure the utility losses from charges. The approach is a financial one, not a utility one, and is not presented in utility-based terms.

44. The theory of government failures explains why competition may not lead to the desired results for public goods, just as the theory of market failure does for private goods. It is possible that there are inherent reasons that one set of failures is more severe than another, but the case for such inherent differences is more subtle than the argument that underlies Myth 8.

45. For example, a rule-based system in which public funds are invested in government bonds or in broad market indexes is relatively easy to monitor and therefore seems to involve limited scope for abuse. In contrast, given the wide variety of ways in which private actors can circumvent the intent of any specific rule, a government regulatory system can be quite complex. Such complexity may increase the potential for corruption, as actors try to "bribe" regulators to approve nontransparent schemes. Such concerns are of particular importance in developing countries, where nongovernmental consumer and investor protection organizations may be weak and unsophisticated.

46. For a contingent claims approach to valuing these guarantees, see Pennacchi (1999).

47. Note that the guarantees transform the system from a pure defined contribution one toward a mixed private defined contribution-public defined benefit system. They thus facilitate some degree of intergenerational risk sharing absent from the pure private defined contribution system.

48. Any government that chose *not* to regulate a privatized system could increase the risk of a crisis; for example, the lack of prudential standards may raise the possibility of a large account provider failing to deliver on its promises to retirees. In any case, if such a crisis hit, the government—despite its ostensible lack of involvement—would likely be forced to provide a bailout anyway.

49. The higher financial volatility in developing economies could be attenuated by allowing individuals to invest in foreign assets. If such investments were appropriately chosen, the returns should then be independent of outcomes in their own country—insulating the individuals from the effects of higher domestic volatility. But this approach raises a number of sensitive issues. For example, in the presence of endogenous growth elements or any differential between social and private returns to capital, investing abroad is not necessarily equivalent to investing at home.

If pension savings are invested abroad, the country benefits from the private return to capital in foreign markets but does not necessarily capture the full potential social return. This effect could thus provide a policy rationale for limiting foreign investments.

50. The authors thank David Ellerman for his insight into this problem. This section relies heavily on his contributions.

51. The voucher funds were creatures of the voucher privatization and are far more numerous and powerful than mutual funds in the West. For instance, in one small country, there are about 10 actively traded companies and over 30 voucher funds (and more than 1,000 voucherized companies with tradable, but illiquid, shares).

52. Given the illiquidity, the current market price is not necessarily particularly illuminating.

53. In practice, in at least one country, voucher privatizations were accompanied by looting, with rapid erosion of the value of shares.

References

Note: The word *processed* describes informally reproduced works that may not be commonly available through libraries.

Abel, Andrew. 1999. "The Social Security Trust Fund, the Riskless Interest Rate, and Capital Accumulation." Paper presented at NBER conference on Risk Aspects of Investment-Based Social Security Reform. Processed.

Abel, Andrew, Gregory Mankiw, Lawrence Summers, and Richard Zeckhauser. 1989. "Assessing Dynamic Efficiency: Theory and Evidence." *Review of Economic Studies* 56(1):1–19

Bateman, Hazel and John Piggott. 1997. "Mandatory Retirement Saving: Australia and Malaysia Compared." In Salvador Valdés-Prieto, ed., *The Economics of Pensions: Principles, Policies, and International Experience.* Cambridge University Press.

Boldrin, Michele, Juan Jose Dolado, Juan Franscisco Jimeno, and Franco Peracchi. 1999. "The Future of Pension Systems in Europe: A Reappraisal." *Economic Policy*, forthcoming.

Burtless, Gary. 1998. Testimony Before the Committee on Ways and Means, Subcommittee on Social Security, U.S. House of Representatives, June 18.

Cangiano, Marco, Carlo Cottarelli, and Luis Cubeddu. 1998. "Pension Developments and Reforms in Transition Economies." Working Paper No. 98/151, International Monetary Fund, Washington, D.C.

Cass, David. 1965. "Optimum Growth in an Aggregative Model of Capital Accumulation." *Review of Economic Studies*, 233–40.

Coile, Courtney, and Jonathan Gruber. 1999. "Social Security and Retirement." Paper presented at NBER conference on Risk Aspects of Investment-Based Social Security Reform. Processed.

Congressional Budget Office. 1999. *Social Security Privatization: Experiences Abroad*. Available at http://www.cbo.gov.

Corsetti, Giancarlo, and Klaus Schmidt-Hebbel. 1997. "Pension Reform and Growth." In Salvador Valdés-Prieto, ed., *The Economics of Pensions: Principles, Policies, and International Experience*. Cambridge University Press.

Council of Economic Advisers. 1997. *Economic Report of the President 1997*. Washington, D.C.: Government Printing Office.

Diamond, Peter. 1998a. "The Economics of Social Security Reform." In R. Douglas Arnold, Michael J. Graetz, and Alicia H. Munnell, eds., *Framing the Social Security Debate: Values, Politics, and Economics*. Washington, D.C.: Brookings Institution Press.

———. 1998b. "Privatization of Social Security and the Labor Market." Presentation delivered at the Massachusetts Institute of Technology (MIT) Public Finance lunch. Processed.

———. 1999. "Administrative Costs and Equilibrium Charges with Individual Accounts." NBER Working Paper No. 7050. Cambridge, Mass.: National Bureau of Economic Research.

Diamond, Peter, and Joseph Stiglitz. 1974. "Increases in Risk and in Risk Aversion." *Journal of Economic Theory* 8: 337–60.

Diamond, Peter, and James Mirlees. 1978. "A Model of Social Insurance with Variable Retirement." *Journal of Public Economics* (10): 295–336.

———. 1986. "Payroll-Tax Financed Social Insurance with Variable Retirement." *Scandinavian Journal of Economics* 88 (1): 25–50.

———. "Social Insurance with Variable Retirement and Private Saving." *Journal of Public Economics*, forthcoming.

Diamond, Peter, and Salvador Valdés-Prieto. 1994. "Social Security Reforms." In Barry Boswoth, Rudiger Dornbusch, and Raul Laban, ed., *The Chilean Economy: Policy Lessons and Challenges*. Washington, D.C.: Brookings Institution Press.

Diamond, Peter, and John Geanakoplos. 1999. "Social Security Investment in Equities I: The Linear Case," NBER Working Paper No. 7103. Cambridge, Mass.: National Bureau of Economic Research.

Diamond, Peter, and Jonathan Gruber. 1999. "Social Security and Retirement in the United States." In Jonathan Gruber and David Wise, eds., *Social Security and Retirement Around the World*. University of Chicago Press.

Duggan, J. E., R. Gillingham, and J. S. Greenlees. 1995. "Progressive Returns to Social Security? An Answer from Social Security Records." Research Paper No. 9501. Department of the Treasury, Washington, D.C.

Dutta, Jayasri, Sandeep Kapur, and J. Michael Orszag. 1999. "A Portfolio Approach to the Optimal Funding of Pensions." Working Paper. Birckbeck College, University of London. Processed.

Easterly, William, Roumeen Islam, and Joseph Stiglitz. 1999. "Shaken and Stirred: Volatility and Macroeconomic Paradigms for Rich and Poor Countries." Michael Bruno Memorial Lecture, XII World Congress of the IEA, Buenos Aires, Argentina.

The Economist. "Economic Focus: Latin Lessons on Pensions." 1999. vol. 351, no. 8123 (June 12): 71.

Feldstein, Martin. 1997. "The Case for Privatization." Foreign Affairs (July/August).

————. 1998. "Introduction," in Martin Feldstein, ed., Privatizing Social Security. University of Chicago Press.

Feldstein, Martin, and Andrew Samwick. 1992. "Social Security Rules and Marginal Tax Rates." National Tax Journal 45: 1–22.

Fox, Louise. 1997. "Pension Reform in the Post-Communist Transition Economies." In Transforming Post-Communist Political Economies. National Research Council. Washington, D.C.: National Academy Press.

Garrett, D. M. 1995. "The Effects of Differential Mortality Rates on the Progressivity of Social Security." Economic Inquiry 33.

Geanakoplos, John, Olivia S. Mitchell, and Stephen P. Zeldes. 1998. "Would a Privatized Social Security System Really Pay a Higher Rate of Return?" In R. Douglas Arnold, Michael J. Graetz, and Alicia H. Munnell, eds., Framing the Social Security Debate: Values, Politics, and Economics. Washington, D.C.: Brookings Institution Press.

————. 1999. "Social Security Money's Worth." In Olivia S. Mitchell, Robert J. Myers, and Howard Young, eds., Prospects for Social Security Reform. Philadelphia: University of Pennsylvania Press.

Greenspan, Alan. 1996. Remarks at the Abraham Lincoln Award Ceremony of the Union League of Philadelphia, Philadelphia, Pennsylvania, December 6, 1996.

————. 1999. "Social Security." Testimony Before the Committee on Budget, U.S. Senate, January 28, 1999.

Gruber, Jonathan, and David Wise, eds. 1999. Social Security and Retirement Around the World. Chicago: University of Chicago Press.

Gruber, Jonathan, and Peter Orszag. 1999. "What to Do About the Social Security Earnings Test?" Issue in Brief #1, Center for Retirement Research, Boston College.

Heclo, Hugh, 1998. "A Political Science Perspective on Social Security Reform." In R. Douglas Arnold, Michael J. Graetz, and Alicia H. Munnell, eds., Framing the Social Security Debate: Values, Politics, and Economics. Washington, D.C.: Brookings Institution Press.

Heller, Peter. 1998. "Rethinking Public Pension Initiatives." Working Paper No. 98/61. Washington, D.C.: International Monetary Fund.

Hemming, Richard. 1998. "Should Public Pensions be Funded?" Working Paper No. 98/35. Washington, D.C.: International Monetary Fund.

Holzmann, Robert. 1997. "Fiscal Alternatives of Moving from Unfunded to Funded Pensions." OECD Development Centre Technical Papers No. 126. OECD, Geneva.

IMF. 1999. *Norway: Selected Issues*. IMF Staff Country Report No. 99/11. Washington, D.C.: International Monetary Fund.

James, Estelle. 1995. "Outreach #17: Policy Views from the World Bank Policy Research Complex." Washington, D.C.: World Bank.

————. 1997. "Public Pension Plans in International Perspective: Problems, Reforms, and Research Ideas." In Salvador Valdés-Prieto, ed., *The Economics of Pensions: Principles, Policies, and International Experience*. Cambridge University Press.

————. 1998. "Pension Reform: An Efficiency-Equity Tradeoff?" In Nancy Birdsall, Carol Graham, and Richard Sabot, eds., *Beyond Tradeoffs*. Washington, D.C.: Brookings Institution Press.

James, Estelle, Gary Ferrier, James Smalhout, and Dimitri Vittas. 1998. "Mutual Funds and Institutional Investments: What Is the Most Efficient Way to Set Up Individual Accounts in a Social Security System?" NBER Working Paper No. 7049. Cambridge, Mass.: National Bureau of Economic Research.

James, Estelle, and Dimitri Vittas. 1999. "Annuities Markets in Comparative Perspective: Do Consumers Get Their Money's Worth?" Paper presented at the World Bank Conference on New Ideas About Old Age Security, September 1999, Washington, D.C.

Kalish, David, and Tetsuya Aman. 1997. "Retirement Income Systems: The Reform Process Across OECD Countries." Social Policy Division, OECD, Geneva.

Kay, Stephen. 1997. Testimony Before the Subcommittee on Social Security of the Ways and Means Committee, U.S. House of Representatives, September 18, 1997.

Leimer, Dean. 1995. "A Guide to Social Security Money's Worth Issues." *Social Security Bulletin*, Summer 1995.

Levitt, Arthur. 1998. Speech at the John F. Kennedy School of Government, Harvard University, October 19, 1998.

Lyon, Andrew. 1995. "Individual Marginal Tax Rates under the U.S. Tax and Transfer System." In David Bradford, ed., *Distributional Analysis of Tax Policy*. Washington, D.C.: American Enterprise Institute Press.

Mackenzie, George, Philip Gerson, and Alfredo Cuevas. 1997. "Pension Regimes and Saving." International Monetary Fund, Occasional Paper No. 153. Washington, D.C.: International Monetary Fund.

Mehra, Rajnish, and Edward Prescott. 1985. "The Equity Premium: A Puzzle." *Journal of Monetary Economics* (March): 145–61.

Merton, Robert. 1983. "On the Role of Social Security as a Means for Efficient Risk Sharing in an Economy Where Human Capital Is Not Tradeable." In Zvi Bodie and John Shoven, eds., *Issues in Pension Economics.* University of Chicago Press.

Merton, Robert. Zvi Bodie, and Alan Marcus. 1987. "Pension Plan Integration as Insurance Against Social Security Risk." In Zvi Bodie, John Shoven, and David Wise, eds., *Issues in Pension Economics.* University of Chicago Press.

Mitchell, Olivia. 1998. "Administrative Costs in Public and Private Retirement Systems." In Martin Feldstein, ed., *Privatizing Social Security.* University of Chicago Press.

Mitchell, Olivia, and Roderick Carr. 1996. "State and Local Pension Plans." In J. Rosenbloom, ed., *Handbook of Employee Benefits.* Chicago: Irwin.

Mitchell, Olivia, and Ping-Lung Hsin. 1997. "Public Pension Governance and Performance." In Salvador Valdés-Prieto, ed., *The Economics of Pensions: Principles, Policies, and International Experience.* Cambridge University Press.

Modigliani, Franco, Marialuisa Ceprini, and Arun Muralidhar. 1999. "A Solution to the Social Security Crisis From an MIT Team." Sloan Working Paper No. 4051. Cambridge, Mass.: Massachusetts Institute of Technology.

Munnell, Alicia, and Annika Sundén. 1999. "Investment Practices of State and Local Pension Funds: Implications for Social Security Reform." In Olivia S. Mitchell, Brett Hammond, and Anna Rappaport, eds., *Forecasting Retirement Needs and Retirement Wealth.* Philadelphia: University of Pennsylvania Press, forthcoming.

Murthi, Mamta, J. Michael Orszag, and Peter R. Orszag. 1999a. " The Charge Ratio on Individual Accounts: Lessons from the U.K. Experience. Working Paper 2/99. Birkbeck College, University of London.

———. 1999b. "The Value for Money of Annuities in the U.K.: Theory, Experience and Policy." Working Paper 9/99. Birkbeck College, University of London.

NASI (National Academy of Social Insurance). 1999. "Report of the Panel on Privatization of Social Security." Available at http://www.nasi.org and as in Peter Diamond, ed., *Issues in Privatizing Social Security: Report of an Expert Panel of the National Academy of Social Insurance.* Cambridge, Mass.: MIT Press.

Orszag, J. Michael, Peter R. Orszag, Dennis J. Snower, and Joseph E. Stiglitz. 1999. "The Impact of Individual Accounts: Piecemeal vs. Comprehensive

Approaches." Paper presented at the Annual Bank Conference on Development Economics, World Bank, April 29, 1999, Washington, D.C.

Orszag, Peter R. 1999. "Individual Accounts and Social Security: Does Social Security Really Provide a Lower Rate of Return?" Center on Budget and Policy Priorities.

Palacios, Robert, and Edward Whitehouse. 1998. "The Role of Choice in the Transition to a Funded Pension System." Social Protection Discussion Paper No. 9812. Washington, D.C.: World Bank.

Pennacchi, George. 1999. "Government Guarantees for Old Age Income." In Olivia Mitchell, Robert Myers, and Howard Young, eds., *Prospects for Social Security Reform*. Philadelphia: University of Pennsylvania Press.

Rothschild, Michael, and Joseph Stiglitz. 1970. "Increasing Risk, I: A Definition." *Journal of Economic Theory* 2: 225–43.

———. 1971. "Increasing Risk, II: Its Economic Consequences." *Journal of Economic Theory* 3: 66–84.

Samuelson, Paul. 1958. "An Exact Consumption-Loan Model of Interest with or without the Social Contrivance of Money." *Journal of Political Economy* (December): 219–34.

Samwick, Andrew, and Jonathan Skinner. 1997. "Abandoning the Nest Egg? 401(k) Plans and Inadequate Pension Saving." In Sylvester Schieber and John Shoven, eds., *Public Policy Toward Pensions.* Cambridge, Mass.: MIT Press.

Siegel, Jeremy. 1998. *Stocks for the Long Run.* New York: McGraw Hill.

Social Security Administration. 1997. *Social Security Programs Throughout the World 1997.* Washington, D.C.: Government Printing Office.

Steuerle, Eugene, and Jon Bakija. 1994. *Retooling Social Security for the 21st Century.* Washington, D.C.: Urban Institute Press.

Stiglitz, Joseph. 1974. "On the Irrelevance of Corporate Financial Policy." *American Economic Review* (December): 851–66.

———. 1982. "Utilitarianism and Horizontal Equity: The Case for Random Taxation." *Journal of Public Economics* (18): 1–33.

———. 1983. "On the Relevance or Irrelevance of Public Financial Policy: Indexation, Price Rigidities, and Optimal Monetary Policy." In R. Dornbusch and M. Simonsen, eds., *Inflation, Debt, and Indexation.* Cambridge, Mass.: MIT Press.

———. 1988. "On the Relevance or Irrelevance of Public Financial Policy." *Proceedings of the 1986 International Economics Association Meeting.*

———. 1998. "Taxation, Public Policy, and the Dynamics of Unemployment." Keynote Address to the 54th Congress of the International Institute of Public Finance, August 24, 1998.

Sundén, Annika. "The Swedish Pension Reform." Federal Reserve Board, September 1998.

Timmins, Nicholas. 1998. "The Biggest Question in Town: America Faces Critical Choices over the Future of Its Most Popular Spending Programme." *Financial Times,* March 20.

Valdés-Prieto, Salvador. 1997. "Financing a Reform Toward Funding." In Salvador Valdés-Prieto, ed., *The Economics of Pensions: Principles, Policies, and International Experience.* Cambridge University Press.

Weaver, R. Kent. 1998. "The Politics of Pensions: Lessons from Abroad." In R. Douglas Arnold, Michael J. Graetz, and Alicia H. Munnell, eds., *Framing the Social Security Debate: Values, Politics, and Economics.* Washington, D.C.: Brookings Institution Press.

World Bank. 1994. *Averting the Old Age Crisis: Policies to Protect the Old and Promote Growth.* Oxford University Press.

2

Comments on Rethinking Pension Reform: Ten Myths about Social Security Systems by Peter Orszag and Joseph Stiglitz

Robert Holzmann, Estelle James, Professor Axel Börsch-Supan, Professor Peter Diamond, and Professor Salvador Valdés-Prieto

Comments by Robert Holzmann, The World Bank

This is an interesting and provocative chapter that raises key issues for debate. However, it has a very strong U.S. orientation and, hence, reveals very little about what happens in the world—in both academic and actual pension reform contexts. Nor is it concerned with how to address the complex and differentiated pension reform issues that the World Bank confronts. Despite these limitations, the chapter helps us to identify important points of contention and areas for future investigation; for example, regarding the possibility of learning from mistakes and cross-country experience, the significance of market weaknesses and failures, and the importance of political failures and the effectiveness of measures to limit them.

I agree with many of the points raised, partly because of the way in which the "myths" were formulated ("necessary," "always," "has no," etc.), and partly because many of the points have been long adopted within and outside the World Bank. Since the publication of *Averting the Old Age Crisis* in 1994, thinking on pension reform implementation has become much more differentiated and sophisticated. Within the World Bank, this is readily evident from a visit to its social protection Web site, which includes a series of discussion papers covering cutting-edge issues in pension reform.

In my comments, I will (i) say a few words on the myths, (ii) address the question of whether or not a multi-pillar system is a useful reference model for the steady-state, and (iii) explain why the multipillar system is also considered a useful reference model for reform.

On the Myths

It is easy to agree with most statements about the myths; because of the way in which the myths were formulated, they are bound to be wrong by the level of generalization. But my understanding is that in the policy discussion and most of the international literature, the points raised to support a *partial* move toward funded, privately managed, defined contribution schemes are argued in a more sophisticated manner. Furthermore, in these discussions not only the comparison between idealized models enters but also the experiences in countries with these models. Despite the caution one has to apply when transposing "historic tendencies in one nation," knowledge sharing is still an important element of learning in economics as well as economic policy.

Against this background, a few remarks on each myth follow:

- Myth 1. Individual accounts per se do not raise national saving, but they may if the transition from an unfunded to a funded scheme is linked with a restrictive fiscal stance, or if the reform creates externalities such as financial market development and economic growth (Holzmann 1997). These reform externalities are likely to be much more important than a change in the national saving rate.
- Myth 2. Rates of return under individual accounts are not necessarily higher. But they may be, if administrative costs can be kept in check, transition costs are low or nonexistent for systems in a start-up phase, or the reform externalities allow for Pareto-improving transition (Holzmann 1999; Homburg 1990).
- Myth 3. Declining rates of return on pay-as-you-go (PAYG) systems do not necessarily reflect fundamental problems. But the high returns typically given to the start-up generation increase the initial demand for the scheme, and political willingness to maintain high benefits renders most PAYG schemes fiscally unsustainable. Then, falling rates, which become negative in some countries (Holzmann 1988), change the relative prices and, as a consequence, the portfolio demand for unfunded/funded provisions, creating pressure for reform.
- Myth 4. Investment of public trust funds in equities will have macroeconomic effects in a world of nonhomogeneous individuals and imperfect capital markets. For this very reason, a (partial) move toward funded schemes should be considered.
- Myth 5. Labor market incentives are not necessarily better under individual accounts. But the conjecture is that it is politically easier

to improve these incentives under a defined contribution (DC) plan than under a defined benefit (DB) plan.

- Myth 6. DB plans do not necessarily provide more of an incentive to retire early, but the empirical evidence suggests that they usually do.
- Myth 7.Competition alone does not ensure low administrative costs under individual accounts. I was not aware of this claim.
- Myth 8. Corrupt and inefficient governments do not provide a rationale for individual accounts. I was not aware of this claim either.
- Myth 9. Bailout politics are not necessarily worse under public DB plans. The government is always a provider/insurer of last resort. But the bailout under a DB plan may be more expensive, since higher commitments have accrued.
- Myth 10. Investment of public trust funds is not always squandered and mismanaged. But the track record is not encouraging, as Iglesias and Palacios point out in chapter 6, and the Canadian reform model, which occurred after decades of poor investment performance, still awaits evaluation and successful implementation in other countries.

On the Multipillar Model

The chapter almost exclusively focuses on the rationale and soundness of the conceptual underpinnings for moving from unfunded, publicly managed DB to fully funded, privately managed, DC systems, but it does not really discuss the overarching proposal of the World Bank, namely the multipillar system as a reference model for pension reform.

Proposing the multipillar makes two assumptions: the model is an optimal one for the steady-state (ignoring transition costs) or for start-up countries, and it is a useful reference point for pension reforms when a monopolistic PAYG scheme is already in place (discussed below).

The arguments for a multipillar system (consisting of a mandatory, publicly managed, unfunded pillar and a mandatory but privately managed funded pillar, as well as supplemental voluntary provisions, including real and financial assets) under steady-state conditions are essentially threefold (Holzmann 1998), in that it allows for:

- A clearer distinction between the redistributive and the income replacement objective of mandatory schemes
- Risk diversification, since not all of the population's retirement portfolio will be subject to the same political, demographic, and economic risk
- Better avoidance of fiscal unsustainability and reduction of negative effects on individual saving and labor supply decisions

Most but not all of these objectives can, in principle, be achieved in a well-structured and publicly managed DB scheme operating under partial funding. But based on the worldwide experience, the conjecture is that the likelihood of this happening is slim. The authors themselves state that "from a risk perspective, the socially optimally system may be a diversified, *partially* funded one." The multipillar system shares this view, but admittedly has less confidence in the public sector to administer a reserve fund, although it does not totally exclude it.

The application of the model for start-up countries has a much larger potential than the authors suggest. In most of the World Bank's client countries, the existing PAYG schemes have low coverage (mostly in the range of 10 to 30 percent), and in many countries provident funds arrangements exist, making less prominent the issue of transition costs.

On Multipillar Pension Reform

When a country has an existing and comprehensive PAYG system, which urgently needs to be reformed for short- and long-term fiscal reasons, its evident negative impact on labor supply and retirement decisions, and its questionable distributive implications, the question naturally arises if a move toward a multipillar system is Pareto-improving, or if the reform effort should not concentrate on a PAYG-only reform.

The needed reforms can, in principle, be addressed by *reforming the PAYG system*, that is, by changing the parameters of the pension system (such as retirement age, accrual factors, length of assessment period, indexation, etc.) and by engaging in partial prefunding in a public reserve fund. The political unattractiveness, however, to engage in a comprehensive PAYG reform—the fiscal and economic gains would be harvested at the time when the responsible politician is already out of office—while undertaking continuous marginal changes creates a time consistency problem. Politicians cannot make a convincing argument that the proposed "parametric" reform is a lasting one (that is, one that puts the scheme on a sound long-term financial basis) and that they have no incentive to change the benefit/contribution structure for political reasons in the future. Given this credibility problem, individuals have an incentive to oppose a "parametric" reform from the very beginning. And examples of marginal parametric reform attempts, many of which failed or came about only after intensive political fighting, are abundant (Demirgüç-Kunt, and Schwarz 1999).

Perhaps a more promising strategy for PAYG reform employs a "paradigm shift"—that is, putting forth a conceptual structure that changes the usual terms of debate. A paradigm shift is inherent in proposals to move to a Chilean-style funded scheme. The close analogue in the PAYG context is the construct of notional defined contribution (NDC) accounts, which China, Italy, Latvia, Mongolia, Poland, and Sweden have enacted or are discussing.

Against this background of the political difficulties of engaging in comprehensive parametric reform and of problems of establishing and securing a reserve fund that is publicly managed, the proposed reform approach toward a multipillar pension system has the quality of a "paradigm shift," provides more credibility, overcomes resistance among broad segments of the population, and may deliver reform externalities. This is the experience in advanced economies such as Australia, Denmark, the Netherlands, Switzerland, and the United Kingdom; it is the experience in Latin America and Eastern Europe where the World Bank is heavily involved (Lindeman, Rutkowski, and Sluchynsky 2000; Queisser 1998).

Yet, while the multipillar pension system serves as a reference model, it is not a blueprint that is applied blindly in all cases. When supporting pension reforms, the World Bank, among other things, (i) takes account of country preferences and circumstances; (ii) applies sound reform criteria (Does the reform meet distributive concerns? Is the macro and fiscal policy accommodating the reform sound? Can the administrative structure operate a new multipillar pension scheme? Are the regulatory and supervisory arrangements and institutions in place to operate the funded pillar with acceptable risk?); (iii) links client assistance with knowledge management, such as through the establishment of a pension reform primer; and, (iv) pursues an active research agenda on the many open problems mentioned in the chapter. As a result, while recent pension reforms in Latin America and Eastern Europe share common characteristics, no two are identical. Accordingly, the World Bank has supported different reform approaches.

The reforms already undertaken and those in preparation will all profit from the conference papers comprising this volume and the attempts by the World Bank to underpin the reform efforts with best knowledge from academic research and best practice experience from client or sponsor countries. Theoretical introspection is very important, but so is hands-on experience reform from countries. This is fully in line with the tone of the chapter and its U.S. background, "It ain't necessarily so. . . ."

References

Note: The word *processed* describes informally reproduced works that may not be commonly available through libraries.

Demirgüç-Kunt, A., and A. Schwarz. 1999. "Taking Stock of Pension Reforms Around the World." Social Protection Discussion Paper 9917. World Bank, Washington, D.C.

Holzmann, R. 1988. "Zu ökonomischen Effekten der österreichischen Pensionsversicherung: Einkommensersatz, Ruhestandsentscheidung und interne Ertragsraten." In Robert Holzmann, ed., *Ökonomische Analyse der Sozialversicherung*. Wien.

―――. 1997. "Pension Reform, Financial Market Development, and Economic Growth: Preliminary Evidence from Chile." IMF Staff Papers 44, No. 2, June, 149–78, Washington, D.C.

―――. 1998. "A World Bank Perspective of Pension Reform." Social Protection Discussion Paper 9807. World Bank, Washington, D.C.

―――. 1999. "On the Economic Benefits and Fiscal Requirements of Moving from Unfunded to Funded Pensions." In M. Buti, D. Franco, and L. Pench, eds., *The Welfare State in Europe*. Cheltenham, UL, and Northampton, Mass.: Edward Elgar.

Homburg, S. 1990. "The Efficiency of Unfunded Pension Schemes. *Journal of Institutional and Theoretical Economics* 146, 640–47.

Lindeman, D., M. Rutkowski, and O. Sluchynskyy. 2000. "The Evolution of Pension Systems in Eastern Europe and Central Asia: Opportunities, Constraints, Dilemmas and Emerging Practices." World Bank, Washington, D.C.

Queisser, M. 1998. "The Second-Generation Pension Reforms in Latin America." OECD, Development Centre Study, Paris.

Comments by Estelle James, The World Bank

The biggest goal of researchers is that other people will think about and debate their ideas. In the policy arena researchers have the equally important goal that governments will implement some of their ideas. In both respects, the team that wrote *Averting the Old Age Crisis* is gratified more than it possibly could have hoped when the book was first published five years ago.

Although, in the spirit of this debate, the chapter by Peter Orszag and Joseph Stiglitz emphasized some of the points of continuing dispute, I would like to start by emphasizing the substantial shift toward consensus among academics and policymakers observed over the past five years. This shift has occurred in part because of the force of events—we have all become increasingly aware of the problems that will be caused by traditional social security systems as populations age and as active progrowth strategies become essential. The flow of information and ideas in numerous books and articles has also helped to shape the new consensus, and I like to think that *Averting the Old Age Crisis* played a role in this intellectual process. The many points on which many economists and policymakers might have disagreed five years ago, but on which they now largely agree, include the following:

- In choosing an old age system, we should take account of its broader macroeconomic and microeconomic impacts, which affect the welfare of the young, as well as its impact on the standard of living of the old. This broad economic impact, indeed, constitutes the core rationale for the multipillar recommendation of *Averting the Old Age Crisis*: funding to increase national saving, private management to maximize the productivity of pension capital, and defined contribution to provide good labor market incentives, especially regarding the age of retirement.
- Some degree of prefunding is desirable in an old age security system. This helps to insulate the system from demographic shock and, if used in conjunction with other appropriate policies (constraints on government dissaving and on consumer credit), can also be an instrument to increase national saving.
- Prefunding is obviously a different concept from privatization. However, once funds are accumulated, someone must manage them, and they must be invested in some portfolio. Most economists now agree that generally the funds that are accumulated should be invested through the private capital markets, in a diversified portfolio, to maximize productivity and rate of return for a given risk. And, the larger the funds are, relative to gross domestic product (GDP) and to

the country's total capital stock, the more important it is to use a decentralized mechanism for accomplishing this in order to avoid distortions and misallocations due to political control. Decentralization also facilitates capital market development and deepening, which is important for many countries. Some disagreement continues about the best type and degree of decentralization, especially in cases where the accumulated funds are relatively small. I will talk more about this important issue later.

- It is important to avoid incentives for early retirement in the structure of the system. That is, early retirement should be penalized and continued work rewarded on actuarially fair terms, and Gruber and Wise (1999) have shown that workers respond to these incentives. This point will become crucial as populations age so that early retirement has an increasing impact on labor force size and system costs. A defined contribution plan that converts the capital accumulation into an annuity through the market automatically accomplishes this. In principle a DB plan can also be designed to accomplish this. However, in the real world very few countries have systems that currently do this, and efforts to change DB systems to do it have almost always met with failure.

- How the transition is financed can have a big effect on its ultimate impact. For example, national saving will not be increased if the transition is financed 100 percent by debt with no other change in benefits or contributions. An increase in saving requires a cut in consumption—either public or private. Thus either taxes must increase, benefits must be cut, or other government spending must decline, as a transition financing mechanism, in order to increase national saving. Partly for this reason, every country that has made the transition from a PAYG system to a partially funded system has used a combination of these methods (plus some debt finance to smooth the distribution of the burden) to finance the transition. Although Orszag and Stiglitz list this as a point of contention, I would list it as a point of consensus.

- Diversification is important to reduce risk. The Orszag-Stiglitz chapter mentions this, and, of course, that is why we recommend a multipillar system with diversified income sources and investments. A system that includes a funded component earning returns from capital plus an unfunded component based on labor income reduces risk through diversification.

- We should look at systems in practice, not only systems in theory. Political economy considerations as well as practical implementation problems may (and usually do) lead systems to turn out somewhat differently from initial expectations. For this reason, continued monitoring and analysis of reformed systems is essential, and second-generation reforms are inevitable. This is part of the work we are doing here at the World Bank, and some of the papers at the conference presented preliminary analyses of these data. Countries that are now in the process of reforming can learn from the experience of those that went before, and countries that reformed early are now improving and fine-tuning their systems. Corrections are ongoing in life. At the same time, in social security as in other aspects of life, the absence of ex post data ex ante should not prevent us from undertaking reforms that, on a probabilistic basis, seem likely to improve the situation.

- Every country is different, and this should and will be reflected in the design of social security systems. Again, the chapter lists this as a point of disagreement. However, I certainly do not disagree with that statement, nor does anyone I know. By now, numerous countries in Latin America; Hungary, Poland, and Croatia in Eastern and Central Europe; a scattering of OECD countries; Kazakhstan and, most recently, Hong Kong, have adopted the general approach outlined in *Averting the Old Age Crisis*: their new systems contain a publicly managed, tax-financed, defined benefit social safety net; a funded, privately managed, defined contribution pillar; and space for additional voluntary retirement saving. But reforming countries have reformed in somewhat different ways, with differing public-private, funded-PAYG mixes, and World Bank advice is always adapted to country circumstances.
- Finally, we all share the common goal of creating an old age system that is sustainable, redistributive toward low-income groups who probably do not earn enough during their working years to support themselves in old age as well, and is favorable, rather than discouraging, toward economic growth. However, we disagree to some extent on the ways to accomplish this.

I will now discuss some ways in which I disagree with the chapter by Orszag and Stiglitz. One basic problem is that they ruled out a discussion of political economy on grounds that each country's politics is different. But politics, like economics, is subject to certain regularities, and I will give examples below of how the political regularities have systematically created problems for traditional DB PAYG systems and for publicly managed funded systems.

A second basic problem is that their chapter deals with a world in which most of the assumptions and evidence come from the United States and, to a somewhat lesser extent, the United Kingdom, and this world presents a situation different from that which prevails in the rest of the world. The chapter is disappointingly devoid of experience—problems, solutions, and data—from the World Bank's client countries. Perhaps this is not surprising, considering that Joseph Stiglitz spent several years chairing the Council of Economic Advisers in the United States and Peter Orszag was on the Council during that time. U.S. conditions and politics inevitably shaped their mindset. But we should all remember that the United States is not the world, especially the world in which the World Bank works. While I personally favor the creation of individual accounts in a multipillar system in the United States, because of the macroeconomic impact mentioned above, the case is even stronger in other countries, especially the countries in which the World Bank operates. It is important to be aware of the ways in which their initial conditions and political economy differ from those in the United States and from those assumed in the Orszag-Stiglitz chapter, adding even more impetus for a multipillar reform. For example:

- The paper begins by distinguishing between how one would design a new system and how one would redesign an already existing mature system. The authors apparently feel the arguments are stronger for a largely funded system with an important DC component in the former case (a new or immature system), but they assert that most countries fall into the latter case (old and mature). Now, that is true of the North American and European countries, but it simply is not true of most of the rest of the world. Recent regressions show that global social security coverage is less than one-third of the labor force.
- If we look at Africa or Asia or Central America, for example, we find that formal systems cover fewer than 20 percent of workers, most of whom are government employees. The private sector has yet to be covered on these continents. Middle-income countries in the southern cone of South America have somewhat greater coverage, but even there less than half of private sector workers are covered. Many of these countries have a large population bulge below the age of 35. These countries have not yet given away a large PAYG windfall because few workers and retirees are covered. But if coverage were suddenly increased in a new or expanded PAYG system, this would imply a large giveaway, and future generations would be saddled with a huge pension debt that does not yet exist. I think it is dangerous to give advice to these countries based on the assumptions that mature systems exist there, as in the United States, when that is patently not the case.
- The chapter assumes that there would be high transition costs upon a shift to a funded system, in large part because of its assumption about the existence of mature systems. The fact is that transition costs

(defined as the existing implicit debt that would become an explicit liability during a transition) would be far less than 100 percent of GDP, sometimes less than 50 percent of GDP, in practically all World Bank client countries outside Eastern Europe. This is because most of the systems in these countries are immature; the few covered workers have only acquired a few years of experience; and the systems are partially funded; and/or they consist mainly of a first pillar that offers a flat or means-tested benefit, to which a second pillar could be added with little or no transition costs. In other words, these costs would be less than in the United States or any existing OECD country. Of course, if these countries continue along a PAYG path, their pension debt and transition costs will grow much larger. These countries have a chance to reform their systems before a large debt accumulates, making a transition more difficult.

- The chapter assumes that most traditional systems have progressive benefit formulas, as in the United States, while this simply is not true. To begin with, in many of the World Bank's client countries, only the upper half or quintile of the population is covered, so any positive transfers, usually intergenerational, go to those who are better off, by definition. Additionally, most DB formulas are not progressive and give larger transfers and rates of return to high earners. Basing benefits on the last years of work in the face of rising age-earnings profiles for high earners and having a low ceiling on taxable wages are examples of such features. (Even in the United States studies have indicated that lifetime transfers are not redistributive to the poor, although on an annual basis they appear quite redistributive.) Moreover, most systems feature idiosyncratic redistributions that benefit special groups without any corresponding efficiency or equity gains. Examples are unreduced benefits to early retirees and low incremental benefits to second workers in a household. These are nontransparent ex ante redistributions, not Pareto-improving insurance against unpredictable risk.

- Often attempts to change DB formulas to make them more equitable and efficient meet with unmitigated failure for political reasons: the beneficiaries are well-defined groups who know they are benefiting and do not want to lose their privileges. Marginal changes, as in the adoption of a multipillar system, can sometimes be more difficult to achieve than changing the system completely in a way that eliminates these undesirable features as a by-product. And it is more difficult to hide perverse redistributions in a smaller, less complicated public pillar that has the explicit and primary objective of providing a social safety net.

- Furthermore, the chapter assumes that the systems penalize early retirement in an actuarially fair manner, as in the United States, or that the systems that do not already do this can easily accomplish it. Actually, few countries in the world outside of the United States and Japan penalize early retirement, and this is one of the most difficult things to accomplish within the confines of a DB PAYG plan. All of us can cite examples from our own experience of policymakers who met defeat when they tried to make their systems more actuarially fair. Moreover, as longevity increases successive governments must repeatedly raise the normal retirement age, so even if today's government is successful, tomorrow's may not be. One of the strongest political regularities outside of the United States is the difficulty in raising the retirement age and penalizing early retirement.

- In contrast, a DC plan that annuitizes in the private market upon retirement automatically accomplishes both of these things. People who retire earlier automatically get lower benefits, which is a deterrent to early retirement, and as longevity increases benefits decline unless people continue to work longer. Significantly, if people decide to retire early, they internalize the costs themselves instead of shifting the costs onto others. So they do not take this option unless the value to them outweighs the cost, and the system as a whole remains financially sustainable. Thus annuitization of a DC plan puts the system on automatic pilot with regard to early retirement, and this is one of its big advantages. In the context of the United States, which penalized early retirement and is raising the retirement age, this may not seem to be a big deal, but in the rest of the world in which most of us operate, we know that it is. Indeed, many policymakers favor DC systems precisely because they automatically create the right retirement incentives and thereby get them and their successors off a very painful hook. (Recently some countries have adopted notional DC plans hoping to emulate this desirable feature of funded DC plans. Unfortunately, when DC plans remain notional or pay-as-you-go, they may continue to be susceptible to allowing early retirement on nonactuarial terms for political reasons—as with Latvia's early minimum pension for women.)

- Stiglitz and Orszag deal with a world in which the total contribution rate is low (12.5 percent in the United States), and contemplated contributions to a funded pillar are very small relative to GDP and other capital stock in the economy. So how these funds are invested is important, but probably not as important as in countries where these funds are the country's major source of long-term capital. In the latter countries, which are the countries in which the World Bank works, funds from a mandatory funded pension plan could grow to more than 100 percent of GDP, and they would be the major source of long-term capital. How this capital is allocated then becomes crucial.

Surely, Orszag and Stiglitz are not recommending that governments should be in charge of the lion's share of a country's investments. That has already been tried, and it failed, as participants from the Former Soviet Union and Eastern European countries are only too well aware.

- It is difficult to separate out "inherent" from "implementation" problems and to avoid political economy concerns in discussing publicly managed funds. But, almost by definition, such funds must either be nondiversified, invested in government bonds, and potentially expanding the amount of government deficits, or invested in the private market, leading to government control of private enterprise. I do not believe that most people want to advocate either course. Even in the United States, if the trust fund were invested in stocks, it could lead to substantial government control over small cap stocks—and in other countries most stocks are small caps. With large amounts of money involved, the Scyllian choice between a growing government debt or backdoor nationalization of a country's private sector could only be avoided by investing the funds outside of the country. Norway is doing that with its Petroleum Fund, but practically no other country is willing to follow this course.

- Finally, the chapter raises the issue of risk and safety, implying that public management is safer than private management. In the United States, where the trust funds are invested in government bonds that earn positive real returns, this argument may apply (although a huge equity premium is being sacrificed in return for a small diminished risk). But in most of the rest of the world, this argument about the safety of publicly managed funds simply does not stand up to empirical examination. In chapter 6, Augusto Iglesias and Robert Palacios show, in a rather large sample of countries with publicly managed pension reserves, that the rate of return on these funds was consistently less than the bank deposit rate or the rate of per capita income growth in these countries. In contrast, privately managed funds generally earned positive returns that exceeded the bank deposit rate or the growth rate of per capita income. (Incidentally, the chapter deals with net returns, after subtracting administrative costs).

- These lower returns either imply a hidden tax on the pension system or a misallocation of capital to lower productivity investments, or both. It seems very strange to me to call these negative, below market returns safe. If I were a worker in one of these countries, I would not feel very safe because I would realize that ultimately either my contribution rate would have to rise or my benefits would fall, or the government would have to tax me in other ways to cover the pension debt when investments were dissipated by politically motivated choices.

Indeed, the latter point is the crux of the issue and the essence of the remaining disagreement. The alternative to public control is private decentralized control, by workers (as in Latin America) or their unions and employers (as in the OECD). As I discuss in a chapter of this volume, on administrative costs, this choice of managers and investment strategies always is and should be constrained by government, to a greater or lesser extent. But, to avoid the risk of low returns and misallocated capital, I believe the evidence indicates that some degree of decentralization and competition, that is, regulation rather than direct control, is essential. This does not eliminate political risk, but it sets up a countervailing force that allows higher returns to be realized, even in countries in which governments malfunction.

References

Gruber, Jonathan, and David Wise, eds. 1999. *Social Security and Retirement Around the World.* Chicago: University of Chicago Press.

Comments by Professor Axel Börsch-Supan, University of Mannheim, Germany

Before dealing substantively with the Orszag-Stiglitz chapter, I will first make a brief introductory remark: Although the chapter claims to be deliberately provocative, I found only one really provocative statement in it, on the bottom of the first page, specifically that the chapter is "nuanced."

Nuance is certainly a matter of perspective. The chapter's narrow-minded view may be helpful in the United Kingdom or the United States, where pension system development has gone far in the direction of private defined contribution (DC) plans. However, the conference concerns the world. In fact, there are many parts of the world—actually a majority of the countries—that have only one monolithic public defined benefit (DB) system, and this chapter does little justice to the many attempts of moving towards more balanced systems that combine elements of public defined benefit and private defined contribution (DC) plans. A nuanced view would take at least a bit of a glimpse at the problems of those countries. As a European, specifically as a German who lives in a country in which, despite all kinds of serious troubles ahead, the reform towards a more balanced system has been repeatedly stalled, I say this with quite a bit of frustration. This brings me to the following substantive points.

Demographic Constraints Are Serious

Demographic changes will increase implicit public debt in a way that is unsustainable even for rich countries. Thus prefunding in the broad sense, as defined in the chapter by Orszag and Stiglitz, is a simple necessity.

This is an important point. The chapter misses this, or at least its fundamental significance for the debate. The chapter actually minimizes this fundamental political constraint by somewhat loosely referring to the illusion that the choice of prefunding or not is only a matter of "intergenerational trade-offs." For many countries, this is simply wrong because the future payroll taxes will reach levels that are unsustainable and will not permit any trade-off.

Again, the perspective is important. In spite of all the discussions in the U.S. Congress, the U.S. demography is relatively harmless. The United States expects to have a dependency ratio in 2030 that is as high as that in many countries today. However, in those countries the dependency ratio will continue to rise rapidly, doubling from this current high level until the year 2030 and seriously constraining policy options.

Corporate Governance of Public Investment

Given that we need to prefund in the broad sense, the remaining core question is whether prefunding should be done publicly or privately. Orszag and Stiglitz advocate public investment. As opposed to the title of the conference, this is not a new idea. It has been done before with results that have been documented quite a few times. Examples are the provident funds in Asia, which have rather low returns even after the correction done in the chapter. Other examples are the partially funded systems in the Middle East that frequently squandered funds in order to finance dubious public investment projects.

But there is a more subtle point, namely the question regarding who should exert corporate governance. In order to answer this question, it is important to get volumes right. Let me pick up the German example. In order to fund 50 percent of Germany's pension claims, the fund would have to be about one-third of current gross fixed capital stock. The political economy of a government running such a significant share of the economy is well known and not favorable. There are plenty of discouraging examples in France, Italy, and Sweden, so I do not have to mention the many countries in the Former Soviet Union and in developing countries.

There is the illusion that the government can passively invest in index funds. This illusion is also shared, by the way, by a proposal recently put forward by Franco Modigliani. This will not work. Somebody has to enforce corporate governance—either the owner of the capital directly or her agents. Direct control is out of the question for most workers and pensioners. So the central question is what motivates the agent, the government in the case proposed by Orszag and Stiglitz. I do not see any compelling corporate governance mechanism that guarantees market rates of return in this case.

Political Risks versus Capital Market Risks

Belittling political risks and being cavalier with political economy questions is another worrisome tendency in Orszag and Stiglitz's argument. I find the discussion in Myths 8, 9, and 10 on the political economy particularly troublesome. While it is correct that the regulation of capital markets is imperfect and subject to corruption and ignorance, it is by no means a logical conclusion that therefore one might as well leave all governance to the state. There is a clear hierarchy and a division of labor. It starts with day-to-day management, continues to the supervisory role of the governors, and finally ends at the establishment of a regulatory environment by the government. The closer the state has been to day-to-day management, the more problematic it has been, as has been proved over and over again in experiences all across the world.

Again, the discussion is very centered on the North American context and misses the reality in most developing countries (and even in large parts of Western Europe) where a large share of GDP is government related and deregulation is slow. To give some actual examples: in Germany a board of state-appointed but independent trustees overseeing a third of the capital stock, as proposed by Orszag and Stiglitz, is wishful thinking in the light of the fact that the social security actuaries have recently adjusted their demographic forecast to match the long-term budget limits of the public pension system. And Germany is not the only country (add certain nongovernment organizations) in which demographic projections are treated as political, not scientific, exercises.

Incentive Effects on Participation and Internal Rates of Return

I will be very brief on Myths 5 and 6, related to economic incentive effects. Orszag and Stiglitz are correct that labor supply disincentives are not necessarily implications of public DB plans. But this is theory. In practice, two significant effects—participation effects and early retirement effects—dominate almost all existing public defined benefit plans, even if they are partially funded.

Concerning participation incentives, evidence in many countries shows that participation declines as soon as public DB plans become voluntary. "Opting out" has been overwhelming in Hungary, the United Kingdom, and the Latin America reform countries. In a similar fashion, public opinion policies on public DB plans yield miserable grades.

The negative incentive effects on participating in public DB plans are governed by the perceived rate of return differences vis-a-vis capital market returns. The chapter by Orszag and Stiglitz is quite correct in dismissing superficial comparisons, particularly if transition costs are ignored. But this does not leave rates of return under PAYG DB plans and fully funded DC plans equivalent. Again, I am missing a more subtle (may I say "nuanced") approach to this question. The equivalence of maintaining the PAYG system and a transition to a fully funded system shown by Breyer (1989), Brunner (1994), Fenge (1995), and others only holds in very simple economies that are frictionless (for example, perfect capital markets) and have a fixed technology. If there are liquidity constraints, diversification constraints, or if the technology changes because productivity is affected by changes in the pension system (Corsetti 1994), these results do not hold and provide room for a genuine difference in the rates of return.

Incentive Effects on Early Retirement and the Political Economy

In terms of early retirement, it should be stressed that the United States is an outlier. Most other countries in the Gruber and Wise (1999) volume have not managed, or did not want, to make their defined benefit plans actuarially fair. This is not by chance but has systematic reasons, namely a link to unemployment policies—the false belief that reducing old age labor force participation will reduce unemployment because labor is a fixed lump—and pork barrels politics—because in many countries the elderly are the largest special interest group among voters (Mulligan and Sala-i-Martin 1999).

Getting quarrels, such as those about actuarially adjustments, out of the day-to-day special interest politics and into the realm of actuaries and insurance managers is an important reason to move away from pure public DB plans—maybe not all the way. Here are exactly the missing nuances that the chapter claims to deliver.

Political Risks versus Capital Market Risks, Revisited

This brings us back to the question of political risks. In being so one-sided, the chapter also misses the point that defined benefits are not defined benefits anyway. It is simply a myth that defined benefit plans carry no risk. And it is simply a myth that any pension system can be risk-free. Public DB plans have an enormous political risk. Social security benefits have been changed up and down for all kinds of reasons in the major European Union countries, as can be studied in the many institutional comparisons available. Once again, this chapter should have expanded its perspective from the United States to include the European, Latin American, or North African experiences.

I provide two examples: in spite of being "defined benefit" plans, in most countries it is not possible to get an official statement of what these defined benefits are for a specific individual. This includes my own country. And taking another example from Germany: during the last eight months, future pension benefits have been increased and reduced again by 15 percent when laws were revoked and administrative rules were changed to fit budget requirements.

On top of this, indexation to inflation is discretionary and subject to pork barrel politics in most developing and even some European countries. Of course, it is not a necessary feature of public DB plans in theory. In reality, however, governments rarely bind themselves in this manner. The historical evidence clearly shows that governments prefer to keep their ability to make discretionary policy.

I do not want to belittle the risk inherent in private DC plans. All things considered, this very much speaks for a multipillar system in which one part is run by the state and might be pay-as-you-go or funded, and another part consists of individual funded accounts. Very obviously—since capital market and political risks are unlikely to be perfectly correlated—a combination reduces overall risk. The balance between political risk and capital market risk is not only country specific (as the chapter correctly and repeatedly points out) but will also vary within countries from rich to poor and according to preferences. It is thus important to give the people some choice of how much the second pillar is investing in public bonds or private equities, very much along the lines of Prime Minister Tony Blair's stakeholder pension idea.

Whom to Trust?

The fundamental disagreement in our debate is on which choices to leave to the people and whom the people should trust. If we take the historical evidence, in most countries—maybe the United States is an exception—governments have a rather bad track record when trusted with running large funds. We have to bite part of this bullet for redistributional tasks because the state provides the only way to organize this. However, it is not necessary to bite all of this bullet, in particular for the nonredistributive bulk of the old age insurance, as this chapter—with too few nuances—suggests.

References

Breyer, F. 1989. "On the Intergenerational Pareto-Efficiency of Pay-as-You-Go Financed Pension Systems." *Journal of Institutional and Theoretical Economics* 145: 643–58.

Brunner, J. 1994. "Redistribution and the Efficiency of the Pay-as-You-Go Pension System." *Journal of Institutional and Theoretical Economics* 150: 511–23.

Corsetti, G. 1994. "An Endogenous Growth Model of Social Security and the Size of the Informal Sector." *Revista Analisis Economico* 9(1).

Fenge, R. 1995. "Pareto-Efficiency of the Pay-as-You-Go Pension System with Intergenerational Fairness." *Finanzarchiv* 52: 357–63.

Gruber, J., and D. Wise, eds. 1999. *Social Security and Retirement Around the World*. Chicago: University of Chicago Press.

Mulligan, C.B., and X. Sala-i-Martin. 1999. "Social Security in Theory and Practice." NBER Working Paper No. 7118. Cambridge, Mass.: National Bureau of Economic Research.

Comments by Peter Diamond,
Massachusetts Institute of Technology

First, I agree with all 10 myths in the chapter—the economic and political advantages of defined contribution individual accounts have been exaggerated. I agree that one should compare politically plausible, well-designed DB and DC systems (excluding economywide earning-related systems) in countries where political plausibility varies for both DB and DC systems and should not compare a well-designed system of one kind with a poorly designed system of the other. The latter sort of comparison may be the stuff of polemics, but it does not belong in good policy analysis.

The politics of DB systems vary across countries, and many countries have been less successful in good design than the United States has been. But DB systems can be improved, and some of the worst features occur at the start of a system and are of little or no relevance to the question of reform. The politics of DC systems also varies across countries, and the quality of design has already been worse in some countries than in Chile. Additional countries and future developments are likely to show more problems.

I want to use this opportunity to discuss an 11th myth—that DC systems are more transparent than DB systems and therefore more democratic. There are issues in pension design where alternative institutions do differ primarily in transparency—the extent to which information is made available and salient. However, in contrasting DB and DC systems, it seems to me that the right vocabulary is that of framing, not of transparency. As we know from cognitive psychology, particularly the work of Kahneman and Tversky (1984), framing has a very powerful effect on thought. It is not surprising that it also has powerful effects on political outcomes. Thus DB and DC systems vary in the focus of what is transparent (or salient), not in the presence or absence of transparency.

DC systems make the financing of benefits particularly salient. This includes making redistribution particularly salient. However, DC systems make the outcomes opaque, measured by benefit levels relative to some measure of needs (replacement rates, measured in some way). Benefits depend on the returns to assets (which are stochastic and with the right stochastic process in dispute) and on the pricing of annuities (which is also stochastic and also subject to dispute about mortality trends as well as future rates of return). But it is not just that individuals find it hard to tell what benefits they will receive conditional on future earnings. It is also that the pattern of outcomes across different individuals is opaque, and citizens care about the pattern of incomes within a cohort.

In contrast, DB systems make individual annual benefits and benefit patterns visible, conditional, of course, on future earnings. That is, a DB system makes clear the outcomes of the system in terms of what the retirement income system is trying to do, which is to replace lost earnings. (The presence of a DB retirement system may also affect the disability insurance program; indeed, it is difficult to integrate well a DB disability system with a DC retirement system.) While DB systems will be adjusted from time to time, so actual benefits are stochastic, that adjustment takes place in the context of the salience of the benefit pattern. But DB systems make the connection between individual financing and individual benefits opaque. (This is also why benefits are generally related to earnings subject to tax, not to taxes paid, another design feature that affects outcomes.)

It is interesting that the contrast in outcomes between public DB and DC systems also occurs in corporate pension systems. Giving past-service credits to long-term employees was common when DB systems were being set up in the United States. Giving analogous lump sums to similarly placed employees when setting up DC systems has certainly been rare in the United States—I have not heard of a single one, although my search has not been exhaustive.

This tension is not unique to the provision of pensions. Every government expenditure has a benefit side and a cost side. While both sides are relevant for policy, no one has found a magical governmental institution that gives just the right salience to the two sides. The earmarking of payroll tax revenues for pension benefits changes the visibility of financing and the distribution of cost bearing, and so changes political outcomes. For example, tariff revenues financed pension benefits for Civil War Union Army veterans in the United States. So supporters of these pensions were big fans of protection. Most analysts believe that the government spends too much on some programs and too little on other programs, although analysts disagree about which programs are which. So the connection between government institutions (both political and administrative) and the evaluation of outcomes varies across analysts.

In democracies, salience affects outcomes. The real question is how much one expects to like the political outcomes that come from different institutions. So the question here is to evaluate the different patterns of redistribution, within and across cohorts, that come with different pension institutions. The conventional wisdom is that DC systems are likely to give more to future generations, and unified DB systems are likely to give more to the poor within each cohort. If true (and the pattern may be more complex since DC pensions automatically cut benefits for longer lived cohorts and DB systems may include some elements that primarily benefit the politically well connected), which is more important? That will depend on how well any particular country will do both types of redistribution under the two different institutions. And it will depend on values.

As an example of how pension design may affect outcomes, let me contrast a unified DB system with a mixed DB/DC system starting with roughly the same funding and the same overall redistribution. If there is a decline in growth, then the underfunded DB benefits will need adjustment. Some of the adjustment may come from taxes. Let us focus on the adjustment that comes on the benefit side. If, for example, the mixed system is like the Pension Security Account (PSA) proposal in the United States—a flat DB benefit with a nonredistributive DC system, then the response is likely to be a phased-in cut in the flat DB benefit. That is, every member of a cohort will have the same absolute cut in benefits. It seems implausible that a unified system with the same financial problem would choose that outcome. Thus a mixed system puts more of the risk of the pay-as-you-go financing on the poor. However, a mixed system may put more of the rate-of-return risk on high earners if the unified DB system adjusts benefits in proportion rather than concentrating benefit cuts on high earners. Of course, a DB system can spread rate-of-return risk over many cohorts, possibly making that risk less of a concern.

It is interesting to consider the analog for Medicare. As a DB system, Medicare is described as giving everyone the same health insurance policy, with financing coming from payroll tax and general revenues. What if we set up Medicare as a fully payroll tax-financed DC system? We could describe it as follows. Everyone is forced to save for his or her retirement medical expenses. Then there are transfers from high to low earners, from healthy to sick persons, and from short-lived to long-lived persons, in order to give each person the amount needed to finance covered medical expenses. This description does not seem to be more transparent, just focused on different issues. It risks losing sight of the apparent purpose of the system, which is to provide everyone with the same health insurance. It might result in a different uniform policy and it might result in transfers that do not give everyone the same health insurance policy. It might result in more funding and less use of pay-as-you-go. Framing can matter.

So, too, individual pension accounts hide how the system provides income relative to past earnings. There is a trade-off —making some aspects more salient makes others less salient. Maybe highlighting who pays for redistribution is the most important thing that can be done. It seems to me that highlighting who has how much relative to their past earnings is highlighting what the system is, in its own terms, trying to do. In the United States, there are individual account proposals that eliminate all redistribution in the system, except that coming from uniform annuity pricing. It is not accidental that people who oppose redistribution favor individual accounts—it would be hard to be taken seriously if one proposed to remove progressivity from the Social Security benefit formula, which is a similar policy.

Institutions that frame issues differently have different patterns of salience or transparency and so will often lead to different outcomes. It is simply wrong that one system is transparent and the other is not.

References

Kahneman, D., and A. Tversky. 1984. "Choices, Values and Frames." *American Psychologist* 39: 341–50.

Comments by Salvador Valdés-Prieto, Catholic University of Santiago, Chile

This chapter can be summarized as an update of a portion of the recent literature on pension reform produced by academic economists in the United States. Unfortunately, it does not provide sufficient attention to the critical pension issues being faced outside the United States.

The chapter devotes a lot of space to theoretical results that have been well known to the economics profession in Latin America for years. For example, the potential for substitution between the public debt hidden in pay-as-you-go finance and explicit public debt issued to finance the transition was well explained in papers by Coeymans (1980) and Arellano (1982), both published in Spanish-language journals. Many macroeconomists in Latin America have understood these issues since the early 1990s.

Even accepting the U.S. focus, the chapter has a narrow focus. As is well known from practice and well established in the academic literature, the critical issues regarding pension policy concern the incentives for politicians to think for the long term versus yielding to the needs of current voters. Almost 25 years ago, Browning (1975) proved that it is rational for politicians to overpromise pensions in a democracy, since the benefits are to be paid by future generations, but the chapter does not mention this literature.

The chapter also fails to report on the attempts by the policy establishment in the United States to improve fiscal institutions, in particular to erect barriers against legislation that results in the use of Social Security surpluses to finance non-Social Security expenditures. The relevance of this debate for pension reform is substantial: its outcome may help to determine whether the savings of public trust funds can be shielded from the tendency of governments to spend those savings. I regret the chapter does not report on the illuminating American experience with fiscal institutions.

The Myths

Regarding the so-called myths, most of them kill strawmen and miss the real policy points. They fail to acknowledge the useful policy lessons that the profession has learned and that have been used by reforming countries.

Myth 1: "Private defined contribution plans raise national saving." Of course, that statement is not correct in general. But the following statement is true: "Moving the pension plan from pay-as-you-go to prefunding offers a unique opportunity to raise national saving."

For decades, pay-as-you-go debts were hidden to the public in the United States, in most rich democracies, and even more so in the countries of Latin America. This is a serious communication and political problem that led overall fiscal policy astray in almost all countries, reducing national saving. In the 1960s and 1970s, the economics profession failed to emphasize that the growth of social security debt could be stopped at the then current level and that society could make an informed decision. Instead, many economists argued that there was no choice but to let social security debt rise for the next three or four decades. Even today, the national accounts published by most countries fail to report second-pillar pension payments as debt amortization and contributions as new debt issues.

Today societies may be given the option to change course, but only if the appropriate information is provided. One of the most effective methods to drive reality home is to shift the social security institution to prefunding. This policy increases the information set for public opinion and opens an opportunity to choose again the appropriate level for the overall public debt. It also offers an opportunity to stop the pension overpromising and the trend towards early retirement that has dominated pension policy in many countries since 1945.

A credible revelation of the true scale of the overall public debt may lead public opinion to accept an increase in consolidated government saving over the coming decades. If this happens, the profession does expect the reform to increase national saving, because the offset coefficient between public and private saving has been shown to be much below 1 by several World Bank studies.

Take the United States as an example: If the current proposals for prefunding Social Security are abandoned for good, will future Congresses keep the promise to "save the deficit for social security?" I do not wish to guess for the United States, but for many countries in Latin America, my answer is no. That is why Myth 1 misses the point.

Myth 2 states that "rates of return are higher under individual accounts." This myth is debunked because, as the transition must be financed somehow, rates of return under prefunding cannot be compared with those under pay-as-you-go financing. In addition, it argues that "diversification undertaken through a public system involves less financial risk for any given individual than diversification undertaken through a private system, because the public system can spread risk across generations."

Consideration of political risk, however, changes that conclusion. Future pension policy is uncertain and risky. It is entirely possible that intermediation of pensions by the government may increase risk, as compared to market intermediation in which property rights are upheld by the rule of law rather than by shifting political majorities. Families can also spread risk across generations, and in many developing countries they probably do so better than governments. A comparison of political and family risks is absent from the chapter, but is crucial in many developing economies.

The Argentinean, Brazilian, Chilean, and Mexican record of stability for state pension policy since 1945 is frankly weak. Even the American record is patchy. If you are lucky, your pension may be overindexed, as in the United States starting in 1972, and you will get a large transfer. Who wants a pension promise whose value depends significantly on which party wins the presidency next time?

The chapter also fails to consider the growth effects of a reform that raises fiscal saving. Recent empirical research at the World Bank suggests that for emerging economies there exists a virtuous circle between saving and growth. In the presence of such externalities, the financing of the transition may offer an opportunity to jump start the virtuous cycle between saving and growth by increasing public saving. And once it starts, the iron link between rates of return and transition finance is broken.

It is clear that a country could use fiscal policy alone to start this virtuous cycle, dispensing with pension reform. But we should recognize that a pension reform offers a substantial *opportunity* to put the option of a long-term tighter fiscal policy on the political agenda, allowing the citizens to take a long-term view. Of course, the value of such opportunities may differ significantly across countries, but this does not preclude that in some countries the value of this opportunity may be high. The chapter fails to mention this important policy point.

When discussing Myth 4, the paper argues that from a risk perspective the socially optimal strategy would be partial funding and partial pay-as-you-go financing, because the latter allows investment in the labor market income of future generations. This is unconvincing. If the government has unique access to an asset that is not traded in the financial markets, then it should simply complete the market. For example, the government should issue long-term bonds with both capital and interest indexed to the labor income of future generations (as measured by tax collections in the future). There is no need to engage in pay-as-you-go financing to complete the financial markets. Moreover, I suspect that the stocks of corporations that sell services to the young already span a portion of future labor income risk.[1]

More important, pay-as-you-go financing produces a "security" very different from the hypothetical security indexed to the labor income of future generations. Future legislation can and does change contribution rates, benefits, and pension ages over time, usually with a short-run perspective oriented to the next election. Thus pay-as-you-go financing is a "security" subject to unilateral modification by the political system, which has a conflict of interest because it knows that the links between pension finance and the budget can affect reelection probabilities. This means that pay-as-you-go financing does not generate a secure "security" but an asset subject to moral hazard by politicians, and this is probably a dominated asset (see Valdés-Prieto 1998). The chapter fails to mention this essential point.

Old and New Issues

I want to avoid devoting all the allotted space to evaluate the so-called myths and instead contribute a Latin American perspective. One way of classifying the main issues in current Latin American debates about pension reform is by distinguishing between the new issues that originated in the wave of pension reforms of the 1990s and the old issues not faced by the reforms and left for later discussion.

Old Issues Not Faced by the Pension Reforms of the 1990s

Among the issues left for later discussion, the most critical is how to increase coverage of independent workers and of people that work at home. In my country, Chile, 30 percent of employment is in the self-employed sector, which is not mandated to participate in social security. Comparable figures are much higher for Mexico and Brazil. Unfortunately, the chapter does not even mention this topic.

In Latin America, a forced saving continues to be perceived as major tax on participation in the covered labor market. Using a large microeconomic data set for Chile, Torche and Wagner (1997) found that half of the contribution rate of 22 percent to all branches of social security in Chile was perceived to be a pure tax. We need to identify low-cost and practical means to reduce the pure tax component in social security contributions.

One reason for this result may be that it is economically unsound for the young to save for old age in the years when labor income is much below expected average lifetime labor income. The young are overrepresented among the self-employed. This has led to proposals to exempt all workers under the age of 30 from the mandate to contribute for old age income. This is the sort of concrete proposal that Latin America expects from the World Bank.

Minimum Asset Allocation Limits

Among the new issues that originated in the wave of Latin American pension reforms of the 1990s, minimum asset allocation limits are important. Many of the mandatory pension funds that have emerged in Latin America are forced to invest at least a certain share or amount in designated asset classes, specifically in government bonds and in domestic securities. These limits should not be confused with prudential regulations and with limits on the level of overall risk pension portfolios may attain, which have more robust rationales.

For example, the minimum asset allocation limits in Mexico require Adminìstradoras de Fondos para el Retìro (AFORE) to hold only fixed-income securities, which effectively forced them to invest an average of 97 percent in government debt as of June 1999.

Here is where Myth 4 by Orszag and Stiglitz could make an important contribution, if expanded to escape a narrow opposition between public trust funds and private pension funds. The result that matters is that investment of mandatory pension funds in equities has positive welfare implications (see Valdés-Prieto 1997).

Such liberalization is unrelated to the method of finance of a transition to funding, because the pension funds would simply exchange government securities for private sector securities with other investors. The World Bank could draw on the experience of Hungary, which has managed this transition by supplying ample information on the overall public debt (as explained by James 1998), to drive this point home in Latin America.

Administrative Charges

The other important issue that emerged in Latin America from the wave of pension reforms of the 1990s is the generally high level of administrative charges.[2] It is a major mistake to project current commission *rates* for several decades into the future, as the chapter by Orszag and Stiglitz does in Myth 7. When the basis of the main commission rates grows over time, that procedure involves unrealistic assumptions regarding the profit of intermediaries, that is, the difference between commission income and production costs in the future, which may be resolved by substantial reductions in commission *rates*. For the same reason, measuring commissions as a "charge ratio" leads to major mistakes.

Charge ratios also lead to major mistakes when there exists a significant component of flat production costs within administrative charges. Under this condition, the charge ratio will be larger when the contribution rate is smaller, as in Mexico (6.5 percent), the United Kingdom (4.8 percent), or Sweden (2.5 percent), even if the absolute administrative charge is lower than in other countries. That is why we should stick to current dollar charges for a comparable basket of services, as in table 2.1.

Table 2.1 shows that charges during 1999 differ substantially across Latin America and that some of the lowest charges are found in industries with decentralized collection and record-keeping and decentralized choice of trustee (Bolivia, savings passbooks at banks, and index equity funds in the United States). Bolivia has administrative charges close to US$25 per year per member, comparable to the charges in the Federal Thrift Savings Plan (FTSP) in the United States.

What industrial organization leads to low charges? Orszag and Stiglitz sidestep this critical question. So let me propose an answer: an organization that leads to a high price elasticity of demand for trustees. This is needed to avoid rent-seeking incentives for firms to engage in nonprice competition, such as offering many portfolios to people who barely understand

Table 2.1. Charges Per Member and Per Contributor, 1999
(Dollars per year at market exchange rates; noncontributing members are almost
free of charges in Latin America)

Industry	Ratio contributors/members	Dollars per contributor	Dollars per member
AFJP Argentina	0.45	239	108
PPP Great Britain (1994)	n.a.	229	n.a.
APFP Peru	0.425	193	82
AFAP Uruguay	n.a.	192	n.a.
AFPC Colombia	0.67	140	94
AFP Chile	0.53	127	67
AFP El Salvador	0.49	93	46
AFORE Mexico	0.854	78	67
Ind. Funds Australia	n.a.	78	n.a.
Equity Index Funds U.S. (1995)	n.a.	68	n.a.
FTSP, U.S.	0.86	31–39	27–34
AFP Bolivia	n.a.	25	n.a.
Chilean Banks (savings passbooks)	n.a.	10	n.a.

n.a. Not applicable.
Sources: Valdés-Prieto (1999); for equity index funds, see Mitchell (1996); for FTSP, see
chapter 7; for Australia, see Bateman and Valdés-Prieto (1999). The figures for Colombia
and Peru are based on an estimate of the true cost of the disability and survivors insurance
that is based on a comparison of number of damages with Argentina.

the differences between stocks and bonds. A high price elasticity of demand
for trustees can be achieved in several ways.

First, Bolivia and Panama did it with a bidding process in which an initial allocation of members is given to those trustees that offer the lowest
commissions. This approach is potentially superior to the monopoly trustee
approach—such as the Swedish Allmän Tjänste Pensionspoäng (earnings-
related supplement) funds recently abandoned by Sweden—because the
workers can be given the freedom to shift between the trustees that won
the bidding. The Bolivian workers that live in the central cities—the majority—are free to choose their trustee.[3]

This freedom is a major advantage because it allows workers to leave
those providers that expropriate the funds, either by exploiting conflicts of
interest or by making deals with the authorities to make social investments or to finance government spending in exchange for regulatory slack.

A second method to increase the price elasticity of demand for trustees
is the mutuality approach, as in the Australian Industry Funds. In this case
the clients themselves set up a trustee organization to search for the

lowest commissions. However, we know that mutualities are subject to the risk of capture by management, so the success of this option depends on the willingness of the members to spend resources to keep management under control. That has been achieved in Australian Industry Funds by giving employers the choice of trustee.

A third method to increase the effective price elasticity of demand is to legislate a ceiling on commission rates, as in Colombia, El Salvador, and Sweden. The ceilings are more complex in Sweden because the authorities are trying to avoid predefining benchmarks and thus want to allow substantial product differentiation—this may raise commissions, as it violates condition (i) below.

When high administrative charges lead to tariff regulation, they become a source of political risk: dissatisfaction with charges may lead the authorities to regulate commissions, creating an ideal environment for collusion in investment decisions between the private trustees and government. Under such circumstances, the government can get the pension funds to be oriented towards social investment or to finance government spending in exchange for looser tariffs.

Tariff regulation increases the risk of worsening investment performance by limiting competition among private trustees, and this risk may be more damaging than the high charges themselves. For example, for current Chilean contribution and commission rates, a modest 40-basis-point drop in investment performance is enough to reduce pensions by 10 percent, eliminating any gain obtained by lowering commissions to the level of the cheapest alternative.

A fourth method is suggested by the other low-cost examples in table 2.1 (equity index funds in the United States and savings passbooks in Chilean banks and Poland).[4] They suggest that a high price elasticity of demand for trustees can be achieved by assuring the existence of close substitutes, which necessitates (i) a limited variety of portfolios and commission rates, to make choice simple, (ii) availability of transparent performance benchmarks for each portfolio, (iii) transparent indicators of the sum of all commission rates, and (iv) allowing switches to other trustees over time, as learning occurs.

All of these conditions seem to be met in equity index funds in the United States and in savings passbooks in Chilean banks. Only the last of these conditions is present in the British personal pension plan market, so we should not be surprised by the high charges it exhibits. The same happens in the American retail mutual fund market for actively managed funds. I submit that in this market the variety of portfolios is so large and time varying that choice is made too complex to yield a high price elasticity of demand.[5] If workers do not know the difference between a stock and a bond, how can they know which is the benchmark for their mid-cap technology fund?

The more expensive Latin American private pension industries seem to meet these conditions, so we expect them to be cheaper than the British personal pension plans and the U.S. actively managed mutual funds. They are somewhat cheaper according to table 2.1, and much cheaper according to data presented by Mamta Murtha, J. Michael Orszag, and Peter R. Orszag in chapter 8. But why are commissions in Argentina or Peru not as low as in Bolivia or Poland?

I suggest two answers. First, condition (iii) is not met in practice. Workers in those industries do not have access to clear and transparent indicators of the sum of all the commissions they pay. Commission rates are expressed as a percentage of wage, looking small, rather than as in Poland where they are presented as a percentage of contributions, which look big. In Chile the account statements sent to workers do not report commissions in a simple format but rather report the *combined* peso amount discounted for disability insurance and commissions and, in addition, do so *separately* for each of the last four months. Most workers do not know how much they pay in commissions every year.

Second, condition (iv) is not met, as other regulations preclude price competition, prevent expansion of competitors, and limit entry, concretely:

- The type of price cut that has proven most attractive to plan members in Latin America is the introductory discount. However, the pension laws make such discounts illegal. Introductory discounts have been forced underground, where they have taken the form of illegal gifts from salespeople to the members that accept a switch of trustee. Thus prohibition has led many of the most informed members to shy away from requesting gifts or introductory discounts, limiting competition in introductory discounts to the more hardened members, who also tend to be the least informed.
- All pension laws in Latin America prevent secret price cuts and require the use of the posted price institution. Plott (1989) summarizes experimental evidence that shows that requiring producers to post their commission rates publicly with the prohibition to change them for a fixed period, as the law requires in Administradoras de Fundos de Pensiones (AFP) markets, is an institution that *raises* observed prices. In addition, Tirole (1988, pp. 262–64) summarizes Stigler's (1964) and Green and Porter's (1984) models to show that a regulation that prevents secret price cuts increases the likelihood of collusive strategies that raise prices. Tirole (1988, pp. 330–32) also summarizes Cooper's (1986) model in which allowing firms in an oligopoly to offer most-favored customer price protection leads to an increase in prices.

- In the last two years, the Superintendencies of Argentina, Chile, and Mexico joined the Peruvian one in introducing regulations that make it difficult for members to switch AFP. These regulations prevent the existing AFPs from expanding market share and prevent new AFPs from entering the market. The result is that commission rates tend to be set either by implicit bargaining with the authorities or by collusion. In both cases they end up being too high.

Summing up, the recent Latin American experience shows that administrative charges can be quite modest in decentralized, privately managed pension systems with individual choice, as shown by savings passbooks in Chile and Poland. To this end, policymakers need to apply the appropriate transparency policies. However, Latin America also shows the dangers of tariff regulation and of capture of regulators to support collusion.

Notes

1. The spanning condition must be tested using a wide variety of stock returns, not the return of a few aggregate stock indices as mentioned in a footnote.

2. I define administrative charges as high when their current level expressed in dollars per member per year is over twice the lowest comparable charges.

3. The Spanish banks that owned the two Bolivian AFPs merged in late 1999, reducing competition in the Bolivian AFP market. In response, the Bolivian government is bringing forward a new bidding stage.

4. Admittedly, current commission levels in Poland are introductory prices. However, the experience in other countries where introductory prices were observed—Chile, Peru and, Mexico—suggests that it is unlikely that charges will double in the long term.

5. In chapter 9 of this volume, Shah and Fernandes show that the ratio of noise to signal in individual fund returns is so large that individual performance cannot be assessed. In order to test the hypothesis that a given fund manager has enough skill to add 2.4 percentage points per year of return, the worker needs to observe the results for at least 32 years before he or she can reject the null hypothesis of no ability at a 95 percent level of significance.

References

Arellano, J. P. 1982. "Efectos Macroeconómicos de la Reforma Previsional Chilena." *Cuadernos de Economía*, No. 56 (April): Santiago, Chile.

Bateman, H., and S. Valdés-Prieto. 1999. "The Mandatory Private Old Age Income Schemes of Australia and Chile: A Comparison." Instituto de Economía, Catholic University of Chile. Processed.

Browning, E. K. 1975. "Why the Social Insurance Budget Is Too Large in a Democracy." *Economic Inquiry* 13 (September): 373–88.

Coeymans. J. E. 1980. "Empleo y Producción con un Financiamiento Alternativo del Sistema Previsional." *Cuadernos de Economía*, No. 52 (December): Santiago, Chile.

Cooper, T. 1986. "Most-Favoured Customer Pricing and Tacit Collusion." *Rand Journal of Economics* 17: 377–88.

Green, E., and R. Porter. 1984. "Non-Cooperative Collusion under Imperfect Price Information." *Econometrica* 52: 87–100.

James, E. 1998. "The Political Economy of Social Security Reform: A Cross-Country Review." *Annals of Public and Cooperative Economics* 69(4): Blackwell Publishers.

Mitchell, O. 1996. "Administrative Costs in Public and Private Retirement Systems." Working Paper 5734. National Bureau of Economic Research. Cambridge, Mass.

Plott, C. 1989. "Applications of Experimental Methods." In R. Schmalensee and R. Willig, eds., *Handbook of Industrial Organization*. North-Holland, Vol. 2, pp. 1140–59.

Stigler, G. 1964. "A Theory of Oligopoly." *Journal of Political Economy* 72: 44–61.

Tirole, J. 1988. *The Theory of Industrial Organization*. Cambridge, Mass.: The MIT Press.

Torche, A., and G. Wagner. 1997. "Previsión Social: Valoración Individual de un Beneficio Mandatado." *Cuadernos de Economía*, No. 103, año 34 (December): 363–90.

Valdés-Prieto, S. 1997. "Financing a Pension Reform toward Private Funded Pensions." In S. Valdés-Prieto, ed., *The Economics of Pensions*. Cambridge University Press.

———. 1998. "The Private Sector in Social Security: Latin American Lessons for APEC." *Proceedings of the APEC Regional Forum on Pension Reform*, Cancun, Mexico, February 1998. Manila: Asian Development Bank, pp. 43–75.

———. 1999. Costos Administrativos en un Sistema de Pensiones Privatizado. Development Discussion Paper No. 677. Harvard Institute for International Development.

3

New Approaches to Multipillar Pension Systems: What in the World Is Going On?

Louise Fox and Edward Palmer

IN 1994 THE WORLD BANK PUBLISHED *Averting the Old Age Crisis: Policies to Protect the Old and Promote Growth* with the intention of surveying the "state of the field" at the time the book was being written.[1] Michael Bruno's opening words summarized the diagnosis of the book: "Systems providing financial security for the old are under increasing strain throughout the world" (World Bank 1994). This message is still relevant today, especially in the developing world. Several factors have contributed to this result. While dependency ratios continue to increase, reform has not been easy to implement, so the fiscal costs of the systems in the developing world have for the most part continued to increase as well. In some countries, economic shocks worsened the fiscal picture by lowering growth and increasing public debt. Finally, the trend in economic policy goals toward lower inflation, tighter fiscal policy, and increased monetary system interdependence has put a sharper focus on implicit pension debts.

Much has happened in the area of pension reform in the short time since the publication of *Averting the Old Age Crisis*. This chapter reviews the more comprehensive reforms since 1994, with a focus on those that generated an improvement in the 1994 choice set. Our review is stylistic rather than exhaustive.[2] Our aim is to highlight new approaches or new answers to the problems mentioned above and identify emerging models. We focus on experiences that may be transferable to the developing and transition economies, the clients of the World Bank.

Nowadays more often than not pension reform discussions refer to "multipillar" systems. What exactly constitutes a pillar? Authors define this term in different ways, trying to capture the key dimensions in the design of national pension systems. Most authors have considered the following elements important in describing systems:

- *Coverage:* Is it universal?
- *Participation:* Is it mandatory or voluntary?
- *Contributions:* Where is the system on the spectrum that has, on one end, a general revenue-financed (perhaps means-tested) benefit, moves to some form of earnings-based formula, defined benefit (DB) scheme, and has, at the other end, a pure individual lifetime account scheme that is defined contribution (DC)?
- *Benefits:* To what extent do benefits (annuities) reflect the life expectancy of the retiree at retirement?
- *Funding:* To what extent do assets cover future liabilities?
- *Management/ownership/governance:* Is it public, private, or some mix?

Categorizing systems on the basis of these criteria is not easy. For example, consider funding. Few pay-as-you-go (PAYG) systems operate without any cash reserves at all, and a few have very substantial reserve funds. Few "funded" systems have the assets to meet all liabilities regardless of economic conditions or demographic changes. Likewise, an employer, a branch (as in the case of automobile manufacturing), or a whole sector (for example, employees of the state, all affiliated unions in a confederation of unions) may require all employees to participate in a pension plan. From the point of view of society, participation is voluntary, but it is mandatory for anyone who wants to be an employee.

In this chapter, we focus on the dimensions of funding and risk in public, mandatory systems, since these have been two major areas in which practice has evolved since 1994. For our purposes, we propose the following definitions of the pillars:

- *Pillar 1:* A large, mandatory public or quasi-public system with inter- and intragenerational redistribution, which can be fully funded (for example, Denmark and the Netherlands);[3] partially funded (for example, Morocco, the United States, and India); or unfunded (for example, Germany and Brazil) and in which a DB or notional defined contribution (NDC) formula determine benefits.
- *Pillar 2:* Fully funded, defined contribution systems in which benefits depend on the assets in the individual's account at retirement. These may be (i) centralized and government-managed provident fund systems, which usually provide lump-sum benefits but may offer an annuity purchase, or (ii) individual financial account systems in which the participants' money is invested in privately managed market funds. Participants may take benefits as a lump sum, use them to purchase an annuity, or withdraw them in phases.[4]

A minimum guarantee may supplement these two pillars. This guarantee, regardless of how it is formulated, is tax-financed, and, by definition, breaks the direct link between contributions and benefits. Some countries (for example, Poland) have called the tax-financed guarantee the "zero pillar." Countries also provide a last resort safety net in the form of social assistance for the very needy. Government-regulated, voluntary or semivoluntary, privately managed pension systems may also supplement pillars 1 and 2. These systems are often referred to as pillar 3 (World Bank 1994). We use this definition of pillar 3 except when the law mandates employers to provide a benefit scheme that in principle covers all (or practically all) employees in the country. We classify these cases as pillar 1 if they are defined benefit schemes (for example, Denmark and France) and pillar 2 if they are defined contribution (for example, Australia), although this classification is not universally accepted.[5] Our reason for doing this is to highlight (i) the universal mandatory character, and (ii) in the case of DB systems, the extent to which the implicit liability is actually public. In this chapter we focus on contributory, publicly mandated pension programs,[6] largely ignoring the zero and third pillars.

Countries may offer contributors only pillar 1, only pillar 2, or a blend. The blend may be a mandatory combination of the two pillars (as, for example, in Poland) or a choice between the two pillars (for example, Colombia). We call countries "blend countries" if this offer is universal. Other countries have pillar 2 pensions for the private sector and a system of DB pensions for the public sector (for example, Indonesia). We do not consider these countries as blends, as they do not offer a combined system to *all* contributors. In effect, with this design, the so-called pillar 1 system is instead an unfunded occupational (pillar 3) system.

In early 1994 (when *Averting the Old Age Crisis* was substantially completed), most of the world had pillar 1 systems (table 3.1). With regard to pillar 2 systems, government-run provident funds constituted the main model. At this time Chile was the only country with a privately managed pillar 2 system.

Chile was not widely received as the best model for the future in 1994. Members of all sides of the political economy spectrum had criticized the Chilean reform. Bonilla and Gillion (1994) raised the issue of system coverage, arguing that pillar 2 systems do not provide enough incentives to cover low-income workers and that only the public system would take on this task. Diamond and Valdés-Prieto (1994) reviewed the experience of Chile and noted the following issues with respect to its application in other countries:

- In countries with a large pension debt, either a politically difficult massive savings effort is required to pay off the debt or the PAYG system continues in a less flexible and more inefficient form.
- The decentralized model that Chile followed has high overhead costs, which can eat up returns.

Table 3.1. National Pension System Architecture, 1994 and 1999

Year	First-pillar only		Second-pillar only		Blend
	DB	NDC	Provident fund	Individual accounts	
1994	OECD (rest)				Australia, Switzerland,
	Latin America			Chile	United Kingdom
	Central and Eastern Europe and Former Soviet Union (FSU)				
	Middle East and North Africa, Africa (most)		Gambia, Kenya Tanzania, Uganda, Zambia		
	Cambodia, China Rep. of Korea, Lao PDR, Philippines, Vietnam Malaysia (public) Indonesia (public)		Asian islands, Papua New Guinea, Singapore Malaysia Indonesia		
	India (public)		Brunei, Thailand India, Nepal,		
	Sri Lanka (public)		Sri Lanka		
1999	OECD (rest)	Italy			Australia, Sweden, Switzerland, United Kingdom
	Latin America (rest)			Bolivia, Chile, El Salvador, Mexico	Argentina, Colombia, Peru, Uruguay
	Central and Eastern Europe and FSU (rest)	Kyrgyz Rep.	Kazakhstan		Croatia, Hungary, Latvia, Poland
	Africa (most) MENA	Gambia, Kenya, Tanzania, Uganda, Zambia			
	Cambodia, Korea, Laos, Philippines, Vietnam	China, Mongolia	Asian islands, Brunei, Papua New Guinea, Singapore		
	Indonesia (public) Malaysia (public)		Indonesia Malaysia		Hong Kong (PRC), Thailand
	Sri Lanka (public)		Nepal, Sri Lanka	India	

Source: World Bank data.

- Individual purchases of annuities may not work out given the problems of moral hazard in these markets, but lump sum payments do not provide much insurance.

Proponents of individual financial account systems began to search for alternatives to the Chilean approach that possess fewer of its negative aspects, while proponents of the PAYG system sought to improve on the 1994 model. Both approaches succeeded. The years following the publication of *Averting the Old Age Crisis* have been ones of blossoming innovation in reform of mandatory pension provision, with an upsurge of ideas for creating financially sustainable mandatory public systems. Within pillar 1, the trend is towards tightening the links between contributions and benefits. The most fundamental and innovative change has been the implementation of NDC schemes to date in six countries: Italy, the Kyrgyz Republic, Latvia, Mongolia, Poland, and Sweden. Within pillar 2, innovation has addressed the high costs of running individual financial account systems.

The chapter is organized into two sections. The first section reviews the main issues and the reforms in five groups of countries—Organization for Economic Co-operation and Development (OECD) countries, European and Central Asian countries with transition economies, Latin American countries, Asian countries, and the middle- and low-income countries of Africa and the Middle East. In our survey we find that many more countries have followed Chile in converting acquired PAYG DB rights into something else. However, the most popular major pension reform turns out to be a blend of pillars (table 3.1). To date only five countries have passed legislation to completely phase out the PAYG system—Chile, three others in Latin America, and Kazakhstan in Central Asia.

The second section analyzes the issues that have permeated the discussion in the 1990s, identifying areas where consensus seems to be emerging and where issues remain unresolved. Here we find that the PAYG system is still alive and well, but pillar 1 reforms have primarily focused on getting PAYG systems to look to the contributor more like DC financial account systems but with little or no funding. This has in essence reduced the differences between the two pillars. We then consider why blends have emerged so strongly as the most popular innovation. We conclude that one of the key driving forces has been the need to finance a high implicit debt in the countries that have reformed. At the same time, the individual financial accounts have gained popularity in pillar 2 reforms, partly because innovations have been made to lower overhead costs of individual accounts.

A number of issues, however, are still open in pension system design, two of which we tackle in our closing section. The first is the issue of managing the risks of public pension systems, where we find that outstanding controversy remains over allocating among individuals and generations the cost of increasing life expectancy and the moral hazard risk of early exit from the workforce. The second issue is whether or not we have achieved a model for low-income countries. Here it is not clear whether the benefits of any system, be it pillar 1, 2, or a blend, outweigh the costs. The concluding sections synthesize lessons for those countries that have yet to reform.

Review of the Major Reforms

This section examines the main issues that the pension systems face in five different groups of countries and what these countries are doing to address them. Some OECD countries have introduced funding, but the main reform efforts have focused on systemic reform and the introduction of notional defined contribution arrangements to the old PAYG systems. A similar situation has prevailed in the transition economies of Europe and Central Asia. Latin American countries have been the most aggressive regarding the implementation of individual financial account systems, often in blend arrangements. Pension systems in Asian countries mainly demonstrate the blend model. Middle-income countries in Africa and the Middle East still have not undertaken major reforms of their pension systems.

OECD Countries

By the late 1980s, it was already evident that OECD countries faced demographic and labor market participation trends that were moving in troublesome directions for pension systems (OECD 1988). The picture is even bleaker a decade later, as survival rates continue to be revised upwards, older workers are still exiting the workforce early, and birth rates remain low. The OECD population will age dramatically in the coming three decades. People over 60 are projected to increase from 20 to 27 percent of the population by 2020 and to 30 percent by 2030 (table 3.2). These expected trends are the result of increased longevity, combined with low birth rates.

The OECD counties mostly designed their DB systems on premises consistent with the industrial economy of the first half-century, when life expectancy was lower and jobs were physically more demanding. In the postwar period, they added generous benefit rules to provide adequate benefits to people unfortunate enough to have lived through two world wars and a deep depression. Optimistic system dependency projections using the high fertility rates of the 1950s and 1960s helped justify these increased benefits. Since that time, however, demographic and social conditions have changed. Not only has life expectancy increased, but fertility has declined. As a result, system dependency ratios deteriorated from roughly 3.5 workers per pensioner in the 1950s to roughly 2.5 by the 1990s and are expected to reach 2.0 in the near future.

Table 3.2. Projected Share of the Population over 60, by Country Group
(percentage)

			Year		
Country group	2000	2010	2020	2030	2050
OECD	19.9	23.1	27.0	30.7	31.2
Transition countries	17.0	18.2	21.5	22.7	26.5
Latin America	7.7	9.3	12.2	16.0	23.5
Asia	7.3	8.6	11.6	15.0	20.7
Middle East and North Africa	7.3	8.1	10.0	12.4	18.1
Sub-Saharan Africa	4.4	4.5	4.9	5.9	9.9

Source: World Bank 1998.

The demographics are not the only explanation of why there are increasingly fewer workers per pensioner. Another reason is that people are leaving the labor force early. Although the retirement age for a full defined-benefit pension in many countries in the OECD is 65, in all countries the de facto average age of exit from the labor force is lower. For some OECD countries it was as low as 56-57 for women and 59 for men by the mid-1990s, and the average age of exit for men has dropped about 3-5 years over the 20-year period from 1976 to 1995 (Palmer 1999a).

Early exit is not justifiable solely on health grounds. On the contrary, the subjectively evaluated health of persons under 70 has improved, and jobs are becoming less physically demanding. For example, in the United States the percentage of workers in physically demanding jobs has declined from around 20 percent in the 1950s to 7.5 percent in the mid-1990s (Steuerle, Spiro, and Johnson 1999). The same authors report that only about 20 and 30 percent of Americans 55–59 and 65–69, respectively, say their health is fair or poor—the vast majority of persons over 60 are in good health. In other words, as economic and social developments have favored working longer, men have been working less. Over the same period, women raised their age of exit by 3-8 years, depending on the country. Nevertheless, in most countries, the labor force participation of women is still below that of men, and the average age of exit for men and women together is still falling (Palmer 1999a).

With the prevailing demographic trends, labor will be in shortage, and this ought to influence employer behavior, including adapting work environments more to the needs of older workers. The timing of exit from the labor force for persons in good health depends on their individual preferences for work and leisure, given their economic resources. Older workers' economic resources depend in part on the overall tax-benefit system. Consequently, it is reasonable to believe that, overall, tax-benefit systems influence the behavior of older workers. A recent set of studies of 11 countries, edited by Gruber and Wise (1999), provides strong evidence that public benefit and tax systems do in fact influence the behavior of older workers. Using the same calculation model for all countries, the studies examined the after-tax gain (or loss) in lifetime wealth of working an additional year from age 55. The results reveal that in countries where the net gain to the individual from staying longer in the workforce is smaller, there are fewer persons age 55 and older in the workforce. This study highlights how a combination of the overall tax-benefit structure and occupational schemes reinforce individual decisions about work and leisure, in favor of the latter.

In sum, people are healthier and living longer, but at the same time the design of tax-benefit systems, together with employer behavior, have reinforced individual preferences to exit the labor force at an early age. Early exit creates a moral-hazard risk for the insurance collective as a whole. The individual actors (employees and employers) behave individually in accordance with the country's system of rules and their own preferences, but the result of this aggregate behavior is to push up the country's implicit debt and future taxes for themselves or their children.

The implicit public sector pension debt has been rising. Recently, Disney (1999) concluded from empirical analysis that most OECD countries have not accumulated sufficient funds in their PAYG systems to cover the extra costs associated with the large postwar baby boomers, let alone the costs that increasing longevity will bring. Countries need to reduce liabilities by tightening up rules or increase funding (taxes and contributions) now to meet unchanged obligations.

What Are OECD Countries Doing?

Three countries have increased funding in their systems by introducing individual account systems. The United Kingdom had already moved in the direction of increasing advance funding in the 1980s by offering people the option to "contract out" of the state earnings-related pension scheme (SERPS) and join private schemes. Reforms in the 1990s strengthened this move. Australia mandated employer coverage, building on existing employer-financed schemes.[7] Sweden, in a series of steps leading to individual choice of fund managers in the year 2000, introduced individual financial accounts on top of its new PAYG notional account system. It already had a large reserve fund in the public PAYG system in 1994 (Palmer 2000). Following the reform, the Swedish quasi-mandatory (central labor-management negotiated) schemes have also largely converted to DC financial account schemes.

These countries form a group with a large element of funding in mandated or quasi-mandated systems. They share this feature with Switzerland, which has mandated, funded, employer-based schemes, and Denmark and the Netherlands, with large, fully funded, quasi-mandated schemes—quasi because they are based on central agreements between management and labor.

Most other countries have focused on reducing liabilities, often in the face of strong vested interests that inhibited systemic reform. The most common liability-reducing reform has been to change indexation formulas. Many countries have gone from wage indexation to less generous price indexation. For example, the United Kingdom converted to price indexation in the beginning of the 1980s. In Japan, this was a component of the cost-cutting package legislated in early 2000. Countries are also raising the full-benefit pension age. As early as 1983, the United States legislated a gradual increase to age 67 to be reached after the turn of the century. Germany will gradually eliminate special (seniority) rules and raise the full-benefit pension age to 65, with a possibility for continued revaluation past the age of 65. The Japanese reform package also proposes gradually increasing the pension age for the earnings-related part of the Employees Pension Insurance (EPI) from 60 to 65 over the period 2013-25 for men and 2018-30 for women.

Countries have also tightened the links between benefits and lifetime earnings and contributions. For example, in 1986 the United Kingdom changed the SERPS benefit to reflect a wage based on a career average instead of the best 20 years. France is changing the calculation basis for a benefit from the best 10 to the best 25 years of earnings and is increasing the number of contributory quarters needed for a full benefit from 150 to 160. Italy went from a 5-year earnings basis for calculating benefits to an entire career (depending on the scheme) for persons still covered by the old system. Italy and Sweden have developed and implemented the notional defined contribution pay-as-you-go account systems, which introduce a full link between benefits and contributions.

NDC PAYG HAS EMERGED IN OECD COUNTRIES

Extending the years of coverage required to receive a full benefit helps bring down costs in DB systems but only goes part way in managing the risks of early exit and increased life expectancy. The NDC PAYG systems legislated in Sweden (1994) and Italy (1995) are designed to manage these risks directly. The appeal of the NDC account system is that it is a PAYG scheme that emulates the principles of a DC scheme but relies on demographic funding. It provides a middle road to the bipolar conflict between traditional PAYG DB systems and fully funded DC financial account systems that continued to dominate the pension debate into the 1990s.

In the NDC PAYG system wage earners pay contributions at a fixed rate, the value of which are accredited their notional accounts—this is the defined-contribution feature of the system. People pay contributions on earnings as long as they work. The previous year's account value is indexed annually with a nominal per capita wage index in Sweden[8] and gross domestic product (GDP) in Italy. Information about changing life expectancy and, given an individual's account record, its effect on an annuity claimed at a specific age is available at any time in the Swedish administrative system. In other words, individual decisions about when and how to exit from the labor force can take into account the parameter of changing life expectancy. In principle, the NDC structure makes it possible to claim any percent of a benefit at any time after a legal minimum age for eligibility. People can combine a full or partial NDC benefit with work (and continue to contribute and acquire new rights) and then get a recalculated benefit at some later date.

The NDC benefit is calculated by dividing the value on the account at the chosen time of retirement with a factor based on unisex life expectancy. In addition to this, the annuities in Sweden and Italy incorporate a real rate of return of 1.6 and 1.5 percent, respectively. This form of front-loading is an alternative to possible wage indexation (from a lower initial level) over the lifetime. Both countries also index annuities to annual changes in prices. Annual indexation in the Swedish scheme includes an adjustment for digressions of actual real growth from 1.6 percent. This keeps the aggregate contribution rate in line with the individual contribution rate of 16 percent.[9]

Proponents of the NDC PAYG formula claim that it represents a paradigm shift in social security thinking (Palmer 2000). By creating a direct link between contributions and the annuity and by basing the size of the annuity on life expectancy at retirement, NDC systems reduce the impact of individual behavioral choice and unexpected changes in longevity on system costs. In the DB framework the burden of the risk is unclear. It may fall on future generations of workers or on present workers before they retire.

Finally, it is important to note the following about NDC account systems:

- By definition, fully funded DC systems insulate against labor supply fluctuations. PAYG systems do not provide natural insulation. But NDC PAYG systems, with demographic reserves and indexation of capital and benefits that follow the growth of the contribution base, yield approximate long-run financial stability (Palmer 1999b). Both funded DC systems and NDC systems rely on good life expectancy projections and require adjustments somewhere when life-expectancy factors are systematically under- or overestimated. Under specific circumstances, other forms of benefit indexation in the NDC system (for example, price indexation) may also work.
- NDC PAYG systems with or without advance funding are subject to the same "political risks" as DB PAYG—"political" management of public funds causing low rates of return, special interest lobbying, etc. For example, in Italy the rate credited to the notional account is

actually higher than the payroll tax earmarked for pensions, while in Poland it is lower. What the NDC provides is a framework for monitoring the costs of these interventions (Fox and Palmer 1999).

- The NDC contribution still has the tax element of any PAYG system if the net rate of return on financial investments (after administrative costs) is higher than the rate of return on the notional account.

In sum, OECD countries have not moved aggressively to address system cost and stability issues. Since the United Kingdom introduced "contracting out" of the earnings-related PAYG SERPS, Sweden and Australia have been the only countries to create a component in the mandatory system with DC-funding through individual financial accounts. NDC PAYG—an explicit, rule-based scheme, with benefits linked to life expectancy—has been the most significant solution for the OECD DB conundrum, and both Sweden and Italy have adopted it. The legislative bodies of other countries (for example, Germany and the United States) have also discussed the idea of creating a benefit formula that is directly responsive to changes in longevity but have yet to adopt it.

The increasing debt implicit in the continued application of the current PAYG rules in many countries will eventually lead to higher contributions for workers and/or higher income taxes for both workers and pensioners. While these same high implicit debts are an obstacle to the introduction of extensive DC funding, the possibility of further innovation in OECD countries should not be ruled out.

Transition Countries of Europe and Central Asia

The transition economies include a large number of diverse countries, from the relatively well-off, such as the Czech Republic and Slovenia, to the very poor, such as Armenia and Georgia. Within countries, the distribution of earnings spread out dramatically during the first decade of transition, and, generally, poverty tends to be high, especially in the rural areas. System dependency ratios dropped from around 2.5 workers per pensioner in the 1980s to around 1.5 in the 1990s.

The transition from centralized to market economies brought new issues to the pension reform discussion and new solutions. Briefly, the new issues were the following:

- *High initial implicit debt.* Acquired rights and commitments to benefit recipients were unchanged after the transition, but the means at the disposal of governments to collect revenues to meet contemporary and future commitments had changed dramatically.
- *Weak administration capacity.* Administrative institutions that could work in a market economy needed to be established.

- *Falling number of contributors.* Following the breakdown of the command economy, the covered wage bill remained relatively high in the wealthier transition countries (central Europe) but fell dramatically in the poorer countries (the former Commonwealth of Independent States, or CIS). This resulted from a fall in economic activity, a decline in female labor force participation, and considerable movement into the informal economy.
- *Many special groups.* Legacies of special privileges for selected groups created problems in moving towards mandatory pension systems suited for the market economy.[10]
- *Low retirement age.* In all the post-Soviet and Eastern European countries but Poland,[11] the full DB pension age was 60 for men but only 55 for women, even though the gap in life expectancy between men and women is 7-10 years, and the labor force participation of men and women up to the pension age is often about the same. In addition, the special privilege of early retirement afforded to many groups lowered the average effective rate of exit from the labor force even more.

The picture emerging in the 1990s was not entirely bleak, however. With the transition came public anticipation and demand for market-oriented change. Since the demographic pressure will come later than in the OECD (table 3.2), a brief demographic window of opportunity for system reform will be available.

WHAT HAVE THE TRANSITION COUNTRIES OF EUROPE AND CENTRAL ASIA
BEEN DOING?

Initially, policy was largely reactive. Countries were forced to trim benefit payments to meet financial resource limitations. The general result was the emergence of flat benefits with price indexation, when this was affordable. In poorer countries, even after stabilization, benefits still depend on whatever means are available, rather than adherence to benefit formulas. As the 1990s progressed, however, policy became proactive.

A first step involved phasing out privileges for special groups. Two approaches emerged. One is to discontinue granting new rights and convert rights already acquired in the old scheme into rights in a reformed public scheme. This is the approach most countries have followed. The other is to transfer acquired rights to newly created occupational schemes. Poland followed this approach, converting the acquired rights of a large group of miners into an occupational scheme (Chlon, Góra, and Rutkowski 1999).

Increasing the retirement age has proven to be an especially difficult issue. Hungary was among the first countries to successfully introduce a gradual increase to a higher normal retirement age (62) for both men and women, and Croatia has followed. These are the exceptions, not the rule.

For example, proposals to equalize the pension ages of women and men in Poland[12] and Russia met vociferous defense (and maintenance) of the status quo. In 1995 legislation in Latvia scheduled an annual increase of the minimum pension age for women by a half year to the age of 60, but amidst protests the next Parliament reversed its decision to allow women to continue to claim small pensions from age 55. As a result most women had claimed an actuarially reduced benefit by age 56, often at the very minimum of what people can live on alone. If married, these women will eventually outlive their husbands by quite a few years. Unfortunately, as Louise Fox and Paulette Castel note in chapter 12, this pattern, which is similar in many of the transition countries, is likely to increase the number of long-term poor.[13]

In the mid-1990s, countries began to work on systemic changes. In legislation passed in 1995 and implemented in 1996, Latvia became the first country to reengineer the first pillar by converting PAYG commitments acquired under the previous regime into NDC PAYG accounts. In 1997 Hungary legislated the next systemic reform, linking contributions to benefits through the introduction, in 1998, of a financial account system to supplement the PAYG system. New entrants were mandated into the financial account system, but current workers were given the choice of either remaining entirely in the PAYG system or entering the financial account system. For a worker in the new system, a financial account with a pension fund replaces one-third of the PAYG system (Palacios and Rocha 1998). During the choice period, people received information to help them decide which alternative was likely to be best for them. In 1997 Kazakhstan became the first (and to date only) transition economy to follow the example of Chile in phasing out the public PAYG system after a transition period of paying off current acquired rights.

Poland passed legislation for an NDC reform of the old PAYG scheme in 1998, topped by a mandatory financial account system that in time is aimed to give a 50-50 split of contributions between the NDC and financial account schemes. With implementation in 1999, Poles under 30 years of age were mandated to participate in the financial account system (with a 9 percent contribution rate), and persons 30 to 50 had the option to join.

In 1998 Croatia chose to reform its PAYG pillar along the lines of the German point system, and in 1999 it legislated a funded pillar on top, to be implemented in 2001.[14] The second pillar is mandatory for persons under 40 and optional for persons 40-49. Latvia followed up its NDC reform with financial account legislation passed in early 2000. In 2001 it will begin to phase in a 50-50 split of a 20 percent contribution rate between the NDC and financial account schemes, mandating participation for those under 30 at the time of introduction and enabling those age 30–50 to choose.

All countries moving in the direction of NDC and financial account systems have retained or created a minimum guarantee of some form.

Kazakhstan, Hungary, and Poland have followed Latin American in providing participants in financial account systems a choice between a limited number of funds, whereas Croatia and Latvia will employ the clearinghouse model,[15] which will enable individual choice among a number of investment funds as the systems develop. Yet another innovation in the Latvian pillar 2 legislation is the option at retirement for the individual to choose between purchasing a market annuity or transferring capital from the financial account into his or her NDC account.

Other countries have developed systemic reforms of their pillar 1 systems without including a pillar 2. These countries have reduced the avenues for early exit, especially among special groups and tightened benefit formulas in earnings-related PAYG systems. Examples include the Czech Republic (one of the first to phase out special privileges), Estonia, Georgia (flat pensions and a jump in the pension age by 5 years in one go), Kyrgyz Republic (an NDC system), Lithuania, Moldova, and Romania. Several of these countries are now considering how to add funding to their systems, using the fiscal space created by the reforms.

Remaining Issues in Transition Countries of Europe and Central Asia

Although there has been a wave of innovation in some of the transition countries, reform has been slow in coming to the majority of the population in this region (mainly because Russia has not yet reformed). The coming decade is likely to bring even more innovation, in both the low- and high-income transition countries.

The challenge for transition countries is to design benefit systems so as to minimize long-term free rider costs by providing incentives for the participation of younger workers on the fringes of the market economy. At the same time, the systems must provide security for current workers on the margins of transition. This implies tightly linking benefits to contributions for younger workers, sending a clear message to those who do pay their contributions and possibly increasing coverage and revenues in the long run.[16]

In parts of the transition region, even if earnings-related schemes are introduced, a majority of the population may be largely or wholly outside the system owing to growing urban informal and rural private agricultural sectors. One of the most urgent questions entails financing the basic needs of the impoverished aged. The situation may become more acute as younger family members leave home to take jobs in more economically dynamic regions. Whether poverty support is provided through some form of guarantee or flat-rate benefit (demogrant), there is a question as to what tax instrument to use to accomplish redistributive aims while encouraging high compliance in the earnings-related schemes.

Latin America

The last five years have seen an explosion in pension reforms in Latin America. This occurred for several reasons.[17] The most important was that the successful stabilization programs of the late 1980s and early 1990s exposed the weaknesses of the PAYG systems, especially in terms of fiscal costs, which high inflation had obscured in two ways. First, benefit adjustments rarely kept up with inflation, which resulted in the constant erosion of the real value of benefits granted to an affordable level. Second, in most systems, benefits depended on the last 3-5 years' earnings, which inflation also eroded. As a result, actual replacement rates were far from the promised replacement rates until inflation stopped. As coverage and covered real wages were not growing rapidly, system deficits emerged. These deficits threatened the gains from the painful stabilization. Latin American systems usually had extra benefits for privileged groups. Ironically, the democratization of the 1980s increased pressure to make these special benefits universal, but this was also unaffordable.

In the 1990s the pressure to reform was strong. At the same time, the Chilean model seemed to be a success. Savings in individual financial accounts were accumulating high rates of return in Chile, suggesting that workers could look forward to good pensions at retirement. Meanwhile, piecemeal reforms in Argentina—the reform leader of the second wave—had failed. An intellectual consensus around the benefits of a second pillar as well as constituencies for reform in the younger generations were developing in the region. Reform leaders liked the microeconomic incentives an individual account system offers, with a lifetime contribution-benefit link (lacking in most of the region's DB systems). They also liked the potential for capital market development, as now stable financial systems sought to tap regional and global financial markets.

WHAT HAVE LATIN AMERICAN COUNTRIES BEEN DOING?

The lead reformer, Chile, basically kept its existing system, which channels 10 percent of wages into pension fund companies, which hold them in individual accounts.[18] A separate body regulates these companies (AFPs), and the government does not participate in the collection of benefits. AFPs must provide a minimum relative rate of return guarantee, and they are restructured if they do not meet this regulation. The government offers a minimum pension guarantee. Acquired rights in the old system were capitalized into no-coupon bonds carrying a fixed rate of interest that beneficiaries redeem at the time of retirement (a continuing liability of the government). Those in the labor force at the time had the option of remaining in the PAYG first pillar, but this pillar allowed no new entrants. Thus the explicit PAYG system will end in Chile sometime in the coming half century.

The first reforms did not follow the Chilean model to the letter. The first reformers were Argentina, Colombia, and Peru, followed closely by Uruguay in 1995 (Schmidt-Hebbel 1999). Mexico and Bolivia joined in 1997, and El Salvador reformed its system in 1998. Most of the early reformers adopted a blend approach. Two kinds of blends emerged:

- The first type is similar to that observed in Europe and is present in Argentina and Uruguay—a PAYG first pillar combined with a modest second pillar. In Argentina, the first pillar is flat, whereas in Uruguay it increases with contributions. The second pillar is optional in Argentina, and contributors can have the earnings-related portion of the pension come from the scaled back PAYG system.
- The second type of blend is a choice of pillars. In Peru and Colombia contributors are either in the first pillar (scaled back PAYG) or the second pillar. In Peru, once in the second pillar, participants must stay there, but Colombia allows shifts back and forth.

Surprisingly, after these blend models emerged, the next reforms were all second-pillar-only reforms—Mexico, Bolivia, and El Salvador. They allowed no choice for new entrants, nor were combinations possible. The Chilean model was moving north.

A Key Issue in Latin American Countries: Second-Pillar Design

Latin America shows a surprising consistency with respect to the system design features. All countries except Bolivia adopted the basic Chilean model for second-pillar design—private pension-fund firms, or AFPs, compete for the right to manage individual accounts. At the outset all countries issued tight regulations with respect to allowable investments (with a heavy concentration on bonds and on national assets), although they have loosened them as systems gain experience. Two main innovations are noteworthy: (i) centralized contribution collection and (ii) integrated supervision of private fund managers.

Argentina was the first country to introduce centralized contribution collection. In the Chilean model employers withhold contributions from employees and pass them on to the pension fund of the employee's choice. In Argentina and Mexico the employer remits the funds directly to the national revenue agency. This innovation emerged as a response to the high costs of the Chilean pension funds (AFPs). It was also supposed to help increase coverage, as one tax agency monitors all payments and can track down evaders. The practice may not be yielding the desired cost savings, however. In Argentina collection costs are even higher and coverage is no better than in Chile (DeMarco and Rofman 1998). Bolivia, however, boasts better results, which likely result from the tax collector being a private firm under contract from the government (von Gersdorff 1997).

Chile created a separate agency to supervise the new AFPs as a part of the reform. The main reason related to doubts about the other financial sector supervisory agencies. The ensuing banking crisis of the early 1980s confirmed these doubts. However, creating separate agencies is costly and flies in the face of the increasing integration of financial markets (Taylor and Flemming 1999). Subsequent reformers have attempted to integrate the AFP supervisory function into existing supervisory agencies (Colombia, Uruguay, and Bolivia).

TWO MODELS ARE EMERGING IN LATIN AMERICA

The Argentinean and Bolivian reforms illustrate well the two different emerging models. Argentina had one of the highest implicit pension debts in Latin America at the time of the reform—in 1990 it had a ratio of the elderly to the working age population (65+/15-64) of 14.8 percent, close to that of Australia or Canada in the OECD, for example. Payroll taxes of 21 percent were not covering system costs, estimated at about 5 percent of GDP. Without a strong fiscal surplus or any prospects of windfall revenues from new, unexploited resources, Argentina had no prospects of moving straight into a fully funded system. It raised the contribution rate to 27 percent, keeping 16 percent in the PAYG system, with the rest in the funded system. It mostly honored acquired rights under the old system and will pay off contributors as they retire (compensatory pension). This is expected to be cheaper than the Chilean approach, which involved the issuance of compensatory bonds, since the rate of return to existing rights is not fixed in real terms in advance, and the pension is only paid to those who live to retirement age. However, the government, not the individual, bears the longevity risk. New PAYG rights are related only to years of contribution and not to the individual contribution wage. The funded system transition is therefore mostly tax financed, with a reduction in future benefits for contributing participants as well.

Bolivia is a much younger country than Argentina, with a ratio of persons 65 and over to persons 15-64 of only 6.3 percent. At the time of reform, pension costs were much lower, at a modest 1.5 percent of GDP. In addition, privatization of energy and mineral resources yielded a fiscal dividend. Bolivia moved completely and instantaneously to a second-pillar system for all participants. Following the practice in Argentina, it will pay acquired rights in the old system at retirement. In addition, Bolivia will pay a special dividend at age 65 to all those aged 21 or higher in 1995 (the Bonosol). This onetime distribution of the privatization funds does not carry forward to future generations. The funds for the Bonosol are in special accounts managed by the private AFPs.

Bolivia also had a relatively thin and inexperienced capital market in 1995. In order to ensure that funds were well managed, the government divided the country into two monopoly AFPs—all other countries in the region have used an open AFP process. International firms competed to purchase these monopolies. The monopoly lasts for five years, after which time the market is scheduled to open up for new entrants (von Gersdorff 1997).

REMAINING QUESTIONS IN LATIN AMERICA

Its success in developing pension reform models has bolstered Latin America as a region. These reforms have succeeded in reducing pension debt and bringing about more fiscally sustainable systems (Schmidt-Hebbel 1999). However, system coverage has remained at about where it was before the reform—with the exception of Bolivia, at about 45–60 percent of the active labor force (Holzmann, Packard, and Cuesta 2001). This has raised questions about these reforms as social risk management systems. Related to the coverage question is the cost of the decentralized system. The magnitudes of the costs and the reasons behind them remain a controversial topic.

Asia

With over half of the world's population, and facing rapid declines in fertility and increasing life expectancy, Asia holds many of the pension system problems for the 21st century. While most of the region is demographically young today, a rapid transition is predicted (table 3.2). For example, in East Asia the ratio of elderly to the working age population is expected to triple over the next 40 years.[19] In Sri Lanka the proportion of those over 60 is projected to rise from the current level of 9 percent to about 20 percent in 2025. This transition will likely occur at a much lower level of income in Asian countries than in OECD or Latin American countries.

Asia has a wide variety of pension systems today (table 3.1). National provident funds are quite common, as are pillar 1 systems. Several countries exempted the public sector from the national provident fund system and instead provide it with an unfunded or partially funded DB system (Indonesia, Malaysia, and Sri Lanka). Coverage varies and is not strongly correlated with level of development. For example, coverage, as a percentage of the labor force, is high in the high-income countries of Malaysia (60 percent) and Singapore (65 percent) and in the low-income countries of Sri Lanka and Mongolia (both over 50 percent). However, it is lower in Vietnam and India (about 10 percent) and the Philippines (28 percent). Most countries in the region continue to rely on informal, family-based systems to support the elderly. These systems will be tested in the future by the rapid rate of demographic transition.

Most of the fiscal pressure in the region comes from the unfunded PAYG systems in the lower income countries. The unfunded civil service occupational pension plans, whose large liabilities the government has, for the most part, not yet costed out, have encountered particular difficulty. For example, in Sri Lanka transfers for civil servant pensions are already one-third of the total government wage bill. Transition economy pension systems in Asia have all fallen into the same difficulties as those in Eastern Europe and the former Soviet Union. Pressures on government budgets from unfunded state-owned enterprise (SOE) liabilities are rising in China, especially in the poorer provinces, and in Vietnam, where contributions already do not cover current outflows. The collapse of the Soviet Union and the resulting fall in income in Mongolia produced a fiscal crisis in this country's pension system. In the other countries with pillar 1 systems, there are substantial reserves, so short-term fiscal pressures are not motivating a major reform.

The most common criticism of Asian pension systems relates to their asset management regimes. Not only do these tend not to be open to public scrutiny or accountability, but they also tend to require a high level of investment in government bonds or publicly held assets, which lowers returns. For example, average real annual returns to assets in plans in Sri Lanka, the Philippines, and Singapore have all been under 2 percent per annum (and negative in Sri Lanka), while income growth during the same period was above this level (Iglesias and Palacios 2000). As a result, benefits from the DC schemes are low, while the funding ratios on the DB schemes are dropping. For these countries, there have been pressures to relax investment rules and offer participants a choice of fund managers.

Malaysia is a notable exception to this trend. Although the system is publicly managed, in 1991 and again in 1995, the government relaxed investment rules, and the share of equities, bonds, and money market instruments in fund assets has risen to over 50 percent. Rates of return have also risen.

Other problematic issues for Asian countries include the existence of separate pension schemes for the public and private sectors. Even where these systems still have reserves, differences in the schemes impede labor mobility. Where separate public systems include SOEs, enterprise restructuring may be hindered. Equity issues may also arise with the lack of a national system, as participants tend to have higher than average incomes.

WHAT HAVE ASIAN COUNTRIES BEEN DOING?

Major reforms in Asia have covered the spectrum of reform possibilities. Thailand and India have gone for blends by adding or strengthening pillar 1 while keeping pillar 2 systems. China and Mongolia are converting the PAYG DB systems into NDC systems. In Hong Kong SAR, the government is adding an individual accounts pillar 2 system.

The reforms in Thailand and India extended DB plans to the formal sector workforce in order to complete the development of a full old age security system. Both reforms were part of overall efforts led by unions to mandate comprehensive social insurance benefits. In both cases substantial funding is envisaged to avoid fiscal crises caused by the demographic transition. This will require public management of reserves of the DB systems for long periods of time. India already had a DB plan for civil servants and a less generous plan for the private sector. In 1995 the private sector employees' plan was substantially upgraded. Thailand had a system of voluntary provident funds as well as a civil service pension scheme. Reforms over the last decade built on this foundation by (i) mandating the establishment of provident schemes in private sector firms over a minimum size and (ii) adding a publicly run, comprehensive social insurance program including sickness, maternity, disability, and old age pension (as of January 1999) benefits. In both cases expanded benefits required higher payroll taxes.

As constructed, the systems of India and Thailand could suffer from the problems of European and Latin American systems. Retirement ages are fairly low (late 50s, and India allows a length of service pension), encouraging early exit. Payroll taxes may encourage evasion, leaving coverage ratios low. Unlike systems in Europe and Latin America, however, both systems are designed to be mostly funded. Investing the funds in high-yield assets and adjusting the benefits to changes in life expectancy could help avoid the type of benefit crisis common in Latin America. This does not seem to be part of the current program, however, leaving cause for concern. India's track record to date on managing funds does not provide much optimism for its system. With most assets in government bonds and the postal savings system, returns have lagged economic growth.

NDC IN ASIA

NDC has proved a popular reform for the transition economies of Asia, despite their very different initial conditions. China established the beginnings of a comprehensive national pension system in the 1950s. However, during the cultural revolution, the government shifted the responsibility for pension provision to the enterprise (with nationally mandated benefits) and spent the funds accumulated in the pooled system. In this context pensions were called "retirement salary." This system has proved to be a major obstacle to reform of the state sector, as well as being an issue in fiscal decentralization (World Bank 1997). Since 1986 China has been trying to return to a national PAYG pension system with intergenerational income redistribution. In addition, China seeks to introduce funding into the system.

In August 1997 China set the framework for the national unification to take place over the next few years. It substitutes a new DB plus NDC PAYG system for the current fragmented system. The DB section is a flat benefit equal to 20 percent of the provincial average wage (called the basic benefit). On top of this flat benefit is a quasi-NDC benefit. The system is not fully NDC because the benefits are not linked to life expectancy. Instead, the balance in the account is divided by 120 to compute the annuity benefit. This approach in effect assumes a life expectancy of 10 years for everyone at all ages and, as a result, (i) may not be stable, and (ii) encourages early exit. There are transition arrangements for those with 15 or more years of service, for the new benefit is less generous than the previous DB rules enterprises were supposed to follow (compliance depends on profitability). Partial funding is envisaged in the pillar 1 system, but how this would happen remains unspecified. China's strong economic growth rate and record of good fiscal management gives some scope for this to occur. Regulations supporting private pillar 3 pensions are also pending.

Mongolia approved an NDC reform in 1999 in the face of a continuing fiscal crisis. It does not have a basic benefit but instead offers a minimum guaranteed benefit equal to 20 percent of the average wage with 15 years of service. Although this reform cut benefits significantly, contributions still do not cover current payouts. However, the return of wage growth and the decline of obligations should reverse this situation over the next decade. Once the current spending level declines as a share of contributions, the addition of a second pillar may allow for partial funding of the system.

Hong Kong: An Emerging Asian-Style Chile?

While it was still under British rule, Hong Kong began considering the establishment of a national, funded pension system to supplement the existing Australian-style demogrant system (which is means tested). After considering the government-run provident fund model, in 1995 Hong Kong opted for a system of individual accounts to be managed by private fund managers. Preparations continued through the return to Chinese sovereignty. The system is scheduled to start in the beginning of 2001.

The Hong Kong system differs from the Chilean model in several important aspects. First, benefits will be lump sum (and tax exempt). As a result, the annuity market is expected to remain thin. Second, the employer will choose and contract the asset manager. Employees may have their choice of funds but only within the employer's contract. This innovation is expected to lower the costs of maintaining accounts and monitoring compliance. It may have coverage consequences, however, as asset managers cannot be expected to race to conclude contracts with small employers (especially those with low average wages). Existing supervisory bodies will handle supervision of asset managers, while a new authority will monitor compliance. Other regulations to control administration costs are currently being formulated. With this organization, Hong Kong is combining the benefit features of the Asian model with the asset management features of the Latin American systems.

If Asian pension systems are converging toward a model, it is clearly a blend. Pillar 1 can take several forms—a classic European DB, a demogrant, or an NDC (transition economies). For now pillar 2 is mostly provident fund and provides mostly lump sum benefits.[20] Hong Kong is the main exception to this trend. Several transition economies are considering converting PAYG obligations to individual funded accounts but have not had the fiscal resources to do so. Major transformations have not yet taken place in provident fund systems.

Africa and the Middle East

African and Near Eastern middle-income countries have not embarked upon major reforms. In part this is because the partially funded DB PAYG systems in countries in North Africa, South Africa, and the Middle East still have enough reserves to get by over the time horizon of the average politician. For example, Jordan's system for private employees has reserves estimated at 16 percent of GDP and saves on average just under 1 percent of GDP per year, although its public system is unfunded. In Morocco all four systems (two public, one private, and one voluntary) have reserves ranging from one-half to four years' worth of benefits. In addition, the countries are still young and rural, and informal old age systems still function. Projections suggest that these systems will also become a fiscal burden without reform but not until well into the next century (Boersch-Supan, Palacios, and Tumbarello 1999).

Pension systems in most low-income countries (countries with a per capita income less than US$700 per year) are in an infant stage. As can be expected, owing to the high percentage of the labor force in agriculture (on average, nearly 70 percent), most systems in Sub-Saharan Africa are marginal in economic terms, often covering less than 5 percent of the labor force and expending less than 1.5 percent of GDP on pensions. The countries are demographically young, with an old age dependency ratio (60/15–64) of 4.4 percent in Sub-Saharan Africa (World Bank 1998).

In many countries, what is called a national social insurance system is actually a public employee's pension scheme. These schemes can be quite generous, with full pensions often offered at 55 with as little as 10 years of service. In the more developed countries of Sub-Saharan Africa, coverage reaches about 10 percent of the total labor force, extending into the formal private sector. In anglophone Africa, the predominant model is separate schemes for the public and private sectors, usually a DB, unfunded civil service scheme, and a funded, DC provident fund scheme for the rest of the formal sector, mostly parastatal and foreign companies (for example, Zambia and Kenya).

Several countries have large reserves for these systems. Generally, a major concern is the management of reserves. Iglesias and Palacios (2000) provide dramatic evidence that assets in low-income countries tend to be mismanaged. In Egypt and Zambia annual compound real returns trailed bank deposit returns by 8–12 percent on average. In Uganda between 1986–94, the real annual compound rate of return was highly negative (–33.1 percent).

Reform is not a major topic on the policy agenda, as most of these countries, especially in Africa, are spending all their energies in a losing fight against hunger and disease in the face of secularly declining prices for commodities, their major exports. Nonetheless, signs of trouble are emerging. For example, in 1998 Kenya spent 100 percent of contributions on administrative costs (Barbone and Sanchez 1999). In Senegal, payroll taxes for the pension system are 14 percent, and total payroll taxes are a whopping 35 percent, contributing to urban unemployment.

ISSUES IN COUNTRIES OF AFRICA AND THE MIDDLE EAST

Countries face two related issues: (i) ensuring long-term equity and sustainability in the face of rapid demographic transitions and (ii) the management of reserves. The demographic transition is happening faster in these countries than it did in Western Europe (World Bank 1994; 1998). For example, in Egypt the share of the population over 60 is predicted to rise from 9 to 18 percent in 30 years, while the same progression took place over a 100-year period in Western Europe. Second, promised replacement rates are much higher than those found in Western Europe in the infancy of public pension schemes. Rates of 40-60 percent after 30 years of contributions are quite common, compared with about 20 percent in European countries before the Second World War. These high rates will rapidly put pressure on the DB schemes. Finally, as the full implications of the HIV/AIDs crisis are felt in the labor force, dependency ratios could rise sharply.

In the poorest countries pension reform is primarily a public sector pay and employment issue, since coverage is so low and the wage economy so small that pension systems cannot possibly be the answer to old age poverty.[21] The poor in these countries continue to rely on private transfers. Pension systems may actually be regressive, depending on the tax incidence and the public sector pay structure. Governments are reluctant to address this difficult problem, preferring to give in to public sector workers' demands for generous deferred compensation. Even where employees contribute, those contributions have in effect gone back into paying their current salaries, as the reserves have primarily financed public sector current expenditure. Strong public sector unions, used to rent-seeking, and powerful but corrupt public sector agencies that "manage" these funds, will make this problem difficult to tackle. At the same time, with a rapidly aging population, elderly poverty is likely to emerge as a critical issue.

Reserve management will continue to be a difficult issue. Improvements in overall governance and in banking regulation and reduced corruption in the public sector will be required to address these problems.

Emerging Models

The last five years offer a wealth of experience in pension reform. Most reforms have been implemented in politically open systems, amid significant debate. Does this imply that models are emerging? This section looks at three areas where pension reforms are beginning to converge in the middle and upper income countries: (i) the shape of the first pillar, (ii) the size of pillars and the financing of the existing pension debt, and (iii) measures to lower administrative costs in multipillar systems.

Building a Better First Pillar

Based on the experiences summarized above, sizable, contribution-related, state-managed, first pillars are here to stay in the OECD, transition economies, and probably most other countries with a share of the population over 60 greater than 12 percent. But the shape of this first pillar is changing. As a result, reform of the first pillar is now seen not only as a prerequisite to the introduction of a second pillar with financial accounts but also as the key overall reform, since it intends to decrease liabilities and thus implicitly increase advance funding.

The most striking feature of the recent reforms of the first pillar is their central direction. They are trying to reduce early labor force exit by tying benefits to individual lifetime account schemes, hoping to replicate the labor market incentives of DC individual financial account systems. This decreases redistribution within the public, earnings-related insurance system, both among age cohorts and within age cohorts.

The large number of reforms in the transition countries has partly driven this result. These countries have had a clear political will to reduce the redistribution in their systems, consistent with the drive to create a market economy and reduce the scope of the public sector. The NDC paradigm is the most explicit attempt to replicate the incentives of a DC financial account system, and transition economies are adopting it. In Latin America the trend is also away from redistributional privileges. Only Argentina has bucked the trend by creating a first pillar more redistributional than the previous system.

How important to economic growth and welfare are the objectives of reducing the labor market distortions of a redistributional DB system? Economic theory tells us that the effect of distortions on individual behavior depends on the flexibility of the labor supply. If people can adapt their labor supply, tax wedges create distortions and affect incentives. People can supply more or less labor, but, provided they have the opportunity, they can also move in and out of the formal economy. Generally, with output, capital, and labor market imperfections, the theoretical results are less clear (Diamond 1997).

There are some important examples of distortions that should be taken into consideration. First, if the rate of return on PAYG contributions is below the net rate of return on other savings, the difference becomes a tax, and if the individual were to choose freely how to use his or her funds, the investment alternative would be the preferred alternative. This is the main argument for restricting the scale of the mandatory public system. Second, high payroll taxes paid by the employer can also raise the effective minimum wage, and possibly reduce the demand for labor—at least taxed labor. Third, if people are forced to "buy" more coverage than they would freely choose (or need in order to stay out of poverty) and cannot borrow to offset this, the net result on their welfare is negative. If they can borrow, but only at a rate that is above the rate of return on paid contributions, an additional tax element emerges. This tax element may be quite high because poor households often face capital rationing. In poor households in middle-income and poor countries, people must be expected to put present needs before future needs. Their discount rate can be quite high, and may rise even more if they have reason to expect much better times for themselves in the future.

As already discussed, for a selected group of OECD countries, Gruber and Wise (1999) use empirical evidence to make a strong case that explicit and implicit taxes on work affect the timing of exit from the labor force. In countries with a higher tax on staying, people tend to exit earlier. Their results demonstrate the importance of the whole system of tax and benefit incentives. The message is that generous systems promote early retirement in OECD countries—on average around eight years earlier than what nowadays seems to be a universal goal of at least age 65. Early retirement for today's pensioners costs future taxpayers, whose wealth profile is unknown. Reformers in the 1990s have approached this problem by implementing individual account systems. However, middle-income countries that have attempted to reduce the distortions through the implementation of individual account systems linking benefits strongly to contributions have not had much success in increasing coverage or participation (Schmidt-Hebbel 1999; Fox and Palmer 1999; Holzmann, Packard, and Cuesta 2001). Most of the reforms are still new, and there is no evidence yet on their effects on the age of exit from the labor force.

Redistribution to the lifetime poor and very low-income pensioners has not been eliminated in countries introducing lifetime account systems. Redistribution to the poor in old age has been made an explicit part of social policy, often financed with general tax revenues from the state budget.

Redistribution commonly takes the form of a minimum pension guarantee that supplements the earnings-related benefit (or provides a full benefit for an individual without an earnings-related annuity) or means-tested benefit. Universal flat-rate benefits from a certain age can achieve the same goal but must be set high enough to achieve their purpose and are thereby distributed to a large number of people who do not need them. Where there is a trade-off, a larger earnings-related scheme for the same money would have been preferable.

Several authors have expressed concern about the effects on poorer women with low wages and interrupted work histories of lifetime earnings-based systems in the middle- and upper-income countries. Even in OECD countries there is some concern that support systems for low earners in old age have been reduced too much. For example, Disney (1996) expresses concern that the reforms in the United Kingdom will push this group into poverty. The purpose of guaranteed minimum benefits is to protect this group. Unfortunately, without massive redistribution, persons who are poor during their working careers are usually poor as pensioners, but hopefully not destitute if the safety net works.

Middle-income developing countries outside of Europe and Central Asia have a distribution of income and wealth that is generally much more unequal than in OECD countries. These countries need to be much more concerned about publicly mandated redistributions to upper-income groups. DB PAYG systems have clearly had that feature in these countries (World Bank 1994). Consequently, reforms of the PAYG system using the models being developed in the countries reviewed here would most likely be welfare enhancing in these middle-income countries.

In sum, there seems to be a political and economic consensus around reforming first-pillar systems to offer labor supply and participation incentives similar to DC financial account systems, but without full funding, while retaining a small safety net. In addition, redistribution through special privileges for select groups is being reduced. The process of improving pillar 1 in the desired direction is moving very slowly, however, especially where benefit outcomes are promised very early in the working life and prove politically difficult to change later. In all groups of countries, there are examples of countries where DB pillar 1 promises are greatly out of line with resources, indicating that we are only seeing the beginning of a reform wave.

Putting the Pillars Together

Countries that have introduced multipillar blends in the latter half of the 1990s have tended to keep large permanent first pillars. This is quite different from the Chilean approach. Chile did not allow new entrants to stay in the PAYG system and capitalized the acquired rights of those who switched into recognition bonds, effectively freezing their present value. This approach (i) ensured that the PAYG system would eventually close (an explicit goal of the Chilean reformers) and (ii) fixed the government obligation to the switchers in real terms over time, as the bonds bear a fixed real interest rate. Many recent reforms have not phased out the first pillar and have not capitalized acquired rights. Even when the second pillar is fully operational, not more than 50 percent of the total contributions within the old age system are designated for second-pillar funds.

There are two reasons why other countries have not followed the Chilean approach. In Chile the government cut spending in the years prior to the reform, yielding a surplus of 5.5 percent of GDP, which it used to cover most of the debt. Only about 1.5 percent of GDP per annum represented a double burden.[22] The OECD and transition countries, as well as some Latin American countries, are demographically much older than Chile was at the time of its reform. As a result, acquired rights of people under the existing schemes are much more significant, and a high fiscal surplus has not been available. For example, Sweden faced entitlements of pensioners and workers together amounting to around 3.5 times GDP at the time it was considering reform. Transition countries have similar implicit debts (Holzmann 1998). This would be a sizable debt to capitalize.

Where some capitalization of debt is considered desirable, it is not obvious that the Chilean model of freezing the rate of return on these acquired rights is the best method. Instead the real rate of return on the recognition bond could be set equal to the rate of change in the covered wage bill, which is the tax base for the system. This is tantamount to retaining the PAYG format. To hedge demographic risks, the value of the bond could be indexed to longevity. This approach resembles the NDC system.

As the slogan for the Polish reform, "Security through Diversity," suggests (Chlon, Góra, and Rutkowski 1999), combining the two pillars in the social security portfolio provides better security. Both pillars are associated with risks, and a mix of the two helps minimize the downside risks inherent in each. A recent paper by Orszag and Orszag (2000) argues that in the face of economic uncertainty on the future value of the debt, a mix of funding and PAYG is the optimal choice.[23]

Countries have used various mechanisms to create room for second-pillar financial account systems. These include the following:

- Reducing PAYG commitments to pensioners, usually by changing indexation formulas
- Reducing PAYG commitments to present workers by tightening benefit rules
- Taking advantage of demographic cycles
- Moving other assets into the pension system to help finance the transition

- Collecting more contributions than are credited to individual accounts, which is just a form of general taxation
- Reducing other forms of government consumption spending (creating a budget surplus to help finance old PAYG commitments)

What are some examples? Preceding the introduction of the chance to opt out of the SERPS, the United Kingdom tightened the PAYG benefit rules and went from wage to price indexation. Croatia, Hungary, Latvia, Poland, and Sweden created room by tightening the benefit rules in the PAYG pillars. The NDC formulas introduced in the latter three of these countries offer worse benefits than the DB formulas they replaced to persons with short work careers (usually people who have not been in the country all their working careers) and younger generations who live longer.[24] Countries have also increased the minimum pension age (for example, Croatia, Hungary, and Sweden), creating liquidity associated with postponed retirement even in actuarial systems. Finally, workers who are mandated or can voluntarily choose to switch to pillar 2 relinquish pillar 1 rights, reducing PAYG costs over time (Palacios and Whitehouse 1998).

In determining the size of the second pillar, future dependency ratios have also played a central role. In the transition countries of Eastern Europe, as we have already seen, there is a "low-pressure" demographic window lasting from 2010 through 2015. With the gradual introduction of the second pillar occurring in Croatia, Hungary, Latvia, and Poland, the burden on younger workers will be relatively light during this period, while the commitments to younger workers will shift over to financial accounts in pillar 2. Some countries may still have to tax-finance some of the transition, but they can anticipate the extent to which this will be necessary while formulating policy.

Finally, some countries are creating a larger second pillar by using privatization assets to fund pensions for current pensioners during the initial stages of the second-pillar operation. Poland, for example, is using privatization assets to help finance the transition, as did Bolivia. In Sweden large PAYG reserves accumulated in past decades will help pay for the baby boomers of the 1940s, helping to keep transition costs within a fixed contribution rate for the NDC PAYG and funded pillar together. To the extent that this does not work out, indexation will reduce NDC rights to workers, implying that—from the point of view of younger workers—the exercise is only meaningful if the rate of return in the financial market (after administrative costs) is greater than this implicit tax. Of course, the main reason why Sweden has introduced a funded pillar 2 is to take advantage of this positive potential return.[25]

Chile, Australia, and Kazakhstan are combining various guarantees with the full-scale transition to advance-funded systems with individual financial accounts. Australia has a universal means and asset-tested income floor. Chile has a minimum pension guarantee for covered workers plus social assistance for the poor who are not covered. In Kazakhstan there is also a minimum pension guarantee for covered workers. There are also some implicit costs of reform that countries may have underestimated, however. In Chile, where coverage is low, the future cost of the guarantee could be substantial, implying an increase in the tax rate on workers. In fact, other countries have likely underestimated costs (future taxes) as well, among them the United Kingdom, as we have already discussed, and Sweden. The reason is that minimum guarantees have been price indexed, and as time passes there will be pressure to increase the floor in these systems.[26] In the blend countries, however, the PAYG system takes pressure off the guarantee and helps make total future costs more transparent.

Lowering Administrative Costs of Individual Financial Account Systems

Probably one of the most important debates around individual financial accounts over the last five years concerns the costs of these accounts, which reach as much as 1-2.4 percent of wages, annually (Schmidt-Hebbel 1999). With these cost levels in mind, Diamond and Valdés-Prieto (1994) asked whether it is possible for system designers to strike the right balance between using the apparatus of the public sector to save costs and taking on the greater risk of political influence on investment decisions.[27]

In the early 1990s, Chile, the United Kingdom, and Australia provided three models of how to design advance-funded systems with individual financial accounts. Chile and Australia seemed to provide the options for mandatory systems, while the United Kingdom could be said to have shown the way for voluntary or "opt-out" systems. In the Chilean model individuals choose from around a dozen authorized private fund managers. Each manager has one fund and offers a choice at retirement between various annuities or programmed withdrawal. The Australian model differs from this in that a large number of fund managers (around 8,000 organizations) may offer a choice of two or more investment funds, but the employers, rather than the workers, choose the fund manager. On the product side there is a choice between annuity products or a lump sum (Thompson 1999).[28] In the United Kingdom individuals themselves are allowed to choose among a great number of investment managers, each of which could have many funds from which to choose (the so-called unit-link model). In addition, insurance products range from lump sum and programmed withdrawals to various annuities. Of the three models available in the beginning of the 1990s, this system provided the greatest freedom of choice to individuals.

To understand what has happened as the 1990s progressed and the current status of the innovations, it is useful to view the separate tasks involved in the administration of advance-funded insurance with individual financial accounts. These include collecting contributions, performing transactions and keeping accounts, managing funds during the accumulation and annuity phases, and providing annuities (actuarial services, customer relations, payments, etc). We examine these one at a time.

CONTRIBUTIONS

Generally, in mandatory individual account plans, employers (and the self-employed on behalf of themselves) remit contributions. The employers can either remit the contributions to the tax authority, along with other taxes, or directly to the investment manager. In the first case, the advantage should be a minimization of costs for businesses and the government. The argument is that if the tax authority is already collecting part of the contribution (to the PAYG pillar) there is essentially no marginal cost of also collecting contributions to the second pillar. The disadvantage is that there may be a lag between payment of contributions and remittance to the investment manager. In the second case, the advantage is that the money goes straight to the investment manager. The disadvantages are that (i) monitoring compliance is much more difficult[29] and (ii) economies of scale in record-keeping are lost. In principle, technology can help to overcome both disadvantages.

Countries introducing individual account systems in the 1990s generally entrusted contribution collection to the government (for example, Uruguay, Argentina, Sweden, Hungary, and Poland). Other countries where second-pillar legislation is being formulated (for example, Croatia and Latvia) are also choosing the centralized model. The cost-efficiency argument has constituted a strong case for putting the collection of all public revenues and social insurance contributions under one roof.[30]

Has this cost-efficiency argument been correct? In Argentina the answer is clearly no, although it is hoped that with the new information system recently installed the situation will improve. There is a lack of analysis of other countries. In Europe (Sweden and the United Kingdom) contributions are only remitted to investment managers annually (with an actual lag of 18–24 months). This occurs in part because employers are only required to remit information to the tax authority on an annual basis (although they make preliminary contribution payments more frequently) and in part because it takes about this long to process and legally establish the final taxable earnings of all citizens.[31] Here, it appears to be the existing legal structures and accompanying accounting systems of the United Kingdom and Sweden, rather than new thinking in this area, that have determined the current course of events. In this case, questions need to be raised regarding financial returns lost.

TRANSACTIONS AND ACCOUNT KEEPING

In Chile, Australia, and the United Kingdom, the investment managers keep the records on individual account balances. This is logical if the country is following the standard insurance model in which the investment manager and the insurance provider are simply two sides of the same insurance business. However, the investment side of the insurance business is traditionally separated from the provision of annuities. Since the market is full of mutual funds, why not let people choose any mutual fund registered to do business in the country? With the voluntary choice of funds, persons with a high degree of risk aversion will be free to choose conservative funds, and persons who want to take greater risks can do so (Srinivas, Whitehouse, and Yermo 2000; Shah 1997). This is the Swedish approach.

In order to minimize transaction costs in investment management, Sweden introduced the idea of the public clearinghouse. The public clearinghouse (PPM) is a public broker that performs net transactions vis-à-vis registered funds (the number of which is, in principle, limited only by the interest of funds themselves in participating in the system). The fund managers have only one customer, the PPM, which keeps the accounts for all individual participants. This limits the costs of fund managers to managing funds and enhances the possibilities to monitor the system. Funds compete by offering the best net-of-cost returns.[32] The clearinghouse manager requires that all funds report fund returns and costs according to the same principles and makes this information available to all participants. Two other countries—Croatia and Latvia—are both working with the Swedish clearinghouse model.

Little empirical evidence is available on the cost savings afforded by this approach. Given published knowledge about costs for various models, Thompson (1999) offered some estimates using standardized assumptions about earnings careers and portfolio returns. Using his assumptions, a system with efficient centralized administration, a clearinghouse approach, a choice limited to a few index funds and centralized annuity provision reduces gross benefits from DC account proceeds by 5 percent, whereas a system with decentralized administration with a Latin American annuity mandate reduces gross benefits by 25 percent. These estimates can be viewed as lower and upper bounds and indicate that there is room for improvement on the costs compared with the initial Latin American results. The lower bound is achieved at the expense of providing minimal choice, which can be questioned. In fact, there are many arguments against having a few big index funds in a small and developing financial environment unless they are competing "world-based" index funds with relatively few investments in the local market.

ANNUITY PROVISION AND PAYMENT

Two models of the administration of annuity provision have also emerged. In all the main models prevailing in the early 1990s, the worker chooses the annuity provider. Even here, however, there are possible limitations on the freedom to move from one provider to another. For example, these may take the form of high costs borne by those who make such a decision.[33]

The Swedish model diverges from the others on this point. In the Swedish model, the government is a single provider of all the annuity products offered. Consequently, the government also administers the payment of the second-pillar annuity together with the public PAYG benefit. On the one hand, the Swedish model, in principle, clearly limits the potential choice of annuity products available to individuals. In contrast, the typical insurance problems associated with adverse selection cannot arise.

In conclusion, the trend has clearly been towards centralization to keep down administrative costs. Central collection by the national tax authority, the clearinghouse for transactions and account keeping, and the government annuity monopoly all work in this direction. As with other innovations, empirical evidence on the effects remains weak.

Open Issues

Given the variety of countries in the world and their economic and social differences, it is not surprising that a number of issues in the design of pension systems are far from settled. Indeed, in some parts of the world (for example, East Asia), the debate is still a very young one. This section looks at two issues that are still the subject of wide discussion and debate around the world. The first looks at (i) the exogenous and endogenous risks to public pension systems, (ii) the sharing of these risks from a social perspective, and (iii) the trade-offs. The second issue focuses on low-income countries, where more than 50 percent of the world's workforce lives, that are not covered by public pension systems.

Who Bears the Risk?

Risk sharing is one of the most controversial aspects of public pension systems. Pension systems are subject to the following main risks to their long-term financial stability and ability to offer income security to participants: (i) long-term demographic shifts, (ii) economic risks (shocks or periods of slow growth), (iii) moral hazard risks (the behavior of individuals and employers, as affected by system design), and (iv) political risks (design features offering short-term political gains that can lead to system financial insolvency). The first two are usually exogenous to the pension system, while the second two are endogenous to it.

In retrospect, it is usually clear who should bear the costs of the exogenous risks after they occur. For example, it is obvious that the postwar generation should have transferred income back to the previous generation, which suffered a world depression and war. Likewise, older generations will bear the costs of the transition to the market economy in Europe and Central Asia, and younger generations will receive the benefits. But how much should be promised to the baby boomers by their children in middle-income countries today is not so simple, nor is it easy to predict the expected real cost. Should the system allocate these risks in advance or allow the electorate to work it out as they become known? Pillar 1 systems offer a range of opportunities for intergenerational risk sharing in the face of major shocks. Without some floor or minimum, pillar 2 systems allocate all the economic risk, short- and medium-term, to the contributor in individual accounts and to the age cohort in provident fund systems.

Demographic risks are difficult to allocate fairly ex ante. DB systems allocate the risk to the "funder"—in PAYG systems, this is the next generation. Again, it is difficult to know in advance whether this will be fair. Yet, if it is unfair, it is difficult to correct. Changes in the indexation system are the only tool governments have once pensioners are near pension age or pensions are in payment, as it is almost impossible politically to lower pensions by other means. Even changing indexation systems can be difficult. DC systems allocate the demographic risks mostly to participants and their generation. Annuities, computed at the time of retirement, reflect changes in life expectancy. If there are imperfect annuity markets, risk pooling may be incomplete, lowering welfare.

The second two risks are a function of system design. We have argued elsewhere that DB systems have a tendency to make these risks worse because of the focus on outcomes rather than costs, whereas individual accounts systems can make the costs of poor design more transparent. In addition, benefits reflect individual labor force participation, which means that the individual—and not other workers in any generation—bears the risk of early exit (Fox and Palmer 1999). Advance funded, privately managed DC systems take a big step towards reducing the endogenous risk of PAYG pension systems (that promises are made without also stating the source of finance), but there are also examples of funded schemes that have gravely misjudged their future liabilities. NDC PAYG moves a big step in the direction of advance funded DC systems.

Critics have complained that public individual account DC schemes force the individual to bear too much risk for too low benefits. It is true that NDC PAYG and funded individual financial accounts have created greater clarity in who bears the risks. The answer is clear: the worker bears the risk. Early exit from the labor force affects the worker's own benefit in a transparent way. This cost cannot be shifted forward to another generation or to members of the same generation, so workers will resist employers' attempts reduce their labor force participation. The worker will be informed and can also determine his or her supply of labor and saving according to personal preferences and the gradually increasing life expectancy of his or her generation (assuming some risk pooling in annuitization). In sum, how the individual risks are to be borne and the costs of insuring these risks, the "rules of the game," are more transparent in DC than in DB systems.

Is this a good risk sharing? Somebody or some generation has to bear these risks. The evidence on DB systems is summarized below:

- In OECD countries, behavior has changed in response to incentives, and workers and employers have collaborated to reduce labor force participation, thus increasing costs to the financiers (those who continue working and the next generations). Few systems have been able to make the current generation adjust to risks once they are realized, even if that generation has the means. Costs are pushed forward onto generations that may not have the means to pay for these obligations.
- In Latin American countries (for example, Argentina), the DB systems hid their full costs until benefits had to shrink dramatically. In this case, the generation paying to insure the risks demanded a change.

Is everyone able to cope with the exogenous risks if the endogenous risks are minimized? Many societies believe the answer is no for the poorest, and they build some safety net or guaranteed minimum into individual account systems. This guarantee is less common in provident fund systems. Blend systems also incorporate safety nets (adding endogenous risks). One thing is clear: in order for a worker to make more informed judgements, he or she must be informed. Especially in transition countries, this aspect has been a problem (Fox and Palmer 1999).

Expanding Coverage in Low-Income Countries and Low-Income Groups in Middle-Income Countries

The risk-sharing issues discussed above take on a new aspect in low-income countries, where coverage is low. In this case, it is rarely the poor who are benefiting, so the arguments for inter- and intragenerational risk sharing cannot be made on social grounds (although they often are). Those who are covered are those within their generation most able to bear the risks, and the arguments for shifting risks forward are certainly not clear ex ante. As a result, the argument for DB systems is quite weak.

Pillar 1 pension systems in low-income African and Asian countries have not, for the most part, presented a fiscal drain of the magnitude that they have in transition and Latin American economies. However, given the predicted rapid demographic transitions, the current DB systems are likely to run into trouble when the endogenous risks come to fruition. Since in many of these countries tax revenues are only 10-20 percent of GDP, even a low expenditure, such as the 1.7 percent of GDP Sri Lanka spends on pensions for the civil service, amounts to 10 percent of budget resources, with a high marginal cost. The income distribution aspects of this transfer have not been analyzed, as these depend on both the incidence of the tax system and the transfer. But it is likely that these civil service schemes are regressive. Conversion to DC schemes would reduce endogenous risks.

Pillar 2 systems are also problematic, as poor reserve management in the provident fund systems has resulted in low benefits. In at least one country (Ghana), the evaporation of reserves in the provident fund system forced the conversion of account balances into PAYG rights during SOE downsizing. China is currently making the same conversion. While we have argued above that pillar 2 systems carry less endogenous risk, that risk is not zero. Public management carries political risk.

Management of reserves in low-income countries with pillar 2 systems is a key issue. Two changes are needed to raise returns. First, the share of government bonds and other investments in the portfolio should be lowered so that government faces the true costs of public borrowing and so that returns increase.[34] Second, management of reserves needs to become more transparent. Is private management a better choice in countries with underdeveloped capital markets? The analysis of Iglesias and Palacios (2000) sheds some light on this question. In their analysis, at every level of national income, private management delivers higher returns than public management. However, Iglesias and Palacios add an important caveat—in countries with poor governance overall (as measured by outside sources such as Transparency International), their model predicts that even private management can yield negative real returns. Note, however, that the governance standard for a prediction of positive returns to private management is fairly low. Egypt and Tanzania, for example, countries with provident funds, are currently above this standard. In addition, the regression model used by Iglesias and Palacios ignores the potential interactive effect of private management on governance. In sum, for young, low-income countries with underdeveloped capital markets, the best starting point for an old age security system seems to be a funded DC system with private management, investing in, for example, a mix of international assets, local bank deposits, and government securities instruments. As local capital markets mature, a more diverse local asset mix could be permitted.

With low coverage rates, pillar 1 systems do not offer security in old age for most of the population today. The argument for preserving traditional pillar 1 systems in low- and lower middle-income countries is that they will grow up to be serviceable old age security systems, perhaps in a robust blend system. The evidence on changes in coverage, based on the upper middle-income countries, is not hopeful for the medium term. Even after reforms, coverage of low-income populations in Latin America has not increased.[35] Looking at the lives of poor households around the world, it is not hard to see why. Savings in pension systems are illiquid and usually earn a real rate of return no greater than 5-8 percent under the best management in developing country markets. Poor households in India regularly pay 50 percent annually for credit through moneylenders and informal credit networks for working capital. Why should such credit-constrained households save for old age in a formal system? In general, household saving for old age is correlated with income. Historically, poor households' income around the world tends to be too erratic to allow the type of life-cycle savings behavior that second-pillar systems encourage. Development of extensive welfare systems correlates with industrialization and income.

This raises the question of whose preferences are being accommodated in the development of full-fledged pension systems in low-income countries. Is there a large unmet demand for contributory pension systems once the true costs are known, or are these systems simply an additional fringe benefit for government sector workers? If the latter, then there is a strong case for low-income countries to concentrate solely on DC occupational systems and not try to create blends at this point. This would reduce the fiscal burden, make the costs transparent, and reduce the risk of public funds being used to bail out these systems at the cost of programs to help the poor (who have no chance of being covered by the systems as currently designed). As countries grow richer, safety net programs for the poor elderly can be introduced (for example, as in Hong Kong). These safety net programs could mature into blend systems. In countries with a high level of inequality, such as South Africa and Brazil, demogrants financed by general taxes have a strong antipoverty effect in rural areas (Morduch 1997). The challenge is to find a level that is affordable without the method of financing causing large-scale evasion and an unfair or undesirable payment burden as a result.

Conclusions

As *Averting the Old Age Crisis* was being prepared, Chile was the model for systemic change from PAYG DB systems to advance-funded systems with individual accounts. The 1990s have been a period of blossoming innovation in reform of mandatory pension provision, but the innovations have taken another course. Few countries have followed Chile more or less to the letter. The 1990s witnessed an explosion of ideas for creating financially sustainable mandatory public systems in different groups of countries in Latin America and the OECD and with economies in transition. What have we learned from the experience of recent years?

First, two-pillar systems combining a PAYG first pillar with a second pillar scheme with funded individual accounts have become popular. New systems of this type have emerged in countries as diverse as Sweden in the OECD; Hungary, Latvia, and Poland among the transition countries; Hong Kong in Asia; and Argentina, Peru, and Uruguay in Latin America. These reforms help reduce the risks of the PAYG system by reducing its size in the long run. They shift the management of funds into the market, offering opportunities for better pensions through higher returns, greater transparency and individual choice. They also diversify the social security portfolio, offering flexibility in an uncertain world.

Second, and related to the first point, the DB system has proved more robust than expected, as some countries have opted to fix their DB systems. This has usually meant increasing the number of years required for full benefits and the number of years counted in the actual computation of the benefit. The idea of introducing a life expectancy factor into the DB formula has also been considered. The goal is to reduce long-term costs. The ability to reduce long-term upside risks for future generations of the DB systems by adding on a second pillar (and simultaneously reducing revenues for and obligations of the DB PAYG system) has probably contributed to its popularity.

The NDC system has emerged as an alternate to the DB system when a country desires to maintain a larger first pillar. It is possible to convert rights acquired under fairly diverse DB systems into NDC systems, with some advance funding to cover demographic fluctuations. Countries that take this step (for example, Mongolia) may do so with the intention of introducing the second pillar at a later time. Countries gain a more direct link between contributions and benefits and account for life expectancy at the benefit payout phase. Key system features, such as indexing obligations to changes in contribution revenues, help to increase long-term financial stability.

Third, countries with funded individual financial accounts have focused on improving old models and developing new ones. Several alternatives for system design have emerged. The focus of innovation has been on reducing costs and providing more individual choice, especially during the investment phase.

Fourth, there are still open issues, such as the type of system that poor and younger middle-income countries should adopt. It appears that we are still no farther along than we were at the beginning of the 1990s. An affordable model with broad coverage has not emerged. The history of richer countries suggests that it may not emerge. Another open issue relates to who bears the risks of increasing longevity and economic shocks in publicly mandated schemes in the more developed countries and the trade-off between sharing risk and moral hazard. The risk that has only recently received attention is the moral hazard risk of the combination of rules, employer practices, and individual and employer attitudes that lead to early exit from the labor force. The generation about to retire (and those who have retired) likes this feature, and future generations do not fully perceive the costs to them. Both NDC PAYG and funded individual financial account systems reduce the moral hazard risk at the cost of less exogenous risk coverage. A blend of PAYG and funding allows a mix of risk sharing instruments and offers more flexibility when shocks occur.

Finally, it is important to emphasize that it is not necessary to go from unfunded PAYG DB to funded, individual account DC systems to create sustainability in the public provision of mandatory old age pensions. Combinations can enhance stability dramatically, as can NDC. Moreover, traditional DB systems can be developed to bring them closer to the DC idea. This is also occurring.

Notes

1. This is a substantially revised version of a paper prepared for the World Bank's conference entitled "New Ideas about Old Age Security," September 14–15, 1999. The authors would like to thank Robert Holzmann, Estelle James, Olivia Mitchell, Peter Orszag, Robert Palacios, Joseph Stiglitz, and conference participants for useful comments on previous drafts. Claus von Restorff provided helpful research assistance. The views expressed here reflect the authors' own and not those of the World Bank.

2. See Demirguc-Kunt and Schwarz (1999) for a more exhaustive discussion of pension reforms around the world.

3. This refers to the mandatory occupational pensions. The social pensions are noncontributory and unfunded.

4. In some countries, these privately managed, decentralized individual account systems are called provident funds.

5. Classifying Australia as pillar 2 is nevertheless problematic, since some employers offer DB. However, the mandate is for DC, and the trend is in that direction.

6. All OECD and many other countries have some form of minimum-income support legislation for the elderly. Although financed on PAYG principles (often out of general revenues), these are usually noncontributory social assistance programs (for example, the United States, Thailand, and Latvia), and we do not cover them in this chapter. Where the pensions are noncontributory but universal or nearly universal (for example, Denmark, Hong Kong, or New Zealand), we consider them first-pillar systems and include them in the chapter.

7. Since1992 employers in Australia have been required to arrange a pension account and contribute a minimum percentage (rising from 3 percent in 1992 to 9 percent in 2002) for employees. People can supplement on a voluntary basis and are covered. Coverage of the self-employed is about

35 percent; full-time employees, 95 percent; all employed, 80 percent (in 1995 for the latter). There is also an income support program for the elderly financed from general revenue.

8. This will be supplemented, however, with a downside brake based on the contribution wage sum, which will affect both the indexation of notional capital and benefit payments (see Palmer 2000).

9. In principle, the Italian system should achieve a long-term equilibrium around the weighted contribution rates of the employed and self-employed if contributions and accrual factors are brought more in line. In practice, the absence of a mechanism to offset chronic divergence from the imputed return of 1.5 percent may lead to financial difficulties. Palmer (1999a) examines the stability conditions of the NDC PAYG system, as does Valdés-Preito (2000).

10. For example, persons who had worked in hazardous occupations for a certain period of time received pensions at an early age (as early as 40) instead of higher wages. Pensions also performed the function of social transfers (or tax deductions) for workers in market economies (for example, a right to retire early as remuneration for being the parent of many children).

11. In Poland the pension ages were 65 and 60 for men and women, respectively, but men and women could retire early with 40 and 35 years of recorded service (work or an equivalent). This, together with the special treatment of some groups (for example, miners), explains why the de facto age of exit with a benefit in the 1990s was around 56 for women and 59 for men.

12. Poland attempted unsuccessfully to introduce a minimum pension age of 63 for both men and women as a part of the 1998 reform.

13. Latvia has recently taken steps to close this loophole (see Fox and Palmer 1999).

14. Croatia, Hungary, Kazakhstan, Latvia, and Poland are all either average or above-average income countries within the group of transition economies (per capita GDP ranges from around US$2,000 in Kazakhstan and Latvia to US$6,000 in Hungary and Poland), with a ratio of the covered wage bill to GDP that is among the highest for transition economies at around 30 percent (Rutkowski 1999).

15. We discuss this model in greater detail the second section of the chapter.

16. There is no evidence yet that the introduction of NDC or funded DC financial systems has led to an increase in the number of persons covered in these countries, although this has clearly been one of the hopes of the reformers. In fact, evidence from other parts of the world (for example, Chile) is discouraging in this respect.

17. This section draws from Queisser (1998) and Schmidt-Hebbel (1999).

18. The other 4 percent of the 14 percent payroll tax is used for survivors and disability insurance and administrative costs.

19. This section draws heavily on Holzmann, Mac Arthur, and Sin (2000) for facts and background on pension systems in East Asia. See also Asher (1999) on Singapore.

20. Singapore provides phased withdrawal options. Members can also withdraw a portion of account balances during working years for other investments (housing finance, medical savings accounts, etc.).

21. During apartheid South Africa and Namibia put in place universal noncontributory pension schemes (demogrants) that continue to operate.

22. Valdés-Prieto (1997, p. 205). Note that this is 3.75 percent of the covered wage bill, assuming covered wages are 40 percent of GDP.

23. The same authors noted that the NDC system provides an excellent choice for partial funding.

24. Of course, younger workers can work longer to compensate for this.

25. Note that as the reform process evolved during the 1990s in Sweden, both blue and white collar private (quasi-mandatory) schemes also converted to individual DC financial accounts, encompassing almost all the private sector employees.

26. However, the argument for separating out redistribution from social insurance is that proposals to change guarantees can be weighed against alternative uses of taxes within the normal political process.

27. See James and Vittas (2000) for a discussion of these costs.

28. Many of the technical details in this section are based on the comprehensive tables presented in Thompson (1999).

29. In countries where there are separate institutions collecting revenues and contributions for mandatory systems, each agency must perform its own audit of an employer's accounts. This creates extra costs for both employers and the public sector. An additional complication arises if the tax base is different for each of the various revenue/contribution systems.

30. It is sometimes argued that the advantage of separating the collection of, for example, general taxes and health care and pension contributions is that potential evaders might be more inclined to pay health care and pension contributions than general taxes. However, this type of tax competition has a negative effect on overall expenditure management.

31. In Sweden, about 90 percent of all returns are processed almost immediately. The lag arises mainly in processing earnings from self-employment.

32. This makes it impossible to compete by offering gifts and (unnecessary) personalized sales services (home visits, etc.). In principle, we should expect advertising to focus on financial information and portfolio strategy, although we will not know until people can make their first choices in the year 2000.

33. Thompson (1999) claims that this can be a problem in the United Kingdom's system. This is not the case in the Latin American systems.

34. If, as we have argued above, poor performing provident funds run the risk of bailouts, this is an even stronger argument for lowering the investment in government bonds, since not only are the current costs of the borrowing lowered but the intertemporal costs are totally distorted, leading to very poor resource allocation.

35. The issue of coverage receives full treatment by Holzmann, Packard, and Cuesta in chapter 13 of this volume.

References

Note: The word *processed* describes informally reproduced works that may not be commonly available through libraries.

Asher, Mukul. 1999. "The Pension System in Singapore." Social Protection Discussion Paper No. 9919. World Bank, Washington, D.C., p. 58.

Barbone, Luca, and Luis-Alvaro Sanchez. 1999. "Pensions and Social Security in Sub-Saharan Africa: Issues and Options." Africa Region Working Paper Series No. 4. World Bank, Washington, D.C.

Börsch-Supan, Axel, Robert Palacios, and Patrizia Tumbarello. 1999. "Pension Systems in the Middle East and North Africa: A Window of Opportunity." World Bank, Human Development Network, Social Protection, Washington, D.C. Processed.

Bonilla, Alejandro, and Colin Gillion. 1994. "Private Pension Schemes in Chile." International Labour Office, Geneva, Switzerland.

Chlon, Agnieszka, Marek Góra, and Michal Rutkowski. 1999. "Shaping Pension Reform in Poland: Security Through Diversity." Social Protection Discussion Paper No. 9923. World Bank, Washington, D.C.

DeMarco, Gustavo, and Rafael Rofman. 1998. "Supervising Mandatory Funded Pension Systems: Issues and Challenges." Social Protection Discussion Paper No. 9817. World Bank, Washington, D.C.

Demirgüç-Kunt, Asli, and Anita Schwarz. 1999. "Taking Stock of Pension Reforms Around the World." Social Protection Discussion Paper No. 9917. World Bank, Washington, D.C.

Diamond, Peter. 1997. "Insulation of Pensions from Political Risk." In Salvador Valdés-Prieto, ed., *The Economics of Pensions.* Cambridge, England: Cambridge University Press.

Diamond, Peter, and Salvador Valdés-Prieto. 1994. *Social Security Reform and the Chilean Economy: Policy Lessons and Challenges.* Brookings Institution, Washington, D.C.

Disney, Richard. 1996. *Can We Afford to Grow Older? A Perspective on the Economics of Aging.* Cambridge, Mass.: MIT Press.

_____. 1999. "OECD Public Pension Programs in Crisis: An Evaluation of the Reform Options." Social Protection Discussion Paper No. 9921. World Bank, Washington, D.C.

Fox, Louise, and Edward Palmer. 1999. "Latvian Pension Reform." Social Protection Discussion Paper No. 9922. World Bank, Washington, D.C.

Gruber, Jonathon, and David Wise. 1999. "Social Security and Retirement Around the World." National Bureau of Economic Research Conference Report. Chicago and London: University of Chicago Press.

Holzmann, Robert. 1998. "Financing the Transition to Multipillar." Social Protection Discussion Paper No. 9809. World Bank, Washington, D.C.

Holzmann, Robert, Ian. W. Mac Arthur, and Yvonne Sin. 2000. "Pension Systems in East Asia and the Pacific: Challenges and Opportunities." Social Protection Discussion Paper No. 0014. World Bank, Washington, D.C.

Iglesias, Augusto, and Robert Palacios. 2000. "Managing Public Pension Reserves: Evidence from the International Experience." Social Protection Discussion Paper No. 0003. World Bank, Washington, D.C.

James, Estelle, and Dimitri Vittas. 2000. "Annuities Markets in Comparative Perspective: Do Consumers Get Their Money's Worth?" Paper presented at the conference "New Ideas About Old Age Security," September 14–15, 1999, World Bank, Washington, D.C.

Morduch, Jonathan. 1997. "Between the Market and the State: Can Informal Insurance Patch the Safety Net?" Processed.

OECD (Organization for Economic Co-operation and Development). 1988. *Reforming Public Pensions.* Paris.

Orszag, Michael J., and Peter R. Orszag. 2000. "The Benefits of Flexible Funding: Implications for Pension Reform in an Uncertain World." Processed.

Palacios, Robert, and Edward Whitehouse. 1998. "The Role of Choice in the Transition to a Funded Pension System." Social Protection Discussion Paper No. 9812. World Bank, Washington, D.C., p. 40.

Palacios, Robert, and Roberto Rocha. 1998. "The Hungarian Pension System in Transition." Social Protection Discussion Paper No. 9805. World Bank, Washington, D.C.

Palmer, Edward. 1999a. "Exit from the Labor Force of Older Workers: Can the NDC Pension System Help?" *The Geneva Papers on Risk and Insurance* 24(4), October 1999. Oxford: Blackwell Publishers.

_____. 1999b. "Individual Decisions and Aggregate Stability in the NDC System." Processed.

_____. 2000. "The Swedish Pension Reform Model: Framework and Issues." Social Protection Discussion Paper No. 0012. World Bank, Washington, D.C.

Queisser, Monika. 1998. "The Second Generation Pension Reforms in Latin America." Aging Working Paper No. 5.4. OECD, Paris.

Rutkowski, Michal. 1999. "The Quest for Modern Solutions: Pension Reforms in Transition Economies." World Bank, Washington, D.C. Processed.

Schmidt-Hebbel, Klaus. 1999. "Latin America's Pension Revolution: A Review of Approaches and Experience." Paper presented at the World Bank ABCDE Conference. Processed.

Shah, Hemant. 1997. "Toward Better Regulation of Private Pension Funds." Policy Research Working Paper 1791. World Bank, Policy Research Department, Washington, D.C.

Srinivas, P.S., Edward Whitehouse, and Juan Yermo. 2000. "Regulating Private Pension Funds' Structure, Performance and Investments: Cross-Country Evidence." Social Protection Discussion Paper. Washington, D.C.

Steuerle, Eugene, Christopher Spiro, and Richard W. Johnson. 1999. "Can Americans Work Longer?" Straight Talk on Social Security and Retirement Policy, No. 5. Urban Institute: Washington, D.C.

Taylor, Michael, and Alexander Flemming. 1999. "Integrated Financial Supervision: Lessons from the Northern European Experience." World Bank Policy Research Working Paper 2223. Washington, D.C.

Thompson, Lawrence H. 1999. "Administering Individual Accounts in Social Security: The Role of Values and Objectives in Shaping Options." The Retirement Project, Occasional Paper No. 1. Urban Institute, Washington, D.C.

Valdés-Prieto, Salvador. 1997. "Financing a Pension Reform toward Private Funded Pensions," in Salvador Valdés-Prieto, ed., *The Economics of Pensions: Principles, Policies, and International Experience.* New York: Cambridge University Press.

Valdés-Prieto, Salvador. 2000. "The Financial Stability of Notional Account Pensions." Processed.

von Gersdorff, Herman. 1997. "Pension Reform in Bolivia: Innovative Solutions to Common Problems." World Bank Policy Research Working Paper 1832. Washington, D.C.

World Bank. 1994. *Averting the Old Age Crisis: Policies to Protect the Old and Promote Growth.* New York: Oxford University Press.

World Bank. 1997. "Old Age Security: Pension Reform in China." Report No. 17090. Washington, D.C.

World Bank. 1998. World Development Indicators 1998, CD-ROM. Washington, D.C.

4

The Political Economy of Structural Pension Reform

Estelle James and Sarah Brooks

MANY POLICIES THAT ARE DESIRABLE for economic reasons have not been implemented for political reasons. This discrepancy between economics and politics has led both economists and political scientists to begin thinking about the political economy of reform. They have already done considerable work on the political economy of macroeconomic reform and trade policy, emphasizing factors such as incomplete information, time inconsistency of preferences, credibility problems, path dependency, and interest groups as major obstacles to reform (Grindle and Thomas 1991; Nelson 1990, 1994; Rodrik 1994; Tommasi and Velasco 1996). There is relatively less work on the political economy of sectoral reform (but see Nelson 1997; James 1986, 1993, 1998b). Using the case of pension reform, this chapter addresses this gap.

Public pension schemes are the largest fiscal program in many countries, and through the world these schemes are in serious trouble. Declining fertility rates and increasing life expectancy have exerted financial pressures on traditional pay-as-you-go, defined benefit (PAYG DB) systems, threatening their sustainability. Thus far, most countries have reacted by altering the parameters (rates of contributions, benefit calculations, and retirement age) of their existing systems. But a growing number of diverse countries, such as Argentina, Sweden, Hungary, and Kazakhstan, have carried out major structural changes, shifting from single-pillar schemes to multipillar schemes that add a fully funded, defined contribution (FF DC) pillar to a downsized PAYG DB pillar. Although funded systems can in principle be publicly or privately managed, the recent wave of multipillar reforms has conferred management responsibility for the second or funded pillar to the private sector, which invests pension funds in the market. Proponents of multipillar systems argue that they are more fiscally sustainable and growth enhancing, due to favorable impacts on labor markets, long-term saving, and financial market development. Opponents dispute these claims.

This chapter does not seek to evaluate these economic arguments about the merits of multipillar systems. Rather, it examines the political economy of the reform process by analyzing the connection between the preexisting conditions in a country and the reforms that are likely to succeed and by describing some of the strategies that policymakers have used to overcome opposition to reform. The chapter addresses three central questions:

- How have political and economic forces influenced the probability of structural pension reform?
- How have these factors influenced the nature of the reform, particularly its public-private mix?
- How have reforming countries overcome resistance from powerful interest groups?

In the first section of the chapter, we use quantitative analysis to answer the first two questions. In the second section, we answer the third question using qualitative case studies of a smaller number of reforming countries in Latin America and the transition economies. In comparison to the econometric analysis, these are able to provide more detailed analyses of political strategy.

Mandatory multipillar systems are a relatively new way of providing social security. Chile was the first country to implement this system in 1981, followed within the same decade by Switzerland and the United Kingdom. Six other countries implemented structural reforms during the first half of the 1990s, and 11 more countries undertook reforms in the second half of the 1990s (figure 4.1). Among the structural reformers, eight are in Latin America, nine in Europe, and three in the Asia/Pacific region. Since structural reform is under consideration in many additional countries, we are not yet at an equilibrium. Therefore, by taking this snapshot, it is more accurate to say that we are analyzing the speed of reform rather than the ultimate probability of reform. Is this process random, or can we predict which conditions are more fertile for reform? We hypothesize that factors such as cultural, linguistic, and geographic proximity to "first movers" play a key role in explaining how reform ideas diffuse across countries via communications and demonstration effects and find econometric support for this argument. Additionally, we expect (and find) that the existence of private financial organizations, such as funded voluntary pension plans, signals institutional interests that speed the adoption of a funded mandatory pillar.

Among countries that have implemented structural reforms, the details vary in many ways. We focus in this chapter on differences in the public-private mix of benefits. The proportion of total expected benefits that stem from the private pillar ranges all the way from 0 to 100 percent. Again, we

Figure 4.1. Diffusion of Structural Reform around the World, 1980–2000

Cumulative number of reforming countries

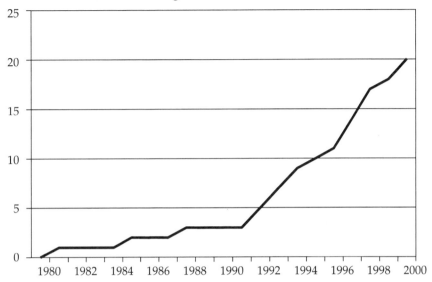

Source: Authors' calculations.

analyze whether this choice is random or follows some predictable order. We hypothesize that path dependency plays a strong role here: legacies from past systems become incentives or constraints on design possibilities for new systems. In particular, we expect the size of the implicit pension debt (the present value of the pension obligations of the government to contributors under the old PAYG system) to play a pivotal role in determining the degree of funding and privatization that can be achieved by reforming countries, and our econometric results strongly support this expectation. Pension reform involves winners and losers. Governments that successfully reform must gain majority support and mitigate minority opposition through a variety of techniques that increase the number of winners, decrease the number of losers, and change people's perceptions about the category into which they fit. We hypothesize that the shape of the new pension system, in particular its public-private mix, depends in part on the fragmentation of power within the political system, which determines how many and which groups must be placated. The first section of the chapter examines quantitative evidence for this hypothesis, and the second section gives examples of many trade-offs that reformers have made to accommodate dissenting groups when political power is dispersed.

The Timing and Nature of the Pension Reform Package

In this section we assess the effects of several variables on the probability and nature of pension reform through econometric analysis. The size of the implicit pension debt is the most important explanatory variable, but several other variables also effect the outcome.

Dependent Variables

In this analysis we examine two dependent variables: (i) the probability that a country has undertaken a structural reform (PROB), and (ii) among those that have done so, the magnitude of expected benefits from the new funded, privately managed pillar relative to total benefits in the multipillar system (%PVT).

PROBABILITY OF STRUCTURAL REFORM (PROB)

The definition of the first dependent variable is fairly straightforward, and we use a probit to analyze it. We considered countries to have adopted a structural reform if the government has mandated the establishment of a privately managed, funded pillar through legislation or other official action or if it has changed the format of its PAYG pillar from DB to notional DC, in which benefits ultimately depend on contributions plus a shadow rate of interest imputed by the government.[1]

PRIVATE SECTOR SHARE (%PVT)

The second independent variable, %PVT, is somewhat more complex. The public-private division of responsibility is clearly a salient feature of new social security systems, but it is also a multidimensional concept, making quantification difficult. Basically, it is evident in terms of the inputs or outputs of the system, that is, in terms of the share of total contributions going to the private pillar or the share of total benefits that the private pillar is expected to generate. Unfortunately, the input or contribution going to the public pillar is often unknown: in some cases (for example, Australia and Chile), the public pillar is financed through general government revenues rather than an earmarked payroll tax, and in other cases (for example, Argentina and Poland), a single payroll tax covers the transition deficit stemming from the old system jointly with the ongoing costs of the public pillar in the new system. Therefore, we employ an output or benefit-based measure of "privateness" in the reformed pension schemes. In this measure we define %PVT as the proportion of the total expected benefit that derives from the private pillar.[2]

Nor are expected benefits, used in this chapter, easy to measure. To develop this variable, we simulate the benefits that a typical worker can expect to get in the long run from the public versus private pillars. For the public pillar benefit, we simply apply the stated rules or formula of the state-guaranteed pension, even though this guarantee is always subject to change in the future. This expected benefit will vary widely among workers. For example, in the case of a minimum pension guarantee, a high earner will get nothing from the state, since his or her private pillar benefit will exceed the minimum, while a low earner (and most women workers) will depend heavily on this guarantee. Similarly, in countries with flat benefits (uniform for all contributors), the public share of total benefits will be much higher for women and low-wage earners generally, while this is not true when the state benefit is positively related to earnings. We circumscribe this hetero-geneity problem by using the "average wage" worker in each country, according to the International Labour Organisation (ILO 1990, 1995, 1997) statistical compendium for 1995 urban manufacturing employment.[3]

The private pillar is more problematic to simulate because the expected benefit will depend on (i) the number and timing of years of payroll con-tributions, (ii) the rate of return to the invested funds, (iii) the rate of wage growth over working life, and (iv) the percentage of the payroll con-tributed. Consider, for example, a 10 percent contribution rate to the pri-vate pillar that is projected to yield a 40 percent replacement rate of final wage. A 1 percentage point increase in the contribution rate will increase the private benefit by 10 percent, or 4 percentage points, while an increase of 1 percentage point in the annual rate of return will increase the benefit by 20 percent, or 8 percentage points. Although the contribution rate is determined by law in each country, the remaining variables must be assumed, and the results of our simulations are highly dependent on these assumptions. In our base case we made fairly standard assumptions: (i) 35 years of payroll contributions, (ii) 4.5 percent rate of return on invest-ments, and (iii) 2 percent yearly growth in wages. In this analysis we make uniform assumptions about these variables across countries (unless the gov-ernment has dictated specific interest rates), but in the real world differences in growth rates, interest rates and average contributory years across coun-tries will also lead to differences in their total benefits and the private share.[4]

Table 4.1 and figure 4.2 display the results of the simulation for the pub-lic and private benefits and %PVT for the "average" worker in each reform-ing country. The private share varies from 0 percent in Latvia and Italy to 100 percent in Chile and El Salvador. Most OECD countries are in the mid-dle. It is clear that significant variations exist in the anticipated role for state versus market mechanisms in the provision of future pension benefits. We explore whether these differences are random or follow some systematic pattern.

Table 4.1. Characteristics of Pension System for Average Worker after Structural Reform
(percent)

Country	First pillar	Second pillar	Total benefit	% Private
Argentina	33	34	67	51
Australia	25	33	58	57
Bolivia	4	42	46	92
Chile	0	42	42	100
Colombia	0	42	42	100
Denmark	28	34	62	56
El Salvador	0	42	42	100
Hungary	43	27	70	39
Italy	81	0	81	0
Kazakhstan	0	38	38	100
Latvia	49	0	49	0
Mexico	3	27	30	91
Netherlands	35	35	70	50
Peru	0	42	42	100
Poland	26	25	51	49
Sweden	35	10	45	21
Switzerland	30	30	60	50
United Kingdom	17	17	34	49
Uruguay	38	25	62	40

Sources: Various reports on each system and simulations described in text.

Independent Variables and Hypotheses about Their Impact

Our major hypothesis concerns the impact of the implicit pension debt (IPD) on PROB and %PVT. For reasons given below, we hypothesize that a large IPD increases the probability or speed of a major reform but decreases the %PVT that will eventually emerge. Other variables may have smaller effects.

IMPLICIT PENSION DEBT

The term "implicit pension debt" has, unfortunately, been used to mean several different things (see Van der Noord and Herd 1994), such as:

> *The stock of obligations accrued to date* (also known as *the termination hypothesis*)—the present value of the accrued rights that current workers have in the old system at the present time
> *Closed system flows*—the present value of the future cash flow deficit, taking into account all future benefits and contributions of current affiliates

Figure 4.2. Public-Private Mix of Pension Benefits

Replacement Rate for Average Worker

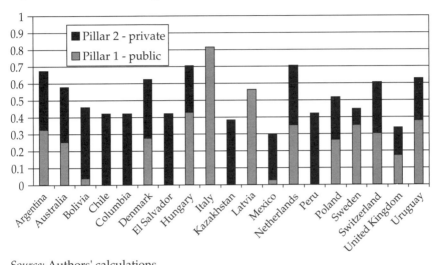

Source: Authors' calculations.

- *Open system flows*—the present value of the future cash flow deficit, taking into account all benefits and contributions of current and future affiliates, up to some specified date.

Each of these concepts has different uses. For our purposes, the first concept is most relevant, since it informs us of the obligations of the old system that remain and must somehow be financed when a country makes a transition from a PAYG public system to a new system with a privately managed, funded pillar. Additionally, the first IPD concept is the one most analogous to the explicit debt that is matched by bonds, which reveals how much the government owes today. By construction, it will be larger in countries with mature systems, older populations, a high level of coverage, and generous benefits. We measure it as a proportion of gross domestic product (GDP).

When part of the old contribution is put into the funded pillar, governments face the "transition cost problem." They must continue to meet their existing obligations by raising contribution rates or other taxes or by issuing bonds, thereby converting the implicit debt to explicit debt. Each of these options, however, has disadvantages. Higher taxes or "contributions" are always unpopular, and the governing party may fear that increasing them will have political costs. At the same time, the government may not want to increase the explicit debt, which is more transparent and readily measured than the implicit debt. Policymakers may fear that a large explicit debt will lower their credit rating or upset financial markets. Some governments face debt limits that are imposed either by their own rules or by external actors such as the International Monetary Fund (IMF) or the European Monetary Union. Furthermore, an explicit debt will raise the government's interest costs. Finally, pure debt finance means that pension reform will not have the positive impact on national saving that is often sought by reformers. These considerations set economic and political limits to the feasible amount of debt financing of structural reform, even though the conversion of implicit to explicit debt does not increase the total public debt.

These constraints on financing a pension transition suggest that a large IPD might have somewhat different effects on the probability and the nature of reform. On the one hand, it may bring social security to the forefront of the political agenda, thereby increasing the probability of undertaking a major reform. On the other hand, once governments have decided to tackle the problem via structural reform, the transition cost problem stemming from a large IPD will dominate and lead to a less aggressive reform. We expect that when governments with a large IPD confront the practical difficulties of financing the reform via debt or taxes, they will choose a small %PVT in order to reduce their short-run cash flow problem by keeping more money flowing into the public PAYG pillar.[5]

Beyond this purely financial argument, a high IPD may also be a proxy for other kinds of path dependencies such as public pressure to retain acquired rights under the old scheme or the strength of an entrenched social security bureaucracy that will resist reform. A high IPD means many pensioners and older workers expect to receive large benefits under the old system and fear that radical change may lead to loss of support for keeping these promises. Social security bureaucracies that managed the old public system may have accumulated power through their monopolistic handling of large sums of money and the employment of large numbers of workers. They are likely to oppose reforms that strip them of this power. The same may be true, in some cases, of labor unions that participated in the administration of public social security systems. This political challenge from older workers and entrenched bureaucrats, proxied by the magnitude of the IPD, strengthens our hypothesis that the outcome for countries with a large IPD will be a less radical reform, or a smaller %PVT.

The next problem concerns the measurement of the IPD. In some cases direct estimates are available, as a result of studies done during the reform process and for other policy reasons (Van der Noord and Herd 1994; Kane and Palacios 1996). For countries for which a precise measure of the IPD is unavailable, we imputed it. Because this variable plays an important role in our analysis, we imputed it in two ways, based on current public pension spending and on the age distribution of the population, to ensure that our results were not sensitive to the imputation method.

In the spending-based method, we regressed IPD on public pension spending (as a percentage of GDP) for the set of known countries and used the coefficients of this equation to impute the IPD of the countries for which we do not have direct observations.[6] Current pension spending is not a precise predictor of total obligations, especially for immature systems with few eligible retirees, but the fit is quite good—our equation explained 78 percent of the variance in IPD. However, this method of imputing IPD might introduce an omitted variable problem: a high level of current pension spending might be correlated with a "taste" for a large public sector, so if IPD leads to a small %PVT, we don't know whether this is due to the IPD per se or to the preferences with which it is correlated. To address this problem we added to the equation a second variable—total government spending on goods and services as a percentage of GDP (GOV), designed to control for taste for public spending. We also used a second method to impute IPD that is more exogenous and less correlated with omitted variables.

One of the major determinants of the IPD is the age distribution of the population. An older population corresponds to more pensioners and workers near retirement and a greater present value of their accrued pension rights. Therefore, as a second method, we regressed IPD on the percentage of the population over age 60 for the set of known countries and imputed IPD for the others based on this equation. Because this measure does not take account of generosity of benefits, it explains only 68 percent of the variance in IPD, slightly less than the previous method. This age-based method has the advantage that it avoids the omitted variable problem discussed above. However, it has the potential disadvantage of introducing a new omitted variable—political pressure coming from older workers and pensioners to retain the current system, which may be correlated with our age-based imputed IPD. This is not really a problem for us, as we interpret a high IPD as operating, in part, through these generational pressures. As we shall see below, most of our results are robust to the choice of imputation method.

GOVERNMENT SPENDING (GOV)

Although economists generally assume uniform tastes, it is possible that some societies have a preference for or political ideology in favor of more public sector intervention in the economy that would also influence the nature of their social security systems. To test this hypothesis, we introduced into the equation government spending on goods and services as a percentage of GDP (GOV), expecting that it might signal such social preferences and, therefore, lead to a smaller %PVT as well as a smaller probability of structural reform.

Explicit Debt (DEBT)

From an economic point of view, the implicit and explicit debt are largely interchangeable (except that legally it may be easier to renege on the implicit debt, which may, therefore, already be discounted). From a political viewpoint, they may be quite different, since the explicit debt is much more transparent than the implicit debt. For many governments the level of explicit public debt is an important factor shaping the choice of policy designs, and international organizations such as the IMF reinforce this predisposition. We, therefore, include DEBT, the explicit debt as a proportion of GDP, in our analysis.

A large explicit debt may make officials in the Ministry of Finance keenly aware of the need for a pension reform that reduces the government's future fiscal obligation. Additionally, the creation of a funded pillar may raise the domestic savings available to hold the national debt on a long-term basis, thereby reducing its reliance on foreign creditors and short-term loans. For example, policymakers in Mexico claimed this was an important motivating factor. At the same time, high levels of debt may become an obstacle to structural reform because of the difficulties in increasing the debt still further to cover the short-run transitional costs of reform. The net impact of explicit public debt on the probability of structural reform is therefore unclear.[7]

The impact on %PVT is similarly ambiguous. On the one hand, high levels of public debt may diminish the %PVT among the reforming countries because of their need to avoid the appearance that they are not creditworthy and to stay within any externally or internally imposed debt ceiling (Brooks 1999; Maxfield 1997). On the other hand, if they expect that creditors will react favorably to radical pension reform as a sign of fiscal responsibility, this effect may be reversed.

Level of Domestic Savings (SAVINGS)

Among the perceived macroeconomic benefits of structural reform are those relating to an enhanced level of domestic savings. Policymakers plagued by low levels of capital accumulation have been attracted by the potential to increase national saving and develop local capital markets through the creation of funded components to their pension systems (Brooks 1999). Also attractive is the possibility of creating a "loyal" source of savings that is committed for the long term, is not subject to capital flight, permits longer maturities on public debt, and reduces dependence on foreign capital. While the theoretical arguments continue on the link between pension reform and aggregate savings, the growth of private savings and financial markets in Chile has been attributed, in part, to its pension reform.[8] We expect that the lower the level of domestic savings as a percentage of GDP (SAVINGS), the greater the value of these potential macroeconomic effects of funding and the more likely a country is to implement a multip-illar pension reform.[9]

The expected impact of a low level of domestic savings on the %PVT is less clear. On the one hand, the desire for more national saving might lead reforming governments to design a scheme with a high %PVT. On the other hand, for countries with little initial saving, partial debt financing of the transition costs of extensive reform might use up much of the available sav-ings, and a low level of savings may signal a high discount rate. As a result, they may choose a pension reform with a lower %PVT. Overall, the expected impact of domestic savings levels on the %PVT in reformed pen-sion schemes is ambiguous.

EFFECTIVE NUMBER OF POLITICAL PARTIES (PARTIES)

Most of the preceding variables have a substantial economic interpretation, albeit with political overtones. We now consider a purely political variable, the degree of concentration of political power, as evidenced by the num-ber of political parties in the country.

Political parties provide the principal means for the articulation of dif-ferentiated interests in a government. These solve collective action prob-lems among politicians and structure the legislative process along distinct partisan dimensions (Cox and McCubbins 1993). The structure of a politi-cal party system, particularly the number of parties it contains, affects the range of interests represented in the reform process and, as a result, the extent of bargaining necessary to build a legislative majority (Sartori 1976).

Multipartism is widely associated with the inclusion of a broad range of interests, including potential "losers," into the reform decision. The extreme version of multipartism, the highly fragmented party system, is associated with unstable political coalitions, credibility problems, and unreliable "veto partners" in reforming governments (Haggard and Kaufman 1992). Accordingly, political theorists have argued that the pro-liferation of political parties in the legislative arena will impede radical reforms. As the effective number of political parties increases, the capaci-ty of the governing party to push through difficult reforms decreases (Shugart and Haggard 1997). The governing party will not always want a radical reform, but if it does, greater dispersion of political power may enable entrenched interests to block reform (Immergut 1992; Tsebelis 1990). We hypothesize that the governing party may be unable to undertake a structural pension reform in the presence of a highly fragmented legisla-tive arena. Where structural reforms are implemented, we expect that frag-mentation requires more extensive negotiations to pass the reform, result-ing in a more moderate design with a smaller %PVT.

Although it is a very rough measure of the dispersion of interests rep-resented in the political process, we use the "effective number of parties" to measure the degree of legislative fragmentation. This variable is measured by $N = 1/\sum p_i^2$, where p_i is the share of seats occupied by the ith party represented in the lower house of the legislature (Laakso and Taagepera 1979; Taagepera and Shugart 1989).[10]

PREEXISTING FUNDED PLANS (PREPLAN)

We hypothesize that the existing institutional structures of pension provision have important effects on the likelihood and success of structural pension reforms. In several OECD countries, large, privately managed, funded pension plans linked to occupational structures existed on a quasi-voluntary, collectively bargained basis even before the issue of mandatory funded plans arose (Ebbinhaus 1998). In many such countries, the mandatory funded second pillar came into being when the government made these plans mandatory for everyone. This was the case with Australia and Switzerland. We expect that the prior existence of funded occupational pension schemes (as represented by a dummy PREPLAN) increases the probability of structural reform because it implies lower transition costs and the existence of political constituencies that favor funded systems (financial institutions that will benefit from managing the funds). For similar reasons it may lead to a higher %PVT, although this is less clear. This is because employers are part of the political negotiation about these employer-sponsored plans, and they may be willing to provide "some" benefits but not "most" benefits.

SPANISH

One of the issues with which we are concerned is the diffusion of new reform ideas. Countries learn about reform ideas and how they work in other countries (the demonstration effect) by media communication, movement of people, and commerce. We would expect that linguistic and geographic proximity would facilitate this learning process. In 1981 Chile was the first country to adopt the multipillar system. We therefore use a dummy for "Spanish as the dominant language" as our simple proxy for speed of diffusion.

OTHER VARIABLES

A variety of other variables undoubtedly help to explain the reform decision in any particular case. For instance, alternative funding sources, such as the preexisting treasury surplus in the case of Chile or privatization assets in Bolivia, may facilitate the adoption of structural reform. Similarly, a total breakdown of the old system (as manifested in high evasion and arrears rates, an effective retirement age that is much lower than the legal age, large system deficits, and government defaults on benefit payments) is likely to facilitate structural reform insofar as it diminishes both the credibility and option of reverting to the old system. In contrast, strong pensioners' organizations or labor unions may impede reform, since these groups may fear that their benefits will be cut in the process (Pierson 1996). Given our small sample size, however, along with the difficulty in obtaining consistent data on these variables for all countries, it is impossible to include all of them in the regression analysis. The second section of the chapter, which discusses key strategies employed by reforming governments to overcome resistance from powerful interest groups, analyzes several of these factors.

Descriptive Statistics

Table 4.2 presents data on the mean values of the main independent variables for three groups of countries: 19 reformers, 44 nonreformers in their regions, and 86 nonreformers around the world. Most striking is the

Table 4.2. Means of Independent Variables for Reformers and Nonreformers

	IPD (spending)	IPD (age-based)	PREPLAN	SPANISH	DEBT	SAVING	GOV	PARTIES
Worldwide (N = 86) non-reformers	87.4	90.8	0.02	0.1	82.4	15.9	15.9	—
Regional (N = 45) non-reformers	121.8	127.2	0.04	0.2	64.4	18.4	16.3	3.9
Reformers (N = 19)	138.8	133.9	0.26	0.4	45.1	19.1	14.9	3.3

Note: IPD is the implicit pension debt, or present value of government liabilities for pension benefits to current pensioners and accrued rights of current workers. This is calculated as a percentage of GDP. PREPLAN is a dichotomous variable coded 1 for the existence of large occupational funded pension system: Australia, Canada, Denmark, Netherlands, Switzerland, United Kingdom, and United States, 0 for all others. SPANISH is a dichotomous variable coded 1 for predominantly Spanish-speaking countries, 0 for all others. DEBT is Central Government Debt, average for years 1990–95, except Chile: 1980. SAVINGS is Gross National Savings (percent of GDP), equal to the gross domestic savings plus net income and net current transfers from abroad. GOV is general government consumption (percentage of GDP), including all current expenditures for all levels of government and excluding most government enterprises. It also includes capital expenditure on national defense and security. PARTIES is a measure of political fragmentation, defined in the text. It is not available for several countries outside the reforming regions, so is excluded from the analyses of worldwide reformers. The Regional set includes regions in which structural pension reform has occurred: Latin America, OECD countries, and the former Soviet Union. The worldwide set includes these plus a sample from Africa and Asia. Sources: IPD for France, Italy, Germany, Japan, Canada, U.K., U.S.: Van den Noord and Herd (1993); IPD for other countries: Kane and Palacios (1996) and authors' calculations; PREPLAN and SPANISH: authors' calculations; DEBT: Global Development Finance (1998) and OECD Government Statistics; SAVINGS and GOV: World Development Indicators (1999); PARTIES: Political Handbook of the World and Parline Legislative Database Worldwide Elections.

increase in the IPD as we move from the worldwide nonreformers to regional nonreformers to reformers (87 percent, 122 percent, and 139 percent of GDP, respectively, when IPD is imputed according to public pension spending; 91 percent, 127 percent, and 134 percent when using an age-based imputation). This is consistent with the expectation that a high IPD "puts pension reform on the agenda," both for individual countries and regionally. Interestingly, an opposite effect is seen for DEBT, which falls from 82 percent and 64 percent to 45 percent of GDP as we move from nonreformers to reformers. This suggests that the transparency of the explicit debt and its use as a measure of creditworthiness may inhibit reforms that will further raise the explicit debt in highly indebted countries. PREPLAN is much higher among the reformers (0.26 versus 0.04 and 0.02) as is the dominance of the Spanish language (0.4 versus 0.2 and 0.1). All of these means values are consistent with our predictions. There is relatively little difference in SAVINGS, PARTIES, or GOV among the reformers and nonreformers. Interestingly, the worldwide nonreformers are most dissimilar from the reformers, with the regional nonreformers in between, suggesting that regional effects may be at work, and other countries within the region are likely to reform before those outside do.

Preliminary Results: Rank Order Correlation between IPD and Public-Private Pillars

As a simplified measure of the relationship between IPD and %PVT, we ranked all reforming countries by their IPDs and compared this with the rank order of their %PVT as well as the type of public pillar in the new system (table 4.3; James 1998b). We classified countries into three groups, according to their %PVT, as shown in table 4.1. The first category has a %PVT of less than 90 percent, and its public pillar usually consists of a modest minimum pension guarantee. The second category has a %PVT between 45 and 60 percent; most of these countries offer a universal or means-tested flat public benefit that is medium in size and is often financed by general revenues. The third category includes those systems whose %PVT is 40 percent or less and whose public benefits are large, positively related to earnings and financed by a payroll tax.[11] We observe a very close inverse rank order correlation between size of the IPD and %PVT.

However, these simple descriptive statistics and rank order correlations do not have the explanatory power of multiple regression analysis, which considers all the explanatory variables simultaneously and treats %PVT as a continuous variable. We proceed now to that analysis.

Econometric Methodology

We carried out two sets of analyses to estimate (i) the likelihood of structural reform and (ii) the degree of privatization in the subset of reformers.

Table 4.3. Implicit Pension Debt (IPD) and Pension Reform

Country	Age-IPD as % of GDP	Spending-IPD as % of GDP	% PVT	Type public pillar
Peru[a]	37	37	HI	—
Bolivia	45	65	HI	F
El Salvador	47	34	HI	MPG
Mexico	48	43	HI	MPG
Colombia	51	44	HI	MPG
Chile	79	112	HI	MPG
Kazakhstan	88	102	HI	MPG
United Kingdom[a, b]	118	118	MED	F
Argentina	125	100	MED	F
Poland	142	241	MED	ER
Australia[b]	145	96	MED	F(MT)
Netherlands[b]	174	198	MED	F
Latvia	175	179	LO	ER
Switzerland[b]	195	215	MED	F(ER)
Denmark[b]	198	170	MED	F
Italy[a]	203	203	LO	ER
Hungary[a]	213	213	LO	ER
Uruguay[a]	214	214	LO	ER
Sweden	226	197	LO	ER

— Peru has not yet implemented a first pillar but will probably have an MPG.
Note: Types of public pillars: MPG = minimum pension guarantee, financed out of general revenues; F = flat (often supplemented with means-tested benefits), financed out of general revenues or payroll tax; F(MT) = flat with eligibility determined by means test; ER = earnings-related, financed out of payroll tax; F(ER) = ER with flat structure (maximum close to minimum). In Bolivia privatization revenues finance flat benefit until these assets are exhausted; shape of first pillar thereafter is unknown.
a. Indicates use of actual IPD, calculated by the following sources: Hungary, Uruguay, and Peru from Kane and Palacios (1996); United Kingdom and Italy from Van Den Noord and Herd (1993). Other countries use spending-based IPD simulated by authors based on current public expenditure (World Bank 1994). Age-based IPD simulated by authors based on 1990 population over age 60 (World Bank 1994). IPD is present value of accrued rights of pensioners and workers, under old system. %PVT is taken from table 1 according to the following groups:
HI = > 90%; MED = 49–60%; LO = 40% or less.
b. Indicates PREPLAN countries.

The first is a probit analysis that estimates the likelihood of a structural reform among two samples of countries: 64 countries from Latin America, Europe, OECD, and the former Soviet Union (the regions from which the reformers came) and 105 countries that added observations from Asia and Africa (all the countries for which we could get the relevant data). We used two samples because we conjectured that regional fixed effects might be at work, that the political economy of reform might be different in Asian and African countries where coverage is low and confined mainly to civil servants, and employees of large enterprises, many of which are state owned. Additionally, we did not have data on PARTIES for the larger sample but wanted to test robustness to sample size for the other variables. As discussed above, we used two alternative methods for imputing one important explanatory variable, %PVT.

The second analysis is an ordinary least squares regression predicting %PVT in the 19 reforming countries included in the analysis. This is admittedly a small sample, driven by the fact that only a small number of countries have thus far undertaken structural reforms. It will be important to rerun these regressions in subsequent years, as the number of reformers grows.

Since some variables used to explain the probability of structural reform are likewise expected to affect %PVT, there is a possibility of bias in the results, owing to covariation in the error terms of these equations. In view of this possibility, we tested for selection bias using a Heckman two-stage selection model, and found no evidence of such bias. We therefore present the results for these equations separately below. The mean values for all variables are presented in table 4.2, the OLS results in table 4.4, and the probit results in table 4.5.

Results: OLS Analysis of %PVT

Our strongest result concerns the determination of %PVT among countries that have undergone structural reform (table 4.4). Recall that %PVT in these countries ranges from 0 percent in Italy and Latvia to 100 percent in Kazakhstan and Peru. Our regressions explain 84 percent of the variance. Clearly, systematic forces are at work, and the nature of reform is not random.

Most striking in explaining these variations is the strong impact of the IPD, which is almost always significant at the 0.1 percent level, whether the spending-based or the age-based imputation methods are used. When IPD is the only explanatory variable in the model, a change from an IPD of 50 to 100 percent of GDP decreases the degree of private provision by 20 percentage points. This is consistent with our predictions and with the simplified picture presented in table 4.3. The close negative relationship between IPD and %PVT is illustrated in figures 4.3a and 4.3b. Choices made about social security in the past limit (but do not completely determine) the feasible set for the future. This is probably our strongest econometric result.

Also of interest is the fact that PREPLAN and PARTIES show up as significant when the age-based imputation is used but not with the spending-based imputation. This suggests that current pension spending already incorporates some of the effects of these institutional variables, thereby hiding their independent effects. It is possible that the existence of more

Table 4.4. Ordinary Least Squares, Predicting Percentage Private

(N=19)	IPD based on public pension spending							
	1		2		3		4	
	Coeff.	t	Coeff.	t	Coeff.	t	Coeff.	t
IPD	−0.004	−5.75a	−0.003	−4.28a	−0.003	−3.23a	−0.002	−2.05c
Preplan	—	—	—	—	0.07	0.61	0.12	0.89
Spanish	—	—	—	—	—	—	0.03	0.16
Gov	—	—	−0.01	−1.59	0.02	−1.56	−0.02	−1.47
Debt	—	—	—	—	—	—	0.001	0.41
Savings	—	—	—	—	—	—	−0.01	−0.8
Parties	—	—	—	—	−0.04	−1.39	−0.04	−1.26
Const.	1.1	11.20a	1.24	9.66a	1.31	9.65a	1.37	4.13a
Adjusted R-sq	0.64		0.67		0.68		0.63	
	IPD based on population > age 60							
IPD	−0.004	−7.10a	−0.005	−4.93a	−0.005	−5.93a	−0.005	−4.59a
Preplan	—	—	—	—	0.22	2.78b	0.23	2.51b
Spanish	—	—	—	—	—	—	−0.08	−0.7
Gov	—	—	0.004	0.39	0.001	0.2	−0.001	−0.09
Debt	—	—	—	—	—	—	0.0004	0.24
Savings	—	—	—	—	—	—	−0.01	−1.23
Parties	—	—	—	—	−0.05	−2.13b	−0.05	−2.06c
Const.	1.2	12.90a	1.17	10.08a	1.3	13.6a	1.52	6.55a
Adjusted R-sq	0.73		0.72		0.84		0.82	

— Not included in calculations.
Note: Percentage private is expressed as a decimal. a - Significant at .1 percent level; b - Significant at 5 percent level; c - Significant at 10 percent level.
Source: Authors' calculations.

Table 4.5. Probit, Predicting Probability of Structural Pension Reform

N = 64: Latin America, OECD, and Former Soviet Union

(N = 19)	IPD based on public pension spending				IPD based on population over age 60			
	1		2		3		4	
	Coeff.	t	Coeff.	t	Coeff.	t	Coeff.	t
IPD	0.01	2.04b	0.01	2.81a	0.01	1.58	0.01	2.05b
Preplan	1.17	2.97a	2.20	3.11a	1.49	2.61a	1.56	2.60b
Spanish	1.14	3.03a	1.51	2.81a	1.56	2.77a	1.60	2.75a
Gov	—	—	−0.09	−1.73	—	—	−0.06	−1.23
Debt	—	—	−0.01	−0.82	—	—	−0.004	−0.69
Savings	—	—	−0.02	−0.75	—	—	−0.01	−0.37
Parties	—	—	−0.13	−1.02	—	—	−0.08	−0.70
Const.	−2.07	−3.49a	−0.40	−0.45	−2.10	−2.84a	−1.01	−1.10
Log-likelihood	−30.60		−26.84		−31.49		−29.41	
	N = 105: Latin America, OECD, Former Soviet Union, Africa, and Asia							
IPD	0.01	3.15a	0.01	3.18a	0.01	2.81a	0.01	2.71a
Preplan	2.00	3.38a	2.39	3.47a	1.56	2.73a	1.67	2.81a
Spanish	1.69	3.92a	1.60	3.27a	1.88	3.89a	1.80	3.45a
Gov	—	—	−0.08	−1.61	—	—	−0.05	−1.09
Debt	—	—	−0.01	−0.90	—	—	−0.01	−0.79
Savings	—	—	−0.02	−0.71	—	—	−0.01	−0.40
Const.	−2.61	−5.26a	−1.21	−1.46	−2.76	−4.67	−1.82	−2.15b
Adjusted R-sq	−32.45		−29.58		−33.37		0.82	

— Not included in calculations.
a - Significant at .1 percent level; b - Significant at 5 percent level.
Source: Authors' calculations.

Figure 4.3a. Relationship between Spending-Based IPD and Private Share of Benefits in Reformed Pension Systems

Percent private

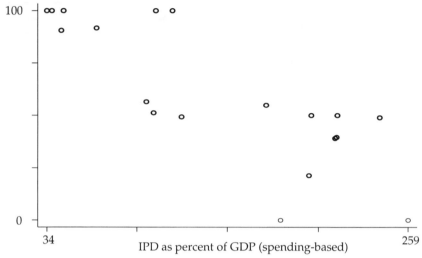

IPD as percent of GDP (spending-based)

Source: Authors' calculations.

Figure 4.3b. Relationship between Age-Based IPD and Private Share of Benefits in Reformed Pension Systems

Percent private

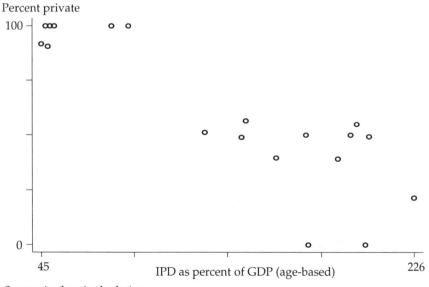

IPD as percent of GDP (age-based)

Source: Authors' calculations.

voluntary funded schemes implies smaller public pension spending, and that more fragmented political parties lead to greater public pension spending ex ante. Thus, when the spending-based imputation method is used, PREPLAN and PARTIES are negatively and positively correlated with IPD, respectively, and the IPD picks up their effects. When the uncorrelated age-based imputation method is used, we find that PREPLAN has a strong independent positive impact, increasing %PVT by 22 percentage points, while fragmented PARTIES decreases %PVT, as predicted. Moreover, both variables affect other features of the reform: in PREPLAN countries the new schemes have been built along occupational group choice lines rather than the individual choice that dominates in countries without powerful preexisting private pension plans. In countries with fragmented political systems, much of the bargaining has been about issues of distributional concern to specific groups, as discussed in the second section.

None of the other variables in the regression is significant in the OLS equation predicting %PVT, whether taken singly or as a group. Despite its possible proxying for "taste for public spending," GOV is never significant, nor does it change the significance of IPD. Anecdotal evidence about the importance of SAVINGS and DEBT is not borne out statistically. Although the implicit and explicit debt are largely interchangeable economically, clearly they have different political effects.

Results: Probability of Structural Reform (PROB)

We find quite a different pattern of explanatory factors in the probit analysis determining the probability of reform (table 4.5). Table 4.6a translates these probit results into reform probabilities. The probabilities are all much higher in the regional sample, consistent with the fact that these are the regions that contain the reformers. But the pattern of significance is quite similar for the regional and global samples and the two imputation methods, so we discuss them all simultaneously. Table 4.7 presents some evidence on the accuracy of our predictions. Overall, we predict the reform–no reform decision accurately for more than 80 percent of the countries. However, it is clear that we are less successful in predicting reform probability or timing than we are in predicting %PVT. In particular, the actual proportion that reformed consistently exceeds our predictions.

The significantly positive effect of IPD on PROB is consistent with the agenda-setting theory of IPD and with the descriptive statistics in table 4.2. An increase in IPD from 50 to 100 percent of GDP doubles the probability of structural reform, and a further increase from 100 percent to 200 percent doubles it again (table 4.6b). The two increases together raise the probability of reform more than 30 percentage points.

DEBT and SAVINGS have no significant impact here, as was the case in predicting %PVT. Nor does the fractionalization of political PARTIES—in

Table 4.6a. Impact of IPD on Probability of Reform

	IPD = mean value	IPD = 50	IPD = 100	IPD = 200
Sample size = 64				
Age-based IPD	0.260	0.118	0.200	0.438
Spending-based IPD	0.252	0.121	0.199	0.425
Sample size = 105				
Age-based IPD	0.096	0.036	0.098	0.395
Spending-based IPD	0.095	0.042	0.101	0.350

Note: The predictions hold PREPLAN and SPANISH constant at their means.
Source: Authors' calculations.

Table 4.6b. Impact of PREPLAN and SPANISH on Probability of Reform

	Preplan = 1	Preplan = 0	Spanish = 1	Spanish = 0
Sample size = 64				
Age-based IPD	0.753	0.210	0.692	0.145
Spending-based IPD	0.818	0.194	0.652	0.147
Sample size = 105				
Age-based IPD	0.561	0.079	0.591	0.050
Spending-based IPD	0.711	0.075	0.529	0.053

Note: The predictions use the partial model, with IPD, PREPLAN, and SPANISH only. All variables are held constant at their means except for the one being varied.
Source: Authors' calculations.

contrast to theory and evidence from the literature on macroeconomic reform. Possibly this is because the numerous variations in the details of sectoral reforms discussed in the second section mute the effects of resistance resulting from fractionalized parties. At the same time, these three variables taken as a group increase the log likelihood and the accuracy of our predictions to a small extent.

Perhaps most interesting is the consistently strong impact of PREPLAN and SPANISH on the probability of reform. In both samples and all specifications, these are significant at the 1 percent level, and each increases the probability of reform by over 50 percentage points (note that none of the countries are both PREPLAN and SPANISH). Two-thirds of the reforming countries were either PREPLAN or SPANISH, while this is true of only 25 percent of the nonreformers in the regional sample and 12 percent in the

Table 4.7. Predicted versus Actual Reform

N = 64: regional	Spending-based IPD – predictions		Age-based IPD – predictions	
Actual	Reform	No reform	Reform	No reform
Reform	10	9	10	9
No reform	4	41	3	42
% of predictions correct	80		81	
N = 105: global				
Actual	Reform	No reform	Reform	No reform
Reform	8	11	8	11
No reform	4	82	2	84
% of predictions correct	86		88	

Note: These predictions are based on the full model. The partial model (with IPD, PRE-PLAN, and SPANISH only) yielded similar results but with slightly less accuracy.
Source: Authors' calculations.

global sample. The influence of PREPLAN is additional evidence of the path dependency of reforms; the existence of voluntary private funded plans in many OECD countries made it easier for them to extend this model by mandating it.

The influence of Spanish is particularly interesting, as it throws light on how reform ideas diffuse across countries. We may not be able to predict "first movers"—why was Chile the first to implement a multipillar reform? This may have been a random event resulting from the conjunction of fertile economic conditions and a receptive powerful political regime. But once a first move has occurred, other countries may learn from it about possibilities and impacts via a demonstration effect. Successful reform in one country increases the perceived probability of success and, therefore, decreases the perceived political and economic costs of reform in other countries. Countries are likely to learn more quickly from others that are linked by geographic, linguistic, or commercial proximity. Thus it appears to be no accident that the majority of Spanish-speaking, Latin American countries have reformed, that non-Spanish-speaking Latin countries have been slower to reform, that most reforming countries with a low IPD were in Latin America and that structural reform in other regions has been far less prevalent.

At the same time, structural reform has not been limited to Spanish-speaking countries; in fact, the majority of reformers are not Spanish-speaking. Since the publication of *Averting the Old Age Crisis* (World Bank 1994), the World Bank's analysis of global social security problems, the World Bank and other international organizations have accelerated the diffusion of ideas via conferences, technical assistance, and study tours. This diffusion process may help explain why actual reformers exceed predicted reformers, and why the transition economies in Eastern Europe are now reforming (and adopting the Chilean model) even though they are not Spanish-speaking and did not have large preexisting private pension plans.

Strategies for Overcoming Opposition to Structural Reform

In the first section we saw that our capacity to explain the shape of structural pension reform, particularly its public-private mix, is much greater than our capacity to predict whether any structural reform will actually take place. While concerns about a growing IPD may put reform on the political agenda in a country and reform innovations may diffuse from culturally proximate countries and through supportive institutions, a large random term remains in determining exactly where these innovations will be implemented. This random term may subsume factors such as the commitment of key policymakers and their skill in building coalitions favoring reform.

Pension reform and other social sector reforms are more complicated politically than "first generation" structural adjustment reforms, both in terms of the political processes required for passage and the conditions needed for long-term success (Nelson 1997). Whereas structural adjustment reforms could be designed by insulated technicians, implemented through executive decree, and rarely target particular groups, social sector reforms directly affect the interests and eventually require the active participation of consumers and producers as well as approval by an elected legislature. These groups are likely to have strong views that policymakers must take into account. Through persuasion, negotiation, trade-offs, compensation, and subtle reshaping of the reform, a majority of stakeholders must be convinced that they will come out ahead, especially in a democracy. But even Chile, which was not a democracy at the time of passage, followed many of the strategies described below in order to gain popular support. Some politicians will be more adept at this process than others, which results in the large random term in the probit analysis discussed earlier.[12]

Generational Politics

Many of the expected benefits of structural reform (for example, sustainability, positive impact on long-term saving, reduced evasion and labor informality, and improved economic competitiveness) are long run benefits and therefore inherently uncertain. If they do materialize, the major beneficiaries will be the younger generation—those under age 40—who will have an opportunity to build up substantial rights in the funded pillar and whose benefits from the existing system are in jeopardy. The young are often in favor of reform for these reasons, and we have seen that reforming countries with a predominantly young population, and correspondingly low IPD, are more likely to end up with a large %PVT. But even the young face considerable uncertainty about the outcome. Although the expected long-run return may be positive, risk is inherent in DC systems, in which pensions ultimately depend on volatile investment earnings. Moreover, this group is difficult to mobilize on pension reform issues, since retirement is many years away and they have more pressing concerns such as finding jobs and raising families.

In contrast, pension reform is a salient issue to older workers, and the most crucial issue to retirees. In some cases, most notably Uruguay, politically potent pensioners' organizations have formed around this issue. In most countries pensioners have the highest voting rates and considerable time to invest in political activity. They often see little perceived gain but potential real cost to them from the reform. They may fear that the privatization of part of the social security system will undermine political support for the public benefits upon which they depend—the "generational compact" will have been broken. If taxes are raised to help finance the transition, they may have to pay part of the taxes without reaping the benefits.

To some degree, then, pension politics is generational politics—the interests of the young versus the old. But more basically, both groups need to be won over. Policymakers who want to enact structural reform must convince the young that they will benefit despite the risk, and they must neutralize the opposition of the older generations by promising that they will not be hurt. This process explains some of the common features found in pension reforms, such as the use of debt finance and the promise of second pillar guarantees.

PENSIONERS AND OLDER WORKERS

Almost universally, pension reforms have protected the rights of older workers and retirees. In most cases older workers (over the age of 50), who will have few years in which to build up individual accounts and who might feel threatened by the uncertainty inherent in financial markets, have been exempted from the new system or strongly encouraged to stay in the old system, and their old-system benefits have been assured. The challenge is to make these promises of protection credible, most convincingly through granting immediate gains, such as the payment of pension arrears (Kazakhstan) or improved public pillar benefits and indexation (Hungary). We saw earlier that countries with many older workers and pensioners (and a large resulting IPD) are likely to retain a large public pillar, thereby demonstrating that contributions will continue to flow in to pay existing pensioners. In almost every case governments have used partial debt financing for the transition, thereby absolving pensioners of the costs and largely passing them on to younger generations that will also gain the most. When tax financing has been used, the largest component has often been the payroll tax, which again absolves pensioners of the cost.

YOUNGER WORKERS

At the same time, governments have taken measures in every case to allay the fears younger workers might have about risk regarding their DC plans in the second pillar. These often involve elaborate guarantees by the state, the employer, or the pension fund. In Hungary the state guarantees that the second pillar will pay at least 25 percent of the first pillar benefit. This protects workers from downside risk and allows them to reap the full potential benefits of high returns. In Switzerland employers choose the investment manager and must guarantee a minimum nominal rate of return of 4 percent over the worker's tenure with them. The state-run fund that has attracted most affiliates in Uruguay guarantees at least a 2 percent real rate of return on all assets. In Chile and most Latin American countries, pension funds keep reserves that are used to recompense individual accounts if their returns deviate substantially (by 50 percent or 2 percentage points, whichever is greater) from the average industry return. Stringent portfolio limits further inhibit risky investments in all Latin American and transition countries that have reformed. These guarantees and portfolio limits have economic costs in terms of nonoptimal investments and moral hazard problems, but these are invisible to most workers. They have the more visible political benefits of allaying fears that workers will lose their retirement savings.

Even with these guarantees, switching into the new system has often been voluntary for the entire generation of current workers, so those who prefer the old system retain their rights to stay there. Besides allaying fears and opposition, this is also a way of reducing the transition deficit, since the total contributions of nonswitchers continue to flow into the PAYG system. Moreover, if switching is voluntary, the government can set a lower rate of compensation for past service, based on the preferences of young and less risk-averse workers. This saves the government money while at the same time ensures that no worker will feel he or she has been made worse off, since he or she has choice.[13] Hungary, in particular, devoted considerable attention to choosing the minimum rate of compensation that would induce the "right" number of workers to switch, consistent with its cash flow deficit limits. But even after careful analysis, the government overpaid, in the sense that more workers switched than was expected or desired.

While governments have designed reform policies to convince both pensioners and workers that they will gain from change, they have also taken active steps to convince them that the status quo is not sustainable, the old system is not functioning well, and under the reversion option of the old PAYG system, they will all lose. In Chile, Jose Pinera, the minister of labor, who processed the reform, went on radio and television weekly to convince workers that they did not want their money to continue disappearing into a "black hole." Hungary and Poland mounted active public relations campaigns, with separate messages targeted to the young and old. In Argentina, Peru, and Kazakhstan, where the government was in arrears in paying pensioners and evasion was rife, the evidence visibly demonstrated that the old systems were not working even without a public relations campaign. By all these means—persuasion combined with promises of continued and improved benefits for existing pensioners, guarantees of benefits from the new second pillar, voluntary switching, partial debt financing of the transition, and emphasis on the poor performance of the reversion option, the existing PAYG system—policymakers have tried to assure broad groups of young and old workers as well as pensioners that they would not be worse off, and most would be better off, after a structural reform.

Institutional Politics

Labor unions, social security bureaucrats, and financial institutions are key stakeholders in the politics of pension reform. The first two groups are often, although not always, in opposition to reform. This may be particularly true of labor unions representing public sector employees, where international competitiveness is not a major issue and labor demand may be perceived as inelastic.

LABOR UNIONS

There are several reasons why labor unions may resist reform. They may be especially responsive to the interests of their older members, with whom mutual loyalty and social networks have been built up over the years, rather than their younger members whose job-based affiliation may be only temporary. Union leaders may also support public spending on education, health, and other services for their members and their families, and may fear that these services will be cut to help finance the transition. In addition, unions often play an active formalized role in running the old social security systems, which gives them substantial power over resources and jobs.

To some extent, the reform can overcome the opposition of unions by giving them a role to play in the new system. In Argentina, for example, in response to intense early opposition from labor, the government offered unions the opportunity to operate pension funds in the new system. While their members would not be required to join these funds, the unions obviously hoped that loyalty would hold. This was a crucial deal that won the support of labor leaders and the votes in the congress necessary to enact the reform. Similar deals were made in Hungary and Poland, where OPZZ and Solidarity (the main unions), respectively, are founders (in international joint ventures) of two of the new pension funds. Indeed, Solidarity, a union that was promarket from the start, was actively involved in the entire Polish reform process, and one of its officials, Ewa Lewicka, became plenipotentiary for social security reform in the final stage. Involving labor unions in designing the reform is probably a shrewd move, but it will only work with unions that are basically sympathetic to the objectives of the reform. This is most likely to be the case with unions representing private sector workers in competitive environments, which perceive low payroll taxes and efficiency as beneficial for survival and growth.

Social Security Bureaucrats

For similar reasons, social security bureaucrats often oppose a structural reform that will introduce competition into the system and take away their monopolistic control over resources. In some cases, their fears have been assuaged by giving them authority in the new system as well. For example, in Mexico and Poland the government gave the social security bureaucracy responsibility for handling collections, record-keeping, and the administration of health and survivors' insurance. Thus, the "privateness" of these reforms, if measured according to bureaucratic decentralization, is much less than privateness as measured according to investment control and benefit provision. This administrative centralization, again, is an option only if the old bureaucracy has the ability and willingness to carry out rather than undermine these functions. In Poland the price of involving the bureaucracy was several months' delay in crediting the early contributions to individual workers and their designated pension funds. In Hungary the old bureaucracy was too outspokenly opposed to structural reform to entrust it with administering the new system.

Private Financial Institutions

In contrast to unions and social security bureaucracies, private financial institutions may have a positive interest in reform. As seen in the first section, countries with large voluntary, funded pension plans (PREPLAN) are more likely to reform. Most developing and transitional countries do not have these plans or other large, well-functioning financial institutions before the reform; in fact, one object of the reform is to help them grow. But where these institutions do exist, they often have particular interests that must be accommodated to gain their active support. For example, in Hungary the voluntary pension funds that existed before the reform lobbied successfully for regulations in the mandatory system that matched their own organizational structure, thereby facilitating their participation in the mandatory pillar. This accounts for the fact that the legal structure of the private pillar in Hungary differs from that in many other reforming countries. In OECD countries as well, the private mandatory pillar was set up to build upon, rather than replace, the large collectively bargained pension system that already existed.

The Politics of Compensation

Generational and institutional interests shape important dimensions of pension reform and help explain how the new system is administered, who can set up pension funds, how the transition is financed, and what guarantees are offered. However, pension reform involves many narrow distributional issues that need to be addressed directly. The government has many tools at its disposal to compensate potential losers, including the power to exempt certain groups from the terms of the reform, to grant cash benefits and tax relief to particular groups, to make political appointments that will further its reform efforts, and to make trade-offs among or link reforms in multiple sectors, depending on its priorities (Edwards and Lederman 1998). Governments have used each of these strategies to build support for pension reform.

EXEMPTION FROM THE REFORM (EXCLUSIONARY COMPENSATION)

Every reforming country in Latin America has exempted certain powerful groups and allowed them to keep their own privileged schemes. Even in Chile, where an authoritarian military regime implemented the new pension system, exempted the military itself—as did every other reforming country in Latin America. The judiciary often receives exemption, in order to ensure that a judicial decision will not render the reform invalid. In Uruguay the reform excluded special regimes for bankers, notaries, and university professors. It is therefore critical to pay specific attention to the political landscape and organizational power of special interests in each country.

Governments often exempt public sector workers from the first stage of the reform. Their pensions, to begin with, tend to be higher than those of private sector workers. They are an older part of the workforce, with more covered retirees. They are more articulate and better organized to maintain their benefits. Since their services face no market test and government directly pays their pensions, they have less to fear from unemployment and lack of competitiveness due to high payroll taxes. In some cases, as in Argentina, local public sector workers have been covered in second-stage reforms, as it became clear that their localities would not have the resources to pay the promised benefits indefinitely.

Mexico offers a prime example of the strategic exemption of public sector workers in its 1995 reform. Technocrats within the Ministry of Finance and central bank had designed a proposal for a Chilean-style pension reform in 1990. Having encountered firm resistance to this plan within the cabinet, they shelved this design. But the following year, the government of the state of Nuevo Leon approached the same technocrats seeking technical assistance regarding the structural reform of the state-level pension system. With the expertise accumulated from their previous studies, the federal reformers lent assistance in designing a Chilean-style pension scheme for the public employees of Nuevo Leon. Organized interests did not become aware of the scheme until after the state assembly had already ratified it. The consequence, according to the federal technocrats, was "brutal." The outpouring of public protests, strikes, and at times violent demonstrations led the state government to repeal the reform before its implementation.

In designing the reform proposal, the technicians had failed to understand the organizational and political power of the public sector unions, particularly that of the teachers. Nuevo Leon has a strong, well-organized teachers' union, which belongs to the state confederation of public sector employees (ISSSTE-Leon). In turn, ISSSTE-Leon is affiliated with the federal public sector union (ISSSTE), which lent both financial and organizational assistance for the protest against the pension reform.

Witnessing these events unfold, the technocrats in Mexico City drew valuable lessons that they applied to the national pension reform effort in 1995. Principally, they realized that where unions are broad and cohesive, their interests must be taken into account in designing the reform. Since the federal umbrella union of public sector employees had been alerted to the reform and had lent support to its undoing in Nuevo Leon, it was clear to the federal reformers that the 1995 pension reform would only prosper if ISSSTE were exempted from its terms. This led Mexico to exempt all public sector workers from the outset and avoid a battle that could have undermined the entire reform.

Direct Financial Compensation

Even after specified groups are exempted and guarantees are offered to others, direct financial compensation has often been used to build support for the reform or to convince workers to switch under a voluntary switching regime. In Uruguay, after five previous pension reform efforts failed, the government devised a new plan that offered a cash subsidy to middle-income participants in the pension scheme. Workers have the option to divide their contribution between the public and private pillar, and those who choose to contribute 50 percent of their 15 percent contribution to the funded DC scheme receive a 25 percent subsidy from the government (providing their monthly income falls below 5,000 pesos or US$500).[14] The new plan was approved, and more than 80 percent of people with the option have chosen to enter the capitalization scheme.

In Chile and Peru direct compensation came in the form of one-time salary increases to offset the added employee tax burden. In both countries the implementation of the market-based pension scheme involved shifting responsibility for contributions to workers instead of employers. An increase in the workers' gross wages when they entered the new system helped to offset the added burden and give them an incentive to switch.

Eliminating early retirement privileges (before age 55 and sometimes before age 50) was a key element of the reform in Poland, helping to make it financially sustainable and free up resources for the second pillar. But the main old trade union federation (OPZZ) was willing to support reform providing that the system maintained a low retirement age for key groups (such as miners) and/or provided direct compensation for those whose special privileges were about to end. The "new" trade union, Solidarity, also supported the miners. The government agreed that once the reform was passed a special commission would be set up to figure out an equitable way to phase out these privileges, and this would involve temporary bridge financing. The compromise solution maintained these benefits in the medium term for middle age workers but got rid of them in the long run, and remunerated the transition group for their lost privileges. One might wonder why workers and unions were willing to go along with an agreement to negotiate after the reform was passed, rather than before, when their bargaining power would have been greater. The fact that Solidarity was in the government and one of its officials was plenipotentiary for social security reform undoubtedly increased the credibility of the government's promise and helped the reform to proceed smoothly through the legislature.

In Bolivia the state assumed responsibility for the unfunded debt of the supplementary pension scheme that had been negotiated by unions to overcome union resistance to the pension and privatization reform. Regulations then required that a high percentage of fund assets be invested in government bonds to finance the resulting deficit.

All of these examples showed how the government used cash compensation to offset lost benefits that were imposed on particular groups by the reform or to encourage voluntary participation in the new scheme.

INDIRECT AND CROSS-COMPENSATION

Governments possess the ability to trade off one policy for another or to link reforms, thereby strengthening both in the process. Thus, if pension reform is a priority issue, the government can compensate an opposition group in some other policy arena without changing the basic pension design. For example, in Mexico the government used tax breaks in other areas to compensate employers for their support of the 1992 Retirement Savings System (SAR), which required an additional 2 percent employer contribution. This was a precursor of the more successful 1995 reform.

In Argentina, the government promised to protect the privileges held by unions in the administration of health care (Obras Sociales) in exchange for labor support for the pension reform. This, along with the opportunity to run pension fund management companies, enabled the Argentine government to gain union support for reform. This strategic negotiation proved critical, despite of the fact that the president's political party, the PJ, held a majority of seats in the congress, which should have been sufficient to pass the reform directly. This incident also illustrates the importance of within-party negotiations. The unions were allied with the PJ, and a bloc of labor-linked deputies in the PJ held up discussion of the bill by refusing to concede the necessary quorum. As the legislative session approached its end, the government faced an elevated risk of losing the entire reform if it did not compromise. As a consequence of this compensatory arrangement, Argentina became the first democratic country to introduce privately managed individual capitalization accounts, although at the cost of "gaps" in the broader market orientation of social services.

As the converse of trading off reforms, coupling of reforms may also help to build coalitions of support. Here again, the Argentine case is instructive, as it linked pension reform and privatization reform. In 1992, President Menem agreed to recalculate the unpaid benefits owed by the government to pensioners and to pay them off using 20 percent of the revenue collected from the initial sale of shares of the state-owned petroleum company, Yacimientos Petrolíferos Fiscales (YPF).[15] Privatization had encountered opposition in the congress, and it only gained acceptance when the government linked it to the solution to the pension dilemma. This arrangement enabled the government to quell the growing hostility from pensioners associations while advancing the march of privatization. By attaching provisions to the oil company privatization, Menem built a coalition of political support for privatization among current retirees who would not have been directly affected by the reform.

Injecting a portion of privatization revenues into the new pension plan also secured support for pension reform in Bolivia. The government used resources from privatization to create a basic pension benefit for all Bolivians over the age of 65, including those not in the contributory system. Additionally, privatization furnished an important source of revenue for financing the transitional costs of pension reform in Peru, Uruguay, and Mexico. In Poland, too, the government will use privatization assets in support of pension reform in a way that was hammered out with Solidarity officials.

POLITICAL COMPENSATION

Broad political rewards comprise another tool that government can use to harness support for reform. Political compensation is a common tool for parties in power, across issues and countries. This may entail the appointment of influential members of one party or interest group to a key position in government, either as a signal to the group that its interests will be taken into account or as a direct exchange for support on a specific issue, such as pension reform.

In Uruguay two of the three main political parties—the National Party (PN) and the Colorado Party (PC) dominated the governing coalition that introduced private pensions in 1995. The third dominant party, the left-wing Broad Front (FA) remained outside the government in opposition. During the negotiation over the pension reform, which occurred in the months between the election and inauguration of the new government, the PN and PC extended an invitation to the leftist New Space (NE) to join the government. Although the PN-PC coalition held the necessary two-thirds majority to pass the pension reform amendment, it offered the NE a cabinet position as well as a seat at the negotiating table. Though seemingly pointless, this maneuver was an effective political strategy for the government, since the NE represented left-wing and union interests. Anticipating that the pension reform would not only have to pass the hurdle of legislative approval, but, potentially, of public referendum as well, the government made the strategic decision to incorporate the left wing into the reform to avoid alienating it.

The government in Hungary agreed to postpone new elections for members of the Pension and Health Insurance Fund Board, which supervised the old system, thereby extending their terms in office and dampening their opposition. This would particularly benefit the trade union representatives, institutionalizing their control over substantial financial resources. This bargain was short lived, however, as a new government came to office the following year and abolished the independent Pension and Health Insurance Funds altogether.

Conclusion

In this chapter we have analyzed the political and economic forces that influence the probability of structural pension reform and help determine the nature of that reform, particularly its public-private mix. We find that somewhat different forces determine the probability of structural reform and the ultimate nature of that reform, although both depend on legacies from past systems that become constraints on design possibilities for new systems.

Most strikingly, a large implicit pension debt from the old pay-as-you-go social security system brings pension reform to the forefront of the political agenda, thereby increasing the probability of structural reform.

Subsequently, however, this same large IPD makes it more difficult to finance the transition to a funded system and to overcome resistance from entrenched bureaucrats and pensioners, thereby limiting the degree of funding and privatization that ultimately emerges. Also, well-established voluntary private pension plans facilitate the move toward a mandatory funded plan, with substantial private management, providing it is shaped in such a way that their role is maintained and extended, rather than displaced. Beyond this path dependency, we find that reform ideas diffuse along lines that depend on linguistic and geographic proximity. Communication, information, and demonstration effects obviously play a crucial role.

While historical and institutional factors have considerable econometric explanatory power concerning the public-private mix of the new system, they are less successful in predicting whether or not structural reform will actually take place. This leaves an important role for the goals, creativity, and ability of individual policymakers to gauge the situations in their countries and come up with strategies that move reform forward. These strategies in countries that have successfully reformed involve shaping the design of the reform package to build a majority coalition of winners from reform, credibly promising pensioners that they will not suffer, postponing some painful adjustments, exempting certain influential groups, compensating groups that fear losses of power or money, and trading off policy concessions or political carrots in other areas. Governments have persuaded pensioners and younger workers, labor unions, social security bureaucrats, and financial institutions to support the reform through these means.

To accomplish this requires key policymakers who hold pension reform as a priority objective and who have the skills needed to negotiate the necessary deals. Country-specific pressures, constraints, and opportunities also influence the exact details of the reforms that finally emerge. At the same time, similar difficulties and solutions occur in diverse places, suggesting that countries can learn from each other about the problems they will encounter and the menu of strategies that have been tried, tested, and prove likely to work. International organizations such as the World Bank can play an important role in helping to diffuse this information.

Notes

1. Latvia and Italy, which have maintained their single pillar PAYG system but with a shift to a notional DC, fall into the latter category. Latvia has passed legislation to establish a funded, privately managed DC pillar in the future but has not yet implemented it. We omitted one of the structural

reformers, Hong Kong, from our analysis because of data gaps. Therefore we had 19 structural reformers in our sample.

2. In ongoing work we explore other possible indices of "privateness"— their correlations and differential explanations. For example, other dimensions that increase "privateness" are the decentralization of collection and record-keeping functions, the delegation of survivors' and disability insurance to the private system, and the requirement that new entrants to the labor market enter a privately managed pillar. In contrast, certain measures increase the state role, such as: exemptions granted from participation in the new system (often given to the military, the judiciary, and other selected public sector workers); the continuation of the old system alongside the new, with workers retaining the right to switch back and forth between them (as in Colombia); the existence of a public DB option in the second pillar (as in Argentina); a public management option for the DC accounts in the second pillar (as in Uruguay and Kazakhstan); and the provision of a guaranteed benefit by the state (as in Hungary). For systems in which workers have the option to choose between public and private arrangements for their second-pillar benefits, we simulate only the private option in this chapter. In a complementary paper, we derive a "bureaucratic privateness" index that summarizes some of these additional ingredients. While the proportion of benefits deriving from the private pillar captures only one dimension of "privateness," it is the most important indicator financially, and the most consistently quantifiable for broad cross-national comparisons.

3. In ongoing work we investigate how %PVT differs for workers of different types and what light this throws on the political economy of reform. For example, in examining %PVT for low earners, we find that the rank order of countries is largely unchanged, but the distribution becomes more compressed as compared with the distribution of %PVT for the average worker because of the greater targeting of public benefits to the poor in countries with a high %PVT.

4. We also experimented with alternative assumptions that lead to higher or lower %PVTs, but they did not affect the significance of variables in our explanatory equation, probably because they affected all countries in similar ways. Therefore, we do not present the results here. In countries where the first pillar takes the form of a notional DC plan, we made similar assumptions about the rate of return and growth rate of per capita wages, plus the additional assumption that growth in total wage bill = growth in GDP = 2.5 percent; we then applied the notional interest rate formula specified by the country's NDC system.

5. A partial transition to a private pension system may take other forms besides a small %PVT: some groups of workers may be exempted from the reform (even in Chile, the judiciary and the military were exempted); only

younger workers may be induced to switch to the private scheme (as in Hungary); or the two systems may continue to operate side by side (as in Colombia). In Hungary the government allowed voluntary switching to the new system, paying close attention to the relationship between compensatory payments and the proportion of workers who were likely to switch. Reformers chose the level of compensation that was estimated to induce a rate of switching to the new scheme that would meet the government's target cash flow deficit (Palacios and Rocha 1998; see second section of chapter).

6. The equation used to impute the implicit pension debt using the spending-based method is: IPD = a + b*(Pubs), where a = 27.9 and b = 14.81. Pubs = percentage of public spending on pensions, taken from World Bank (1994a). Values of the coefficients and constant are based on regression of known sets of implicit pension debt values and levels of public pension spending. This equation explains 78 percent of the total variation in IPD levels. Using the age-based method, the equation is: IPD = a + b*(Age), where a = -10.71 and b = 10.35. Age = percentage of population over age 60, taken from World Bank (1994a). $R^2 = 0.68$. In our regressions with the spending-based measure, we used actual rather than imputed values of IPD, where these were available.

7. An anecdotal example of the inhibiting effect of DEBT on reform comes from a recent round of pension reforms in Brazil in which policymakers postponed a plan for a moderate structural revision that would have eventually reduced its huge IPD—in large part due to the medium-term constraints of financing the transition. Citing the risk of speculation that would follow the issuance of new explicit debt to pay for such measures, officials in the Ministry of Finance and central bank insisted that the government put aside the structural reform model until its borrowing constraints eased. In contrast, in Mexico the peso crisis of 1995 forced the government to liquidate much of its outstanding explicit debt (mainly through privatization), which left it in a good position to issue new explicit debt as a means to finance its structural pension reform.

8. For the economic debate on the presence of these macroeconomic effects, see Arrau and Schmidt-Hebbel (1994), Agosin, Crespi, and Letelier(1996), Haindl Rondanelli (1996), Holzmann (1996), Cifuentes and Valdés-Prieto (1997), Corsetti and Schmidt-Hebbel (1997), Schmidt-Hebbel (1997, 1999a, and 1999b). For a summary of the issues and related literature, see World Bank (1994) and James (1998a). The impact on national saving seems to depend on two factors: the extent to which decreased voluntary saving offsets the new mandatory saving in the funded pillar and the degree to which the government finances the transition through increased taxes and spending cuts rather than increased borrowing.

9. In Mexico, for example, the desire to increase domestic savings took a central place in President Zedillo's 1995 National Development Plan,

which listed pension reform as a primary means to achieve that end. In addition, the introductory text of the 1995 pension reform law in Mexico identifies "the enhancement of domestic savings" as a goal of the system (Solís and Villagomez 1997). In contrast, countries with higher levels of domestic savings may be more likely to frame the question of pension reform around the more modest objective of correcting long-term actuarial imbalances in the benefit-contribution ratio of their pension scheme— a goal that may be achieved through parametric changes.

10. Scholars of legislative systems explain this variable by suggesting that "if one had to give a single number to characterize the politics of any country that employs competitive elections, it would be the number of parties active in its national assembly" (Taagepera and Shugart 1993, p. 455). While the number of political parties does not provide full information on the functioning of the legislative system, it has been closely related to the ability of governments to carry out economic reform (Haggard and Kaufman 1992) and how long cabinets last in parliamentary systems (Lijphart 1994). The "effective number" of parties tells us the number of hypothetical equal-sized parties that would have the same effect on the fractionalization of the party system as have the actual varying sized parties. The advantage of the "effective" parties (over the actual number of parties) is that it establishes a systematic way to distinguish the significant parties from the less meaningful (or influential) ones. By being squared, each party is weighted in such a way that very small parties add relatively little to the score (Taagepera and Shugart 1993). This measure of political dispersion has the weakness of failing to capture fragmentation and bargaining that are often necessary within a dominant single party system, a factor which played an important role in shaping the Mexican reform.

11. Switzerland offers an earnings-related benefit that is very compressed, and most workers are close to the maximum level, hence it functions almost as a flat benefit. In Bolivia the government uses privatization proceeds to pay every Bolivian over the age of 65 a small flat benefit that is less than 10 percent of the average wage; it is unclear what kind of first pillar Bolivia will have when the privatization proceeds are exhausted.

12. Most of the examples come from the field work of Sarah Brooks in Latin America and Mitchell Orenstein in the transition economies.

13. Mexico appears to be an exception since all workers had to join the new system with no compensation—but this went together with a government guarantee that their pensions, upon retirement, would not be lower than would have been the case under the old system. It is likely that most workers over age 45 will utilize this guarantee and will revert to their old system benefits, financed by the government. Kazakhstan is another exception, although this time the government did not provide such a guarantee. As a result, pensioners and older workers mobilized against the

reform both before and after it was passed. Given their lack of representation, however, this opposition was not particularly effective in changing the law.

14. For a worker whose income was 1,000 pesos, 15 percent of 500 pesos is directed to the DC pillar, while the worker still gets credit for 750 pesos in calculating the pensionable wage in the DB to which he or she is entitled in the public pillar.

15. According to the Constitution, the government was responsible to pay pensioners benefits equivalent to 70–82 percent of their salary in activity. But the government claimed it did not have the money to pay this obligation. The use of privatization revenues solved this constitutional dilemma and also gained support for pension and privatization reform.

References

Note: The word *processed* describes informally reproduced works that may not be commonly available through libraries.

Agosin, Manuel R., Gustavo T. Crespi, and Leonardo S. Letelier. 1996. "Explicaciones del Aumento del Ahorro en Chile." Centros de Investigacion Economica. Santiago, Chile: Banco Interamericano de Desarrollo.

Arrau, Patricio, and Klaus Schmidt-Hebbel. 1994. "Pension System and Reform in Developing Countries: Country Experience and Research Issues." *Revista de Analisis Economico* 9(1): 3–20.

Brooks, Sarah. 1999. "Social Protection and the Market: Pension Reform under Capital Mobility." Paper delivered at the Annual Meeting of the American Political Science Association, September 3, 1999.

Cifuentes, Rodrigo, and Salvador Valdés-Prieto. 1997. "Transitions in the Presence of Credit Constraints." In Salvador Valdés-Prieto, ed., *The Economics of Pensions: Principles, Policies, and International Experience.* Cambridge University Press.

Corsetti, Giancarlo, and Klaus Schmidt-Hebbel. 1997. "Pension Reform and Growth." In Salvador Valdés-Prieto, ed., *The Economics of Pensions: Principles, Policies, and International Experience.* Cambridge University Press.

Cox, Gary, and Matthew McCubbins. 1993. *Legislative Leviathan: Party Government in the House.* Berkeley: University of California Press.

Ebbinhaus, Bernhard. 1998. "The Second Pillar Between State and Market: A Comparison of Occupational Pensions in Britain and Germany." Paper presented at the Conference on the Varieties of Welfare Capitalism, Cologne, Germany, June 11–13, 1998.

Edwards, Sebastian, and Daniel Lederman. 1998. "The Political Economy of Unilateral Trade Liberalization: The Case of Chile." In J. Bhagwati, ed., *Going Alone: The Case for Relaxed Reciprocity*. Washington, D.C.: MIT Press and American Enterprise Institute.

Grindle, Merilee S., and John W. Thomas, eds. 1991. *Public Choices and Policy Change: The Political Economy of Reform in Developing Countries*. Baltimore: Johns Hopkins University Press.

Haggard, Stephan, and Robert Kaufman, eds. 1992. *The Politics of Economic Adjustment*. Princeton University Press.

Haindl Rondanelli, Erik. 1996. "Chilean Pension Fund Reform and its Impact on Saving," IBC Discussion Paper No. 96-2. University of Miami, International Business Center, Coral Gables, Florida. Processed.

Holzmann, Robert. 1996. "On Economic Usefulness and Fiscal Requirements of Moving from Unfunded to Funded Pensions." Working paper. Saarbruucken, Germany: University of Saarland.

Immergut, Ellen. 1992. "The Rules of the Game: The Logic of Health Policy-Making in France, Switzerland and Sweden." In S. Steinmo, K. Thelen, and F. Longstreth, eds., *Structuring Politics: Historical Institutionalism in Comparative Perspective*. New York: Cambridge University Press.

ILO (International Labour Organisation). 1990, 1995, 1997. *International Labour Statistics*. Geneva: International Labour Office.

James, Estelle. 1986. "The Private Nonprofit Provision of Education: A Theoretical Model and Application to Japan." *Journal of Comparative Economics*, 10 (September): 255–76.

_____. 1993. "Why Do Different Countries Choose A Different Public-Private Mix of Educational Services?" *Journal of Human Resources* 28: 571–92.

_____. 1998a. "New Systems for Old Age Security: Theory, Practice and Empirical Evidence." *World Bank Research Observer* 13 (August): 271.

_____. 1998b. "The Political Economy of Social Security Reform: A Cross-Country Review." *Annals of Public and Cooperative Economics* 69(4): 1–35.

Kane, Cheik, and Robert Palacios. 1996. "The Implicit Pension Debt." *Finance & Development* 33(2): 38–41.

Laakso, Markku, and Rein Taagepera. 1979. "Effective Number of Parties: A Measure with Application to West Europe." *Comparative Political Studies* 12: 3–27.

Lijphart, Arend. 1994. *Electoral Systems and Party Systems in Twenty-Seven Democracies 1945–1990*. Oxford University Press.

Maxfield, Sylvia. 1997. *Gatekeepers of Growth: Central Banking in Developing Countries*. Princeton University Press.

Nelson, Joan M., ed. 1990. *Economic Crisis and Policy Choice: The Politics of Adjustment in the Third World*. Princeton University Press.

_____. 1994. *Intricate Links: Democratization and Market Reforms in Latin America and Eastern Europe*. New Brunswick, N.J.: Transaction Publishers.

_____. 1997. "Social Costs, Social Sector Reforms, and Politics in Post-Communist Transformations." In Joan Nelson, Charles Tilly, and Lee Walker, eds., *Transforming Post-Communist Political Economies.* Washington, D.C.: National Academy Press.

Palacios, Robert, and Roberto Rocha. 1998. "The Hungarian Pension System in Transition." Social Protection Discussion Paper No. 9805. World Bank, Washington, D.C.

Pierson, Paul. 1996. "The New Politics of the Welfare State." *World Politics* 48 (January): 143–79.

Rodrik, Dani. 1994. "What Does the Political Economy Literature on Trade Policy (Not) Tell Us That We Ought to Know?" Working Paper Series No. 4870. Cambridge, Mass.: National Bureau of Economic Research.

Sartori, Giovanni. 1976. *Parties and Party Systems: A Framework for Analysis.* New York: Cambridge University Press.

Schmidt-Hebbel, Klaus. 1997. "Pension Systems: From Crisis to Reform." EDI Conference, World Bank, Washington, D.C. Processed.

_____. 1999a. "A Review of Chile's Experience with Pension Reform." Annual Conference on Economic Development. World Bank, Washington, D.C. Processed.

_____. 1999b. "Does Pension Reform Really Spur Productivity, Saving and Growth?" Processed.

Shugart, Matthew Soberg, and Stephan Haggard. 1997. "Institutions and Public Policy in Presidential Systems." Irvine, Calif.: Center for the Study of Democracy. Processed.

Solís Soberon F., and A. Villagomez. 1997. "Domestic Savings in Mexico and Pension Reform." In M. Serrano, ed., *Mexico: Assessing Neo-Liberal Reform.* London: Institute of Latin American Studies.

Taagepera, Rein, and Matthew Soberg Shugart. 1989. *Seats and Votes: The Effects and Determinants of Electoral Systems.* New Haven: Yale University Press.

_____. 1993. "Predicting the Number of Parties: A Quantitative Model of Duverger's Mechanical Effect." *American Political Science Review* 87(2).

Tommasi, M., and A. Velasco 1996. "Where Are We in The Political Economy of Reform?" *Journal of Policy Reform* 1(2): 187–238.

Tsebelis, George 1990. *Nested Games: Rational Choice in Comparative Politics.* Berkeley: University of California Press.

Van der Noord, Paul, and Richard Herd. 1993. *Pension Liabilities in the Seven Major Economies.* Paris: OECD.

_____. 1994. *Estimating Pension Liabilities: A Methodological Framework.* OECD Economic Studies No. 23.

World Bank. 1994. *Averting the Old Age Crisis: Policies to Protect the Old and Promote Growth.* Washington, D.C.

5

Improving the Regulation and Supervision of Pension Funds: Are There Lessons from the Banking Sector?

Roberto Rocha, Richard Hinz,
and Joaquin Gutierrez

THE FINANCIAL PROBLEMS FACED BY pay-as-you-go (PAYG) pension schemes around the world have led several countries to curtail public pension benefits and promote supplementary private pension provision by encouraging a voluntary (third) pillar through tax incentives and/or by introducing a mandatory (second) pillar.[1] The desire to achieve a high rate of coverage in private pension provision has led an increasing number of countries to introduce a second and mandatory pillar, not only in Latin America but also in Europe. Within the next decades, these private pillars are expected to provide a significant share of retirement income in many countries. As a result, there has been a growing interest in analyzing the institutional and regulatory framework of the pension industry and assessing whether the industry will be able to meet the expectations of workers and policymakers.

In analyzing the regulatory framework for the pension industry, it is important to identify the types of risks to which the industry is exposed, assess whether the regulatory framework in most countries is prepared to cope with these risks, and whether there is room for further improvements. In examining these questions, it may prove useful to ascertain whether there are lessons to be learned from other areas of the financial sector, especially the banking sector.

Banks and pension funds are different is several aspects, and many elements of banking regulation have been introduced to address risks specific to the banking industry, including the risk of systemic crisis and failures. However, there may be general lessons to be drawn from the intense effort to strengthen bank regulation in the recent decades and also specific elements of bank regulation and supervision that may be both relevant and applicable to pensions. These include regulations on the provision and pricing of guarantees, regulations addressing the quality of corporate governance, and the techniques that have been developed to ensure effective supervision of a large number of institutions.

This chapter reviews the regulatory framework for pension funds and examines whether there is scope for improvements in pension regulation, particularly in light of regulatory and supervisory developments in the banking industry. The chapter is structured as follows. The second section summarizes the literature on banking regulation and supervision, identifying the areas of consensus and the trends in regulation and supervision across countries. The third section summarizes the literature on the regulation of pension systems. The fourth section examines the scope for improvements in pension regulation, identifying possible lessons from the banking sector to the pension industry. The fifth section provides a summary and draws conclusions.

Regulation and Supervision of the Banking Sector

The banking sector has always received more attention than other sectors of the financial system. This has been due to the dominant position of banks in the financial system, the particular structure of their assets and liabilities, and the huge leverage with which banks operate. Banking activities typically involve the transformation of short-term liabilities into long-term assets (loans) that are difficult to value and monitor. The combination of high leverage in banking and the structure of bank liabilities imply a substantial degree of exposure of capital to various types of risks and the possibility of contagion effects triggering a chain of bank runs and failures.

The specter of massive bank runs and failures with disruptive consequences for economic activity and the perception that social costs of failures may well exceed private costs have traditionally led to a great degree of intervention in the banking system. In addition to the existence of central banks providing lending of last resort, governments have tried to reduce the probability of bank runs by introducing explicit deposit insurance.

Deposit insurance may reduce the likelihood of bank runs, but it also generates moral hazard, aggravating the principal-agent problem in banking. There has been an extensive discussion on the best strategy to deal with moral hazard and reduce the incentives for excessive risk-taking. The set of measures that have been proposed to enhance prudent banking in the presence of deposit insurance can be grouped into four classes. The first involves measures designed to reduce the scope of insurance and improve its pricing. The second entails quantitative regulations designed to ensure minimum levels of capital and liquidity and limit risk concentrations. The third deals with qualitative standards designed to strengthen bank governance. The fourth covers measures to strengthen supervisory capacity and minimize regulatory forbearance.[2]

Reforming Deposit Insurance

Various measures have been proposed to directly offset the moral hazard effects of deposit insurance by enhancing incentives for more market monitoring of banks and improving market discipline. These measures include capping the statutory insurance limits at lower levels, introducing more coinsurance, making more use of market-priced subordinated debt, ensuring extensive disclosure of the banks' financial conditions, and making insurance fees more risk based. An increasing number of countries are introducing most of these measures.[3]

Quantitative Prudential Regulations

Quantitative prudential regulations are rules that aim at diversifying the risks that banks assume, preserving a buffer of tangible capital to absorb potential losses and ensuring minimum levels of liquid and safe assets. The most widely adopted regulations include the following:

- Minimum entry and capital adequacy rules that reflect the risks that banks undertake
- Appropriate limits on risk concentrations with individual borrowers and groups of borrowers
- Limits on other types of financial risk concentrations in investment and trading
- Asset classification and provisioning rules establishing the fair value of the bank's assets, contingencies, collateral, and capital
- Minimum liquidity requirements

Qualitative Prudential Regulation

A growing perception exists that even the best quantitative regulations are not sufficient to avoid the recurrence of crisis. Quantitative rules can neither be sufficiently customized to the conditions of individual institutions and the realities of some countries (the "one size fits all" problem) nor replace good bank governance. Thus, there is a growing awareness that quantitative regulations must be complemented by a set of qualitative rules specifying the rights of shareholders, the tasks and responsibilities of boards and senior management, the auditing functions, and the adoption of mechanisms to manage the most fundamental types of risks. These qualitative standards intend to place the primary responsibility for compliance and supervision where it belongs: on the banks themselves or, more concretely, on their boards, external auditors, and shareholders.

Internal and external audits are seen today as particularly important elements of the corporate governance of banks and also have importance for bank supervision, since they can provide a first independent assessment of the integrity of the institutions. The measures that most countries have introduced to strengthen the audit function include obligatory rotation of external auditors, obligatory reporting to independent directors' audit committees, obligatory assessment of the integrity of controls and systems, and previous shareholder and supervisory approval to the removal of auditors. Some developed countries have gone even further, essentially replacing external audits for onsite examinations. In these cases, however, bank supervisors must be able to influence the audit programs and have full access to their outcomes.

Bank Supervision: Basic Strategy and Building Blocks

Although there are significant differences in the organization of bank supervision across countries, it is possible to identify a four-stage evolutionary process characterizing the development of bank supervision. As shown in box 5.1, the first stage consists of developing minimum capacity to assess compliance with quantitative regulations. The second stage follows a financial crisis and is characterized by a more interventionist approach and concentration of powers in the supervisory agency. During this stage, supervisors are more actively involved in failure resolution.

Box 5.1. Stages of Evolution in Bank Supervision

Stage 1	*Stage 2*	*Stage 3*	*Stage 4*
Develop own capacity to enforce compliance	*Develop own capacity to resolve problems*	*Develop banks' capacity to manage risks*	*Develop market capacity to share supervision burden*
Focus on monitoring key financial indicators for compliance: minimum capital, earnings, liquidity, asset quality, arm's length loans.	Focus on resolving problems and failed banks, weeding out bad banks and bankers. Strengthen independence, supervisory powers, and capacity.	Focus on assessing the quality of banks' risk management procedures and methods. Improving stability by strengthening risk management.	Focus on making all market players more responsible for their decisions. Strengthen board and audit functions. Augment disclosure; introduce subordinated classes and co-insurance.

Finally, the last stages follow an increasing understanding that a stable banking system needs to have prudent bankers following best financial practices. At this point, the regulatory and supervisory frameworks shift to a more qualitative and broad-based approach—that of providing better incentives for prudent banking and distributing responsibilities more evenly among market players.

Irrespective of the stage of development, banking supervision in every country comprises three basic building blocks: licensing or ex ante supervision, ongoing supervision and enforcement and resolution procedures, and ex post supervision (Basle Committee 1997). These basic blocks are clearly integrated, although countries may need to put more emphasis on one of these blocks depending on their specific conditions and stages of development.

Licensing of Banks. Licensing plays an important role in ensuring the viability of new banks and the integrity and fitness of those who manage them. A well-performed licensing function is not restricted simply to screening applicants and providing licenses based on certain criteria but is also empowered to authorize all major changes in the original license. This should embrace changes in the control of institutions, additions to the list of permissible activities, appointment of directors and auditors, changes in the composition of capital, and related party transactions.

Ongoing Supervision. While the process for ongoing supervision varies from country to country, supervisors use several methods or tools for such purposes, including off-site surveillance, on-site examinations, contacts with internal and external auditors, and interviews with senior management. The basic objective of off-site surveillance is to monitor the condition of individual banks, provide early identification of problems, and target scarce supervisory resources to areas of greatest risk. Off-site surveillance provides an ongoing tool to evaluate financial performance between on-site examinations. Off-site surveillance systems are highly dependent on the quality of the reported information. Facts crucial for the supervisory process, such as loan portfolio strategy, the quality of loans, or the bank's internal policies can only be effectively evaluated through on-site supervision.

On-site examinations usually involve an assessment of asset quality, earnings, liquidity, and the depth of management systems and controls. On-site examinations can take different forms, depending on the sophistication and experience of the supervisors and the degree of development in the banking system. In more sophisticated systems, supervisors go beyond simply determining banks' financial condition to assess the manner in which banks manage risk. Alternatively, supervisors may decide to rely in different degrees on the external and internal auditors of banks. Bank supervisors also use management meetings to verify how well the business is doing, management's basic strategy, and how well policy is implemented.

These meetings may also replace parts of on-site supervision in developed banking systems.

Intervention and Problem Resolution. In several countries, supervisors handle failing banks, while in others specialized agencies, such as a deposit insurance fund, resolve banks' failures. There are still other countries in which ordinary courts hold this responsibility. Whether resolution is or is not a formal responsibility of the supervisory agency, supervisors are usually involved in the resolution process, especially in the preliminary steps that precede the withdrawal of a bank license. For the purpose of minimizing costs, supervisors must closely watch the capital position of each institution, which is not a straightforward task, because loan assessment is a subjective exercise. There is a growing recognition that supervisors should take action at a much earlier point than when regulatory capital is depleted. To this end, several countries have also introduced rules limiting the scope for regulatory forbearance by supervisors. These "prompt corrective action" rules typically include thresholds on the level of the capital adequacy ratio, with each threshold triggering a set of predetermined actions, leading ultimately to the closure and resolution of problem banks before their capital declines to negative levels.

The Legal Structure and Scope of the Supervision Agency. The particular location, legal status, and scope of banking supervision have been subject to considerable debate. Frequently discussed points include whether the bank supervision function should be located inside the central bank, the necessary degree of formal legal independence that it should possess, and whether it should be formally integrated into agencies with other supervisory functions (for example, for insurance and capital markets). Advocates for the location of bank supervision inside the central bank point out the synergies between the monetary policy and regulatory functions, the advantages of the independent status of the central bank, and the economies of scale. The critics of this solution stress the potential conflicts of interest that may result from the concentration of functions. When supervision is located outside the central bank, there is an awareness that it must be endowed with the necessary regulatory and enforcement powers, but there is no consensus on whether it should have the same status of independence usually enjoyed by central banks.

There has recently been a growing discussion as to whether the different supervisory agencies should be merged into a single integrated structure. Proponents of this solution stress that the increase in the number of financial conglomerates and the blurring of the boundaries between products make separate supervisory bodies increasingly ineffective and argue that an integrated agency can achieve much greater efficiency. It is on the basis of these considerations that several countries in the Organization for

Economic Cooperation and Development (OECD) have adopted full or partial integration of their supervisory agencies. The critics of integrated supervision stress that major differences remain in the nature of business of banks and other financial institutions, the structure of their assets and liabilities, and the risks that they assume. They claim that these differences justify a differentiated approach to regulation and supervision, although with all the appropriate coordination channels.[4]

The Regulation and Supervision of the Pension Industry

In examining the pension fund industry, it is important to keep in mind the great variety of pension funds across countries and even within a single country. There are defined benefit (DB) and defined contribution (DC) funds; closed (occupational) and open funds; funds constituted as profit-oriented joint stock companies and funds constituted as nonprofit mutuals; funds with and without boards, including a variety of rules on board composition within the first group; and mandatory and voluntary funds. The existence of a great variety of funds is easily appreciated by realizing that there may be multiple combinations of these different characteristics.

The chapter places more emphasis on the analysis of DC funds because most countries have shown a general trend of shifting from DB to DC funds and also because most of the new second pillars that have been introduced in the last two decades operate on a DC basis. However, the chapter examines the different legal constructions of pension funds, since these differences have important implications for regulation and supervision.

Governance Structures for Pension Funds

In examining the governance structures of pension funds, it is useful to classify pension funds into four broad classes: (i) accounts in banks or insurance companies, (ii) participating endowment insurance funds, (iii) pension funds run by management companies, and (iv) foundations/trusts/mutuals. Most private pension arrangements fall into one of these four broad classes, particularly into the last two classes. There are some additional arrangements, such as the system of book reserves, but these types of arrangements will not be examined, since they exist in a small number of countries and are generally considered to be an unattractive option.

Pension plans in banks or insurance companies are common in most developed countries. These plans are defined contribution and are treated essentially as another form of policy or deposit, although several of them have additional restrictions and performance obligations. Pension plan members are not represented in the boards of these institutions unless they also happen to be their shareholders. They may be able to vote with their feet and change plans, although frequently subject to considerable restrictions and penalties. The quality of corporate governance in these cases depends fundamentally on the quality of the regulatory framework for insurance companies and banks. The lack of clear segregation of assets in these cases is a key regulatory issue.

Participating endowment insurance funds are allowed in some OECD countries and constitute the third pillar in the Czech Republic. This type of fund is constructed as a separate joint stock company, with shareholders and plan participants. As in the case above, there is a board, but plan participants are not represented in the board unless they also happen to be shareholders. Also, plan members may be able to change funds, although usually subject to restrictions and penalties. The quality of governance depends on the legal and regulatory framework for joint stock companies and for this type of fund in particular. This type of construction is more transparent than simple policies or accounts in insurance companies and banks, since the fund is separately constituted. However, this type of fund also suffers from the problem of lack of asset segregation (between participants and shareholders).

Open funds without boards and run by a management company are the only permitted structure in most of Latin America. In other countries, this structure is permitted but is not the only one. These funds operate as mutual funds without voting rights. They are usually managed by parent entities engaged primarily in financial services. These management companies typically invest the resources directly, making strategy and selection decisions in house. They also perform individual account maintenance functions and often serve as intermediaries in the purchase of annuity contracts. Participants are generally permitted to switch accounts among a limited set of companies, resulting in a "managed competition" type of market discipline.

These funds are defined contribution, but the regulatory framework frequently imposes some performance obligation on the asset manager. The quality of governance depends fundamentally on the regulatory framework for management companies. Since there are no boards, fund members do not have voting rights and are expected to exert discipline by voting with their feet. Shifting is usually allowed with few, if any, restrictions and penalties. The advantages of this type of construction, relative to the two described above, include much greater transparency and clear asset segregation, since the assets of the pension fund must be held separately from those of the management company. The main problems observed in most countries include the intensive marketing activity, large marketing costs, illegal selling practices, and excessive switching (Queisser 1998; Srinivas, Whitehouse, and

Yermo 2000; Vittas 1998). Regulations and supervisory activity have attempted to address these problems, but with only limited success.

Foundation/trusts/mutuals with boards are very common in the OECD and are usually occupational based but can also be open. Occupational plans are constituted as trusts or foundations and are one of the main forms or pension provision in most developed countries. The board is legally responsible for administering the fund but does not typically directly engage in management activities. These types of organizations are more characteristically constituted as an organizing nexus for members with some type of affiliation (an employer or trade union). The assets of the fund are separated from the sponsor, and management and administration are undertaken through various contractual arrangements. When of sufficient size to be practical, some of the fund management activities may be undertaken in house. Board members may be appointed by an employer or directly by the members or a trade union (or both).

Occupational plans can be either DB or DC. In DC funds the employer's only obligation is to contribute specified amounts to the pension fund. Thus the employer may exercise little diligence in seeking efficient fund management due to the lack of additional financial obligations. However, at least three factors usually mitigate this principal/agent problem. First, the senior management of the employer usually belongs to the plan and has a personal interest in seeing that it is well managed. Second, employers typically compete in the labor market in offering a benefit package and lose competitiveness if the value of the pension benefits offered is discounted in response to weak management. Third, the boards of many occupational funds operating on a DC basis have split representation (employers and employees), which contributes to a better alignment of investment policies with the interests of plan members.

In DB funds the employer normally guarantees the benefit and also contributes to a general guaranty fund. This gives the employer a strong financial interest in the performance of the fund because poor performance will increase the employer's costs. Whereas this built-in incentive for performance may be a positive feature of these plans, there are also a variety of problems associated with DB plans. These plans can be a significant source of rigidities in labor markets, since employers seek to bind valued workers with benefit formulas that disproportionately value a longer period of employment. Guarantees can also create substantial moral hazard issues, particularly when the employer faces significant liquidity or solvency problems. In such circumstances, the employer may undermine the funding status of the arrangement by promising future benefits in lieu of cash wages and fail to restore the financial viability of the fund. More seriously, senior management may take their benefits out of the fund before the employer goes into liquidation. DB plans are generally more complex to regulate and supervise and could stretch the institutional capacity of some emerging countries if implemented on a large scale.

The potential principal-agent problem in occupational funds may also depend on whether the plan is sponsored by a single employer or by many employers. The presence of a single employer as an interested sponsor holding responsibility for the quality and results of asset management has often helped to ensure that these plans operate efficiently. Multi-employer occupational plans may prove more problematic. In contrast to single-employer arrangements, in which the equity of the sponsors can effectively substitute for capital, some types of multi-employer plans may lack a financially liable and interested sponsor. Although the board of the plan may be held legally liable for the consequences of fraud and negligence, there may be no practical mechanism to ensure accountability for their decisions and secure financial assistance from the sponsors.

Although the performance of occupational-based funds may be affected by a potential principal-agent problem, the extent of this problem should not be exaggerated. A serious problem would have to be reflected sooner or later on the main performance indicators, namely, returns and costs. As shown in figure 5.1, the average return of private pension funds in the United Kingdom, the United States, Ireland, and the Netherlands (countries where occupational arrangements dominate the pension industry and where portfolio composition is subject to few restrictions) have been

Figure 5.1. Pension Fund Returns in Selected OECD Countries

Percent

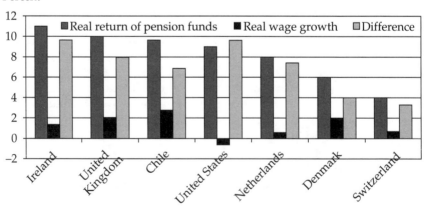

Real Wage Growth and Real Returns on Pension Funds (1984–1996)

Source: OECD (1997).

comparable or higher than the returns generated by Chilean funds over the same period, especially if measured in relation to wage growth. The returns in Switzerland and Denmark were lower, but this was in part due to restrictive investment regulations, rather than governance problems.[5]

Occupational plans also operate with lower costs than open funds run by management companies, largely because of the absence of marketing activities. As shown in table 5.1, the differences among the costs of different plans is primarily determined by the type of contract (that is, whether the plan is occupational and operates with group contracts, or whether it is open and offers transferable individual accounts) and not by the type of benefit (DB or DC). Note that for the younger systems in table 5.1 (Argentina, Chile, and Australia) two ratios of charges to assets are provided—the actual and the long-term equivalent (as calculated by Whitehouse 2000). The long-term equivalent is more relevant for comparison with mature systems. Although some of the costs of occupational plans are hidden (subsidized by the sponsor), these hidden costs tend to be limited to subsidized rental space and salaries and fees of board members and directors and are probably small in comparison with the large marketing costs of open plans, which account for roughly half of total costs in many countries.

Finally, in addition to trusts and foundations, there are also pension funds with boards operating as mutuals (the fund is a nonprofit entity and

Table 5.1. Charges of Different Private Pension Plans in Selected Countries

Country	Year	Type of fund/contract	Type of benefit	Charges/assets (percent)[a]	Charges/ contributions (percent)
Argentina	1999	Open/Individual	DC	5.8 (a); 1.2 (lr)	23
Chile	1999	Open/Individual	DC	1.4 (a); 0.8 (lr)	16
Australia	1999	Occupational/Group	DC	1.2 (a); 0.5 (lr)	9
Australia	1999	Open/Individual	DC	1.5 (a); 2.0 (lr)	29
Ireland	1998	Occupational/Group	DB	0.7 (a)	12
South Africa	1997	Occupational/Group	DB	0.5 (a)	7
Switzerland	1997	Occupational/Group	DC	0.44 (a)	6.6
U.K.[b]	1998	Occupational/Group	DB	0.2–0.5 (a)	8–12
U.K.	1998	Open/Individual	DC	1.2 (lr)	24

a. (a) represents the actual ratio and (lr) the long-run equivalent as calculated by Whitehouse (2000).
b. The two numbers for the costs of occupational funds in the United Kingdom are the weighted and unweighted averages.
Sources: Whitehouse (2000); Government Actuary's Department (U.K.); Irish Pensions Board; Australian Supervision Agency; South African Financial Supervisory Agency; Argentine Supervision of Pension Funds; Vittas and Queisser (2000).

the board is elected from the members). This is the situation in Hungary, where both open and employer-based funds operate under this legal structure. However, the existence of a board with legal obligations does not necessarily imply that members are represented and control the operation of the fund. In the case of the open funds, it is very difficult for the board to change the asset manager, because the asset manager dominates the board and was the reason most of the members joined the fund in the first place. Therefore, the open funds in Hungary operate de facto like open funds without a board and run by a management company (as in Latin America). The employer-based funds more closely resemble the Anglo- Saxon trusts because of the closer link with a sponsoring employer and a board that may play a meaningful role. However, the employer-based funds account for a very small share of the second pillar.

Identifying the Risks of Pension Funds

As with any type of financial institution, the regulation of pension funds originates with the identification and assessment of risks. Although fund members are subject to a great variety of risks, these risks can be grouped in three major classes: (i) portfolio or investment risk, (ii) agency risks, and (iii) systemic risks.[6]

Portfolio risk contains unsystematic or diversifiable risk and systematic or market risk. Proper portfolio diversification eliminates the unsystematic risk, leaving only the market risk. One of the main objectives of regulation is to ensure that portfolios are well diversified, while also eliminating some very risky and illiquid assets from the range of investment opportunities. Plan members are still subject to the risk of fluctuations in the market, even after proper diversification. This could be due to a variety of factors, such as normal fluctuations in asset prices, episodes of bubbles and crashes, and unexpected jumps in inflation. The exposure to market risk tends to decline with increased extension of the time horizon and the holding periods, but an element of risk always remains (see chapter 11 of this volume; Krishnamurthi 1999). There are proposals to deal with market risk, but most of these proposals involve complications and some negative side effects (as examined below).

Agency risks arise when the interests of fund administrators and asset managers are not fully aligned with the interests of fund members. The complex portfolio strategies associated with long-term investment horizons, the informational asymmetries between fund managers and members, and the low levels of legal and financial sophistication of many fund members create room for incompetence, inefficiencies, and abuse. The types of agency risks depend in good part on the legal and governance structure of pension funds (as described above), but all these types of funds are exposed, in one way or another, to agency risks.

The most immediate and obvious agency risk is the potential for fraud, misfeasance, malfeasance, or outright theft of assets. High-visibility incidents, such as the Maxwell case in the United Kingdom, the diversion of union pension funds in the United States by organized crime syndicates in the 1960s and early 1970s, and, more recently, the disappearance of self-designated "pension funds" in the former Soviet Union have repeatedly brought this problem into sharp focus.

The well-publicized cases where the fund's assets are transferred to personal accounts in exotic locations are the most obvious manifestations of agency risk, but there are other, more subtle channels, through which fund administrators and asset managers can siphon value away from plan members. Self-investment, investment in related companies, directed fee arrangements, and kickbacks constitute other examples. There is also room for a reduction in net returns, through large overhead costs and fees. There are many opportunities for this problem in pension fund management because of the multiple types of fees that may be charged, including administrative, asset management, and transaction fees, as well charges associated with annuitization.

Finally, systemic risks arise from the links between the pension industry and other areas of the financial system (and the economy as a whole). Although pension funds have minimal liquidity concerns related to a "run on the bank," they may be affected by banking crises that can result in a sharp collapse in asset prices, negatively affecting some cohorts and leading to the insolvency of several banks. To the extent that fund managers are subsidiaries of banks, there is an overall erosion of capital protection in the pension industry. For the same reasons, the industry is also subject to negative spillover effects from other industries, such as the insurance industry. Finally, a general economic downturn can also deteriorate the financial status of sponsors (in occupational plans). Among employer-sponsored arrangements, sectoral losses in employment leading to early or bunched retirements may result in payout requirements that are coincident with negative investment returns and a loss of contributions.

The Regulation of Pension Funds

Although private pension regulatory regimes are consistent in their attempt to address the various risks identified above, they vary in the manner in which they handle risks. This variation originates with a number of factors, including the historical evolution of the system, the particular legal structure of the pension funds, the state of institutional and regulatory development of capital markets and of economic development in general, as well as unique political and cultural environments. It is possible, however, to identify the main components of regulation found in most countries, which typically include licensing (authorization) criteria, governance rules, asset segregation rules, independent custodian, external audit/actuary, disclosure requirements, investment regulation, guarantees, minimum capital and reserves, and regulations on costs and fees.

Licensing criteria are adopted in most every country, although the conditions for licensing can differ substantially across countries and institutional models. Countries allowing only open funds operated by management companies generally focus on the capital and professional credentials of the management company. The supervisors in these countries typically seek to limit agency and systemic risks by imposing extensive licensing procedures in conjunction with capital and reserve requirements, as well as "fit and proper" tests. This limits entry to a relatively small number of entities, making in-depth oversight practical, and provides a significant source of security, albeit possibly at the cost of implicit rents on capital.

Systems utilizing the trust/foundation approach impose less stringent licensing requirements and rarely require capital or reserves, although they may verify the qualifications and reputation of trustees. This approach to licensing is a reflection of the voluntary employment origins of the system, which relies on minimizing costs and entry barriers to attract participants. It also represents an implicit reliance on the capital of sponsoring employers to secure assets. Other methods, such as bonding requirements in the United States for parties handling assets, are less restrictive than those applied in Latin America.

Governance Rules. In occupational funds, the boards usually play a number of important functions: setting broad investment strategies, delegating responsibility for the management of funds to a range of service providers, and monitoring performance. Clear rules on board composition, voting rights, and duties and responsibilities of board members can help improve fund governance and minimize agency risks. For example, the 1995 Pension Act in the United Kingdom clarified and enhanced the role of trustees and greatly emphasized education of trustees. However, the importance of the board in occupational schemes in the OECD also depends partly on the particular legal setting. Trust laws typically impose a greater reach of personal liability for responsible parties than do commercial codes, often penetrating corporate liability shields and permitting the attachment of personal property. In continental Europe, several countries attempt to reduce agency risks by mandating split representation in the boards.

In open funds operated by management companies, the governance rules apply to the management companies themselves, since the funds typically have no boards. The management companies must be exclusively dedicated to pension fund management; they cannot delegate or subcontract their management functions, and they can each manage only one pension fund. The quality of governance depends in great part on the quality of the rules applicable to the boards of management companies, that is, rules concerning self-dealing and conflicts of interest, the responsibility of board members, and the exposure of board members to personal liability. In the countries where open funds have boards (Hungary, for example), the management company typically dominates and appoints the board and plays a more limited role in practice. In this case, the rules applying to the management company will be critical in determining the quality of governance.

Asset segregation rules aim at separating the pool of fund assets from the assets of the sponsor/management company in order to protect members' balances and vested rights and limit systemic and agency risks. Asset segregation is obtained by construction in open funds operated by management companies and is also obtained in most occupational funds through the requirement that assets be held in a separate legal entity, such as the Anglo-American trust fund (except for the book reserve system, which requires insolvency insurance). Asset segregation does not hold in pension plans operated internally by insurance companies and/or banks (nor in endowment insurance funds). Although good prudential regulation of banks and insurance companies should protect the assets of plan members, there is definitely more scope for negative spillovers from banking and insurance crisis (systemic risk) in these cases.

External custodian rules are also essential to limit agency risks. Under adequate custodian arrangements, the administration of the fund and/or asset managers never directly hold legal title to the assets of the pension fund, limiting the opportunities for fraud and theft by requiring a separate party with defined responsibilities to execute all transactions. Custodians can also help enforce prudential regulations by refusing to effectuate transactions that violate investment guidelines and other rules. For the custodian protection to be effective, however, it must control the flow of payments from members to the funds/asset managers without interruptions. Some systems allow gaps in such a control, opening room for misappropriation of funds.

Disclosure requirements involve a number of important rules, such as asset valuation rules, the frequency of asset valuation, and the distribution of relevant information (for example, on returns, costs, levels of capital and reserves) to fund members and the general public. Disclosure requirements are generally regarded as an essential component of regulation across all the sectors of the financial system. In the pension industry, however, disclosure requirements vary substantially across countries and models.

Disclosure requirements are very important in mandatory DC schemes, particularly those allowing unrestricted choice. Open funds in most Latin American countries are subject to extensive disclosure requirements, which usually include daily asset valuation on a "mark to market" basis, distribution of account statements to members several times a year, and the publication of detailed information on the industry by the supervision agency in quarterly and annual bulletins. Such an extensive disclosure of information is designed to enable workers to make informed choices, put competitive pressure on asset managers, and allow switching on a fair basis. The disclosure requirements themselves are an attractive feature of these systems, although marketing efforts seem to drive the extensive switching across funds more than objective comparisons of returns and costs (Queisser 1998; Srinivas, Whitehouse, and Yermo 2000; Vittas 1998).

Disclosure requirements in OECD countries are generally less extensive. In some countries regulators impose disclosure of information, albeit mostly through annual reporting, and also permit greater discretion in terms of valuation. The reliability of these reports is assessed through external independent audit requirements because it is not feasible to review the large number of regulated entities. In some countries there are no legal requirements to disclose information (OECD 1998). The less extensive disclosure requirements in the OECD probably derive from the occupational nature of the pension industry. Funds are less pressed to publish frequent and detailed individual statements in systems that restrict individual switching. It has also been argued that under these systems, there may also be a rationale for allowing some deviation from mark-to-market valuation rules. Valuation techniques based on projected revenues from assets and other interest accrual methods smooth fluctuations in asset prices and may enable funds to hold a larger share of equity in their portfolios. Thus, it has been argued that this is one reasons why British funds generally held more equity and obtained higher returns (OECD 1998).

Despite these justifications for more flexible disclosure rules in occupational funds, it is still surprising that some OECD countries do not impose any legal obligation to disclose information, since members must be informed about the situation of the fund in order to be able to exert discipline and control over the fund's situation and reduce agency risks, irrespective of whether the fund is occupational or not and whether it operates on a DB or DC basis.

External audits of pension fund accounts are required in every country, although the scope and quality of external audits may vary substantially from country to country. In underdeveloped legal and institutional environments, the external audits do not provide an independent and objective assessment of the fund's situation, and the legal responsibilities of auditors are not clear and/or enforceable. In other countries, external audits not only provide an accurate and independent assessment but also constitute the most important tool of supervision. Auditors are required to report any problems to the supervisor and are legally liable for failure to do so. External actuaries play a similar role in DB schemes or DC schemes with guarantees.

Investment Regulations. The stated objective of investment regulations in most countries is to ensure diversification and minimize agency, systemic, and, especially, portfolio risks. The regulations typically involve ceilings on holdings by issuer, type of instrument, risk, concentration of ownership, and asset class. Whereas the first four restrictions are considered as non-controversial prudential rules, restrictions by asset class constitute one particular area of regulation that has generated more controversy.

There is a group of OECD countries that does not impose restrictions by asset class, other than the prescription that the portfolio be managed prudently in this regard. The regulatory framework in these countries (which are mostly the Anglo-Saxon countries and the Netherlands) is said to follow the Prudent Man Rule, or Prudent Investor's Rule, which simply requires that those responsible make investment decisions while exercising diligence and considering the specific circumstances of the fund. The usual adjunct is a dictate for diversification and a duty of loyalty (sole consideration of the members' interests). This rule usually permits higher risk assets to be included in a pension portfolio so long as the risk is hedged elsewhere in the portfolio.

In contrast, a second group of OECD countries and all Latin American countries impose restrictions by asset class. Investment regulation in these countries has been labeled "quantitative" or "draconian" (OECD 1998; Queisser 1998; Srinivas, Whitehouse, and Yermo 2000; Vittas 1998).[7] These regulations typically specify the maximum amount that pension funds can invest by asset class, although some countries also specify ceilings on individual assets and even minimum holdings of assets (typically government bonds).

There is evidence that real returns of pension funds in prudent man environments have been higher than the returns of funds operating in more restrictive environments, essentially because of a larger share of equity in their portfolios (Davis 1995; OECD 1998), although investment restrictions cannot entirely explain the difference because these were not binding in many countries. It is clear that investment restrictions may be counterproductive in principle, since they may prevent diversification and expose fund members to a greater degree of portfolio risk. However, it is also understood that investment restrictions may be initially justified in countries with underdeveloped institutional and regulatory structures and shallow asset markets. The draconian approach is also simple and easy to police. The prudent man approach requires a greater element of judgement by the supervisor and necessitates a substantial interpretive effort to assist practitioners in understanding how the general principles will be applied. It is consequently associated with greater uncertainty for all parties. While in principle it should preclude outlying investment behavior, in practice the courts in the United States have been reluctant to reverse even highly risky investment behavior solely on the basis of prudence, unless losses have been realized.

The literature on pension fund regulation generally concludes that investment restrictions may initially be justified in emerging countries introducing private pension schemes, particularly those introducing a mandatory second pillar. However, there is also a consensus on the need for these countries to relax the restrictions over time in accordance with the development of institutions and instruments and improvements in the depth and liquidity of securities markets and the overall legal framework. The long-run objective would be the adoption of the prudent man approach in which minimal restrictions are imposed. The experience of Chile in this area is regarded as a positive example for other reforming countries.

A more recent and controversial issue in the area of investment regulation relates to the debate on single versus multiple portfolios. The portfolios of pension funds in most countries are already reasonably diversified, and the degree of diversification has been increasing with the relaxation of investment restrictions in many countries and the increase in the share of equity and foreign assets (Davis 1995; OECD 1998). However, it has been argued that the overall degree of diversification is still insufficient because the portfolio composition across funds tends to be similar due to a strong herding effect.[8] Even in countries where switching is allowed, workers do not have a meaningful choice among risk-return combinations because all the available portfolios are essentially identical. Thus young and old workers are forced to hold the same portfolio, which is suboptimal for both, because young workers would favor portfolios that exploit risk and liquidity premiums (with a larger share of equity), while older workers would require portfolios with less risk and greater liquidity (with a larger share of short-term, fixed income assets). Although several pension funds calibrate their investment policies to the average age of the fund members, it could be argued that the portfolio would still be suboptimal for members of different ages. To help solve this problem, it has been proposed that workers be offered a choice of more than one portfolio (for example, Srinivas, Whitehouse, and Yermo 2000). This issue will be examined in more detail in the next section.

Guarantees. Most countries that have introduced a second, mandatory pillar have also introduced some form of guarantee on second-pillar returns. In Latin America and Central Europe, most minimum return guarantees have been expressed in relative terms, although there have been several variations around this theme. These minimum return guarantees have been defined relative to the average return of all pension funds, to a broader market benchmark, or to a combination of both. They can also be expressed in nominal or real terms. For example, Chilean funds have to achieve a minimum return equal to 50 percent of the average real return of the industry, and Argentine funds must achieve a minimum return equal to 70 percent of the average nominal return of the industry.[9] The minimum reserves and equity imposed on the asset manager usually back these guarantees. The level of minimum reserves is usually stated as a fraction (1–2 percent) of the size of assets under management. In the case of insolvency of the asset manager, there is usually an explicit guarantee from the budget.

Other countries have introduced minimum absolute rates of return, expressed either in nominal or real terms. Switzerland provides a minimum nominal return of 4 percent per annum, backed by a central guarantee fund. This guarantee has amounted to a minimum real return of around 2 percent per year, given the low levels and stability of inflation in Switzerland. Hungary has introduced a minimum second-pillar benefit that is defined in relation to the first-pillar benefit. This benefit can be expressed in terms of a minimum rate of return, although the rate of return is age-specific. Under baseline assumptions, this guarantee is equal to a reasonable 0 percent real rate of return for young workers, calculated over the working life, but a much more ambitious 4 percent real rate of return for workers in their forties. A central guarantee fund and the imposition of minimum reserves on the pension funds back the guarantee. The minimum reserve of pension funds is used when the returns are lower than 85 percent of a benchmark portfolio.

The introduction of guarantees always raises three interrelated issues. The first is the types of risk that the guarantee is expected to cover. The question here is whether the guarantee is excessive or not. The second is the amount of capital backing the guarantee. Critical here is whether the capital buffer is consistent with the probability of the guarantee being called and the size of the exposure. The third is the changes in behavior triggered by the guarantee. The key point is the extent to which the guarantee itself modifies behavior in perverse ways (moral hazard).

Relative guarantees such as those introduced in Latin America attempt to deal primarily with incompetent/inefficient asset management, fraudulent behavior, and other agency risks. They do not attempt to deal with market risk. Also, the typical construction in Latin America puts private capital at risk to some degree with the exposure (that is, the reserves and equity of the asset manager are a fraction of the assets managed) before the government guarantee is called. Therefore, the guarantee is not overly generous and does not seem to induce excessive risk-taking behavior by asset managers. The problem that has been observed in Latin America is the herding behavior of pension funds; as mentioned before, herding in Latin America seems more intense than herding among pension funds in the OECD.[10]

Absolute guarantees such as those introduced in Switzerland and to some extent in Hungary attempt to deal with market risk as well, by introducing some measure of intergenerational risk pooling (as in DB schemes). Both countries back this guarantee by a central guarantee fund (supported by mandatory contributions from all pension funds) but without putting private capital at risk first. Swiss funds are not forced to constitute minimum reserves or capital. Hungarian funds are forced to hold minimum reserves of 0.5 percent of the size of individual accounts, but these reserves are imposed at the level of the fund itself, not the asset manager.

These constructions are, in principle, flawed because they provide access to the resources of a central guarantee fund without putting private capital at risk first. The scheme has operated in Switzerland, apparently without major problems, partly because of the implicit links with the sponsor and the reputation and goodwill factors. Single-employer funds usually provide resources required for the fund to reach the minimum 4 percent (sometimes pressed by the supervisory authority), and open funds (managed by insurance companies or banks) also provide the resources necessary for the fund to reach the minimum, in order to safeguard their reputation. Therefore, the system seems to operate relatively well without explicit legal backing because of recourse to more implicit forms of private capital protection.

In the case of Hungary, the guarantee is less generous for younger workers but more generous for older workers. It is fortunate that most of the workers in the new Hungarian system are under the age of 35, but the probability that workers in their forties will trigger the guarantee is not negligible. As mentioned before, the other problem is that the minimum reserves have been imposed at the level of the pension fund, not the asset manager. If these reserves need to be used, they may be replenished from new contributions, rather than from the resources of the asset manager, implying that there is no effective link with private capital. Therefore, this construction also depends on more implicit links with the sponsors, which are large companies in the case of employer-based funds, or large banks and insurance companies in the case of open funds. Although these sponsors are usually well-established organizations with their reputation at stake and will probably back their pension funds, the protection still lacks an explicit legal base.

Capital/Reserve Requirements. The notion of capital does not have meaning in funds constituted as trusts, foundations, and mutuals, since these legal entities do not have shareholders, although the liability assigned to the sponsors of these arrangements often serves as a proxy. In pure DC schemes providing no minimum returns, there is no rationale to constitute capital, except in the form of voluntary reserves, agreed by the members and designed to smooth fluctuations in yearly returns. DC schemes may also voluntarily adopt portfolio strategies that involve an implicit target rate of return and smoothing of short-term returns. This can be achieved by use of immunization strategies that smooth the impact of short-term fluctuations in interest rates and/or use of derivatives to limit the impact of equity price fluctuations on the pension fund.

If the fund has an explicit obligation to produce minimum returns, then it becomes essential to impose capital requirements commensurate with the obligation. As mentioned before, in Latin America these requirements are imposed on the management company.[11] Two countries with mandatory DC schemes have constituted central guarantee schemes to which all funds have to contribute. The asset managers/management companies in these countries do not need to constitute capital and reserves. The foundations in Switzerland do not need to constitute reserves either, whereas the Hungarian mutuals do. The Hungarian construction is possibly slightly better than the Swiss, since it signals to fund members that they need to exert discipline on the asset manager. However, asset managers/sponsors do not have their capital explicitly at risk in either country.

Restrictions on fees are a common feature in Latin American and Eastern European systems. Chile, for example, permits only certain categories of fees, prohibiting exit charges, asset-based management fees, and performance fees. In contrast, commissions for selling agents and annuity conversions are held to a prescribed level. Hungary places limits on the fees that the fund may charge for administration but places no specific limits on what it may pay asset managers. Trust-based systems generally do not explicitly regulate fees. In the United States, the general prudence requirements indirectly regulate fee levels through a provision in the law that specifies only that they be "reasonable." It is debatable whether regulation of fees in the pension industry (and in the financial sector more generally) can be enforced and whether it produces the desired effects (assuming that they can be enforced). Regulation of costs may lead to the shifting of costs to other unregulated categories and a loss of transparency. Prescribed limits may also result in a clustering of expenses at the maximum. The reasonableness approach, in contrast, is difficult to enforce because it is associated with systems with many funds (700,000 in the United States).

The Supervision of Pension Funds

The supervision of pension funds incorporates the same three basic aspects relevant to the oversight of banks discussed in the previous section: (i) licensing activities, (ii) ongoing monitoring, and (iii) remedial and punitive problem resolution. However, consistent with the greater diversity of system designs and regulatory approaches outlined above, there is greater variation in these supervision programs than among those for banks. In general, the pension supervisory programs reflect the regulatory frameworks that they are designed to implement.

In this respect, supervision of pension funds may generally be categorized as following two basic models. The first model is characterized as proactive (Demarco, Rofman, and Whitehouse 1998; Vittas 1998) and is associated with systems based on a small number of open funds, such as those operating in most Latin American countries. This approach emphasizes the first two building blocks, limiting participation in the system through strict licensing criteria, imposing extensive reporting requirements, close off-site surveillance, and regular on-site examinations. It is closer to the bank supervision model followed in most countries.

The alternative supervisory model is associated with systems that use the trust/foundation form of organization. Supervision within this model is labeled as reactive, because the supervisor usually intervenes only when problems are reported, either by trustees, fund members, external auditors, actuaries, or other relevant players (including other supervisors). Pension supervision is more remedial in nature, or more oriented toward the third element of problem resolution. The system essentially relies on other active players monitoring the funds and also on credible deterrents to violations of the laws.

This fundamental difference in these styles of supervision originates from the basic organization of the industry. Among the most important organizational features are the number of funds, the less restrictive practices in occupational-based systems, and the level of development of capital markets and legal systems. The management of assets via other highly regulated financial intermediaries (banks and insurance companies) and the development of independent auditing institutions are of particular significance. The nature of pension funds as second levels of intermediation enables regulators to rely more on other supervisory institutions to provide the first line of defense against fraudulent practices. A tradition of independent audits with a high degree of integrity also permits supervisory authorities to rely on this mechanism for monitoring and deploy their resources toward corrective actions. As with regulatory frameworks, a key differentiation in the applicability of these models is the level of development of the economy. A reactive approach is only feasible in the context of developed economies with well-established and reliable financial and legal institutions.

Despite the importance of supervisory institutions and programs to the security of private pension systems, at present there is very little literature on the various institutional arrangements and operations of pension supervisory agencies. The methods in use, however, may be generally categorized as follows.

Licensing of Funds. The range of methods for the approval of funds to operate is one of the more widely varied areas of supervision. In most Latin American and Central European countries, with systems based on a small number of open funds, licensing constitutes one of the primary activities of the supervisory agencies, which may often have a distinct unit devoted to this process. Prior to the granting of licenses, funds are required to provide extensive documentation regarding their compliance with minimum capital levels, reserves, or other financial criteria. The legal forms of organization of the fund management, business and marketing plans, investment policies, and the qualifications of relevant staff are also scrutinized.

Representing the other end of the spectrum, countries such as the United States do not require any specific license for employer-sponsored pension funds. The requirements to operate are indirectly established, through written documents that set forth terms of the trust and benefit formulas and designate individuals with specific responsibilities. However, these are not required to be submitted to any government authority for approval, only to be made available to participants and supervisory authorities on request. The only action similar to licensing is the application of preferential tax treatment to the appropriate tax authorities. Many other OECD countries fall within this range. Australia requires no license for the fund to operate but requires approval of the trustees.

Monitoring and Inspection. The core of most supervisory programs is the monitoring of the activities of funds. This involves two main components: the review of reports on the financial status of pension funds (off-site surveillance) and the conduct of on-site reviews. In proactive environments, supervisors utilize reports to monitor portfolio composition and other structural requirements in effectively a real-time environment, taking preemptive action on the basis of the information. Supervisors operating in the reactive mode generally receive financial reports after more extended periods, often annually, and use the data to select funds with indications of potential problems for more in-depth review.

On-site inspections are often the most visible element of a supervision program, and supervisory agencies will typically devote substantial resources to these kinds of activities. Differences lie in the objectives, scope, and frequency of these reviews. Proactive systems structure these reviews as audits, in which there is a systematic attempt to review all aspects of the funds activities, tracing contributions through to individual accounts, verifying the completeness and accuracy of financial statements, and evaluating adherence to investment limitations and other requirements. These inspections are undertaken on a regular schedule, with all funds reviewed at least annually, with the objective of making a full assessment of compliance.

Alternatively, reactive arrangements often entail on-site inspection on an ad hoc basis in response to a complaint or specific indication of a problem. Examination tends to be more specific, focusing on a set of transactions, the flow of individual contributions, or fee arrangements. Once such a review is initiated, however, it may lead to the examination of other issues. This mode is partly a practical response to the need to cover a myriad of funds with limited resources, but it also reflects the reliance on independent auditors to undertake in-depth reviews of the institutions. Some supervisory programs also include random investigations designed to provide a cost-effective deterrence presence. In these kinds of regimes, establishing effective systems for processing complaints and developing algorithms for the automated review of annual reports are critical to the success of the endeavor.

Problem Resolution. The application of sanctions for remedial and punitive purposes is usually the most difficult part of any supervisory program. In countries employing more proactive systems, there is a heavy emphasis on preemptively addressing compliance issues, by providing supervisory agencies the authority to direct funds to make changes in their operations. The corrective actions in reactive systems more closely resemble civil or commercial legal proceedings. In these systems, letters or more formal legal complaints are more likely to be the predicate to corrective action. In addition, some supervisors, perhaps most notably in the Netherlands, have also relied on moral suasion in the form of exposing problem institutions to bad publicity, which has apparently been effective in correcting problems. Virtually all systems provide access to the courts to resolve the most contentious problems and contain a check on the authority of the supervisors.

A final key aspect of supervision is the placement of the authority. While all approaches necessitate political independence in the regulation of pension funds, there are systemic differences in the placement of this authority. Latin American countries have generally established independent institutions, reflecting the underlying construct of pension funds as special-purpose financial institutions. Most others have established the authority as a distinct unit within a larger public institution, placing regulators under the broader auspices, most commonly, of Finance or Labor Ministries, or Insurance Regulatory Authorities (see OECD 1998). Two recent East European reforms (Poland and Hungary) have essentially split the difference, creating supervisory authorities that operate with a reasonable degree of independence but that ultimately report to ministries. Consolidating regulators is a greater imperative in systems that are more interactive with other regulated financial intermediaries. The integration of supervision activities in the United Kingdom and some Scandinavian countries represents the furthest extent to which this concept has been advanced.

Scope for Improvements and Possible Lessons from the Banking Industry

Before examining the scope for improvements in pension regulation, and the possible lessons from the banking sector, it is useful to review some of the major differences between banks and pension funds. As mentioned

before, banks are highly leveraged, involved in substantial maturity transformation, and hold assets that are difficult to value and monitor. The
high leverage in banking and the structure of bank liabilities imply a substantial degree of exposure to these risks and the possibility of contagion
effects triggering a chain of bank runs and failures. Pension funds function
with substantially longer time periods than banks and other intermediaries,
with the typical participant having a relevant investment horizon measured
in decades rather than months or years. They are also prohibited, with relatively few exceptions, from borrowing and leveraging their portfolios,
which tends to minimize their liquidity requirements.

Although systems subject to extensive switching across funds (as those
in Latin America) may shorten the time horizon somewhat and create the
need for some additional liquidity, it remains true that pension funds are
not subject to contagion effects and runs, at least not directly. In systems
dominated by occupational funds, there is little, if any, risk of massive withdrawals in the presence of a crisis in the financial sector. In systems dominated by open funds, there can be withdrawals from individual funds in
principle but not from the system as a whole. Systemic failures are not likely for the same reason, except in hypothetical case in which the funds are
subject to high minimum returns imposed on an annual basis and there is
a major capital market crash, depressing asset prices substantially and for
a protracted period. No country seems to be exposed to this type of extreme
situation. These are very fundamental differences between banks and pension funds that determine major differences between the two regulatory
frameworks (for example, in terms of the imposition of liquidity requirements, access to lender of last resort facilities, the complex machinery of loan
classification and provisioning, and the complex measurement of capital).

At the same time, while pension funds are not subject to systemic runs
and failures, they can still suffer the effects of a major financial crisis in other
ways. It is important however, to examine further what the worst possible
scenario for the pension industry would be, how the industry would be
affected, and the possible regulatory options to deal with it.

The worst possible scenario for pension funds is essentially the same scenario for banks and other financial intermediaries. The economy is subject
to a major macroeconomic shock, generally following a period of rapid output growth. The period of expansion is usually accompanied by steep
increases in asset prices and possibly unsustainable asset price bubbles, particularly in equity markets but also in other markets such as real estate. A
balance of payments crisis usually triggers the shock and typically provokes
a policy response that includes a real devaluation, a fiscal adjustment, and
an initial contraction of credit.

The shock and the policy response usually cause an immediate rise in
interest rates and a contraction in economic activity, concentrated in the sec-

tors that were overexpanded and overleveraged. Several enterprises become insolvent, and bank portfolios deteriorate rapidly, leading to bank insolvency as well. A loss of confidence, which triggers runs on banks, is frequently observed in these cases. Irrespective of whether there are bank runs or not, asset prices decline, and if the period of expansion is accompanied by asset price bubbles, the new equilibrium levels may be substantially lower. Moreover, the decline in asset prices may involve an initial undershooting—prices decline initially more than their new lower equilibrium level.

A financial crisis can affect pension funds in two fundamental ways. First, the pension funds may experience a major decline in the value of their portfolios. Second, they may be subject to negative spillover effects from other areas of the financial and real sectors. The spillover effects are potentially more severe in cases where there is no clear asset segregation, that is, where the pool of pension assets is not separated from the assets of financial intermediaries and companies.

The decline in the real value of pension funds' asset portfolios implies a commensurate decline in the accumulated individual balances and in future pensions, but the impact of this decline needs to be examined, considering the long holding periods with which pension funds operate. Most of the cohorts that experienced a decline in real asset prices as a result of a financial crisis probably benefited from sharp increases in prices in the previous years. The long holding periods imply a smoothing of periods of price level fluctuations and even of sharp price level bubbles and bursts.

The effect of long holding periods can be appreciated by examining the average real returns of pension funds in the OECD over the last three decades. As shown in figure 5.2, the average real returns of pension funds in the OECD were negative during the 1970s. During this decade, the world economy was subject to two oil shocks that caused a sharp contraction in economic activity and unexpected price jumps. Equity markets were depressed during the period, and pension funds also realized sharp capital losses in their portfolio of long-term fixed income securities. On the other hand, during the 1980s and 1990s real returns were extremely high, probably driving the overall average return over the three decades to around 5–6 percent per annum, some 3–4 percent above average wage growth during the same period. These averages mask significant differences across countries. Pension funds subject to less restrictive investment regulations achieved higher returns.

The smoothing effect of long holding periods is generally reassuring, although it must also be recognized that fluctuations in asset prices may lead to differences in replacement ratios across cohorts with the same level of income, even after considering the long-run averaging effect. In a simulation with U.S. data on asset returns covering 125 years (1970–1995), in

Figure 5.2. Annual Real Returns in OECD

Percent

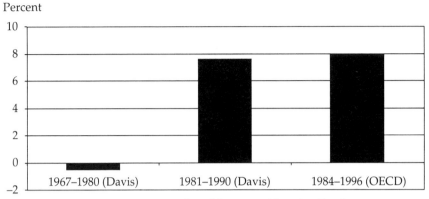

Average Annual Real Returns of Pension Funds
in Sub-Periods, Selected OECD Countries

Sources: Davis (1995); OECD (1997).

chapter 11 of this volume Alier and Vittas find that the average return on a balanced portfolio (consisting of 60 percent equity and 40 percent fixed income assets, and held for a period of 40 years) would have ranged from around 2.5 percent per year in the early part of the century, to more than 8 percent per year in the post-World War II period. These differences in average rates of return would have translated into significant differences in replacement ratios—a 10 percent contribution rate would have generated replacement ratios ranging from a minimum of 22 percent to a maximum of 70 percent.

These simulations should be examined with caution, since they probably overestimate the likely differences in replacement ratios across cohorts generated by real systems. For one, Alier and Vittas also show that only 11 percent of the cohorts would have received replacement ratios under 30 percent of final wages. Achieving a 30 percent replacement ratio with a 10 percent contribution rate is a better result than that provided by most PAYG systems in demographically mature countries. Secondly, the dispersion in replacement ratios would be reduced if the first decades of the century were excluded from the sample. Thirdly, many pension funds already apply asset management techniques designed to smooth the fluctuations in returns over time, and the scope for smoothing returns has increased with increasing portfolio diversification, the development of derivatives, and other hedging techniques.

Although Alier and Vittas' results probably overestimate the likely differences in replacement ratios, they do illustrate the potential effects of market risk on retiring cohorts and raise two important questions for regulators. The first question relates to the size of workers' exposure to market risk and whether there are instruments to deal directly with this type of risk. The second concerns whether or not there are other regulations that would strengthen the governance and management of pension funds and their capacity to cope with these and other risks. In examining these questions, possible lessons from banking regulation will be identified.

Coping with Market Risk: Possibilities and Pitfalls

The exposure of the average retiring worker to market risk depends in the first place on the relative size of the private pillars of retirement provision, particularly the size of the second pillar. Multipillar systems already contain an element of risk diversification, since the implicit returns on the first pillar contributions are weakly correlated with the second pillar returns.[12] The new second pillars that most Central European countries and many Latin American countries have introduced generally account for 25–50 percent of total mandatory contributions (Chile being the exception rather than the rule in this regard). Therefore, the multipillar construction dilutes the exposure of the average worker to market risk. It is important to have this in mind because most measures available to reduce market risk involve complications and negative side effects.

Assuming that pension funds exhaust the potential for risk reduction by proper portfolio diversification (including investment in foreign assets), portfolio risk is reduced to market risk. There are five possible ways to deal with this risk: (i) introduce DB schemes, (ii) introduce guarantees on minimum second-pillar returns and/or benefits, (iii) allow multiple portfolios, (iv) allow deferral of annuities, and (v) introduce variable annuities or a sequence of fixed annuities. These different solutions are examined below.

Introducing DB Schemes. DB schemes deal with market risk by introducing an element of intergenerational risk pooling. However, DB schemes also generate several complications in the labor market and are much more difficult to regulate and supervise. The penalties imposed on early leavers also weaken the intergenerational risk pooling in practice, and their effects may worsen when the sponsor faces financial difficulties. Most importantly, it would be very difficult to implement a mandatory, privately managed second pillar on a standardized DB basis. In fact, the tightening of regulation in voluntary DB schemes in the United States and the United Kingdom and the increasing costs of compliance for employers are the major reasons behind the trend of shifting from DB to DC in the two countries.

Guarantees on Second-Pillar Benefits. Guarantees on minimum second pillar returns/benefits also introduce an element of intergenerational risk pooling. Examples of these type of guarantees are the Swiss minimum 4 percent nominal return (around 2 percent in real terms) and the Hungarian minimum second-pillar benefit, which is equivalent to a minimum lifetime real return of 0–4 percent, depending on the age of the worker (around 2 percent on an age-weighted basis). A central guarantee fund, to which all funds must contribute, backs both guarantees. The introduction of absolute guarantees on second-pillar benefits generates complications similar to those generated by deposit insurance and guarantees in general. As mentioned in section 2, the main lessons from the experience with deposit insurance in the last decades is that the guarantees should be partial and backed by risk-based capital requirements and risk-based insurance premia. The constructions above do not seem to contain most of these elements.

A guaranteed real rate of return of 2 percent applied on an annual basis can hardly be seen as partial. Although the rate itself is lower than the average real return in the OECD over the last three decades, its application on an annual basis is problematic. It allows workers to share periods of boom in asset prices without sharing the downside risk, actually leading to a return above the long-run market average. This guarantee would either prove unsustainable or would need to be financed by very large contributions to the guarantee fund or through the imposition of large fees by the asset manager, thereby reducing the overall net return. An alternative but equally undesirable outcome would involve a very conservative portfolio selection and low returns for fund members.

The Hungarian construction for young workers is better in this regard, since it establishes a minimum real return of around 0 percent, computed over the whole working life. However, this construction introduces other problems, primarily the difficulty of linking the guarantee with capital protection from asset managers/sponsors. This link can only be easily established when the minimum return applies to the level of the fund, not the individual. The Hungarian system tries to cope with this problem by also imposing a minimum annual return on the funds, relative to a market benchmark, but the reserve requirements are imposed on the pension fund itself (a nonprofit mutual), not the asset manager. As mentioned before, neither of the two constructions places private capital explicitly at risk nor defines the insurance premia on a risk-related basis. The contributions to the central guarantee fund in both countries are flat and around 0.4 percent of contributions.

Designing an absolute guarantee on second-pillar benefits that reduces the exposure of individuals to market risk, proves financially sustainable, and minimizes moral hazard is a complex task. It would probably have to include the following elements: (i) a minimum return on individual second-pillar contributions, applied over the working life that would have to be sufficiently low to be sustainable and maintain the worker's interest in

monitoring his or her pension fund, (ii) a minimum performance obliga
tion on the asset manager/sponsor (measured in real return) that would
have to be sufficiently low and computed over a relatively long period, say,
36 rolling months or longer, (iii) the imposition of explicit, possibly risk-
based capital/reserve requirements on the asset manager/sponsor backing the minimum return, and (iv) the imposition of risk-based insurance
premia on the asset managers/pension funds.

The complexity in design can be further appreciated by noting that it
would not be easy to differentiate capital requirements and insurance premia according to risk. Attempting to establish a relation between capital
requirements and insurance premia on the one side, and portfolio risk on
the other side, could lead pension funds to avoid equity, contradicting
some of the main objectives of a second pillar. The regulators could limit
themselves to differentiating institutions according to capital strength
and/or quality of management, but it is not clear to what extent the institutions would accept ratings heavily weighted by the supervisors' subjective evaluations.

On balance, absolute guarantees on second-pillar benefits seem to raise
more costs and complexities than benefits and should generally be avoided, especially in countries where the private mandatory pillar is a component of a multipillar system and accounts for less than half of contributions.
If absolute guarantees are deemed as essential, they should be kept sufficiently low and computed over a relatively long period. Explicit capi-
tal/reserve requirements at the level of the asset manager/sponsor should
match the guarantees. When a guarantee fund is created, consideration
should be given to differentiating insurance premia, although the criteria
for differentiation should probably be restricted to capital and quality of
governance/management.

Multiple Portfolios. As mentioned before, the introduction of more portfolio choices to workers provides an alternative mechanism to deal with
market risk. The assumption underlying this solution is that workers will
make informed portfolio choices and will hold progressively lower shares
of equity as they approach retirement. Under this construction, workers are
expected to bear fully the consequences of poor investments, and the government is not expected to intervene if the outcomes are not favorable.

Whereas the proposals for the introduction of multiple portfolios may
have some merits, it is not clear that the gains would offset the costs. First,
it is generally recognized that multiple portfolios would tend to increase
the costs of administration and compliance. Although these costs would
tend to decrease with developments in electronic technology, they could
still prove a burden in some emerging countries.

Second, the welfare gains depend on how many individuals the single
portfolio effectively constrains. It does not affect high-income individuals,

since they have a large volume of individual savings and can build their own voluntary asset portfolios in a way that offsets any constraints. Low-income individuals do not have individual savings to offset these constraints, but the retirement income of low-income workers in many countries comes primarily from the first pillar (PAYG) benefits, especially in the cases where the first pillar is large and redistributive. The welfare gains from multiple portfolios would be relatively modest in these cases. Therefore, they would be concentrated among the average-income individuals and could still be substantial or not, depending on the size of mandatory portfolios in total pension wealth (including the first-pillar benefits), the extent to which these individuals are already offsetting these restrictions through voluntary savings, and income (and age) distribution.

Third, the gains would also depend on whether individuals would make informed decisions about the composition of their portfolios. In this regard, the experience with 401(k) plans in the United States, which now typically provide at least four to five choices to participants, is rather mixed. Although it is reassuring that the share of equity is negatively correlated with age, the patterns of asset composition still differ significantly from prior expectations—relatively large numbers of young workers seem to hold small amounts of equity, and relatively large numbers of old workers seem to hold large amounts of equity (Srinivas, Whitehouse, and Yermo 2000). Market surveys of workers participating in these plans also indicate that the average level of financial sophistication is rather low (Vittas 1998).

Fourth, given the long holding periods (30–40 years), the size of the gain of a strategy that involves declining equity shares (say, from 80 to 20 percent of the portfolio) relative to a balanced portfolio (with 50–60 percent invested in equity) is not clear.[13]

Finally, the strategy of multiple portfolios to deal with market risk faces one additional constraint in the case of new second pillars. It is generally recommended that new private pillars in emerging markets start with conservative portfolios and gradually build their holdings of equity and other riskier assets, since capital markets mature in depth and liquidity. Therefore, one cannot expect that young workers will be holding large shares of equity in the early years of implementation. Expecting workers to hold less equity in the final years when they cannot hold large amounts in their first years implies a relatively low proportion of equity over the working life, which defeats some of the objectives of a second pillar.

Multiple portfolios can still be seen as an elegant and efficient construction in sophisticated environments and within the context of voluntary arrangements. To be effective, it requires the development of a regulatory framework that allocates liability for investment decisions among members directing their accounts and fund administrators conducting all the other activities, which imposes a substantial new layer of complexity on any system. It also requires an extensive and ongoing program of education for fund members. Both of these considerations limit the applicability to well-developed systems serving sophisticated populations. Introducing multiple portfolios in mandatory pillars and less sophisticated environments requires a more careful assessment of costs and benefits.

Deferral of Annuities. The deferral of annuities allows retiring workers to postpone the conversion of their accumulated balance into an annuity, thus preventing an unfavorable year to give rise to lower annuities. This is a measure that provides some flexibility without distorting incentives and should be allowed under any regulatory framework. It has obvious limitations, however, for not all workers can afford postponing their annuities.

Variable Annuities or Sequenced Purchase of Fixed Annuities. Variable annuities (or phased withdrawals) could allow workers to diversify market risk to a significant extent. Workers retiring in a bad year could experience a sharp recovery in the real value of their pensions during the retirement period, when markets would be expected to recover. In chapter 11 Alier and Vittas show that variable annuities could significantly raise the minimum and average replacement ratios—in their simulations, the conversion of half of the final balance into a variable annuity could double the minimum replacement ratio, from around 20 percent to around 40 percent. The problem with variable annuities, however, is that they expose retirees to fluctuations in replacement ratios during the retirement period. One alternative solution to deal with market risk without exposing workers to fluctuations in replacement ratios is the gradual purchase of fixed annuities (for example, five annuities, purchased gradually five years before retirement). This solution would also raise the minimum replacement ratio and reduce dispersion, although its effects would be much smaller in comparison with variable annuities.

In sum, most attempts to limit market risk may cause more harm than benefit and should be generally avoided or very cautiously introduced. Among the potential options available, allowing deferral of pensions and developing different annuity packages are probably the ones with the least negative side effects. Multiple portfolios may prove an elegant construction for voluntary pillars in sophisticated financial systems. Their introduction in mandatory pillars in less sophisticated financial environments requires a more careful evaluation of costs and benefits. Absolute guarantees raise even more substantive questions, except for guarantees limited to fraud and theft. When absolute guarantees are introduced, regulators should ensure they are sufficiently low and backed by the capital of asset managers/sponsors, particularly in the cases where there is also a central guarantee fund. In these cases, regulators should explore the scope for introducing risk-based insurance premia, but the criteria for differentiating premia should not distort portfolio strategy to the detriment of fund members.

Improving the Regulatory Framework: Other Lessons

Portfolio Diversification. Pension funds that are restricted to a narrow range of investments may find themselves with excessive holdings of a few asset categories and greater vulnerability to real and financial shocks. Therefore, before considering the introduction of guarantees and other measures to deal with market risk, policymakers should ensure that the potential for portfolio diversification is fully explored.

Means of limiting this risk lie in the adoption of less restrictive investment regimes, when the development and security of capital markets establish conditions that make it feasible. Unlike banks, pension funds have much longer investment horizons and fewer liquidity constraints to limit their capacity to manage risk through broad diversification. Permitting limited entry into market segments (for example, foreign equities and venture capital) that offer the potential for increased yields and portfolio diversification provides the potential to avoid exposure to the kind of crises banking systems have experienced. However, it is also clear that permitting these investments would need to be contingent upon utilization of risk-management strategies that would complicate the job of regulators. A careful phasing of the relaxation of restrictions and the imposition of hedging requirements would be critical to the success of such an approach.

Valuation and Auditing. Even pension systems involving relatively few institutions and proactive supervision must ultimately depend on reliable valuation methods and an efficient auditing function. This issue is potentially of even greater concern for countries envisaging hybrid systems, combining a larger number of employer-based and open funds. In this regard, there are some lessons from banking regulation that may find application in the pension industry. One lesson relates to the degree of independence of auditors from management. In order to prevent interference from the management of pension funds or asset managers from diminishing the quality and integrity of the auditing function, it would be useful to introduce an obligatory rotation of auditors; make external auditors directly accountable to the boards, as opposed to management; restrict the ability of management to fire the auditor without board and supervisory approval; and force the auditor to report to the supervisor the reasons for resignation or termination. The second lesson deals with the integration of external auditing in the supervision process. Supervisors should be empowered to influence the scope and depth of the external audits and should have full access to all the audit results. The third lesson deals with the legal liability of external auditors. The potential power of external audits in the valuation and monitoring of funds' activities is only realized when auditors face clear penalties for failing to discharge their functions, which are also enforced.

Regulation of Fees. There is debate on whether regulation of the level and/or the structure of fees may have a significant impact on marketing activities and the switching across funds. Reducing the intensity of marketing activities and the large marketing costs may require a more fundamental change in the industry's structure. In a pension system, this could be accomplished through mixed or hybrid approaches, incorporating voluntary private alternatives (either individual or employment based), and facilitating the entry of occupational schemes in the second pillar as well. Greater participation of occupational schemes in both the voluntary and mandatory pillars, and the greater threat of entry by these institutions, could increase the market contestability that the industry in some countries seems to be lacking. Needless to say, this would require changes in the regulatory framework to accommodate the existence of two or more different types of institution.

Building Supervision Capacity. Proactive supervision in banking has emerged as a result of banking crisis and failures and attempts to identify and correct problems at an early stage before they become too costly to solve. However, proactive supervision itself can be costly. Moreover, even proactive approaches have not been able to avoid episodes of bank failures. Although these failures have been partly due to regulatory forbearance caused by political pressures, there is also a growing awareness that proactive supervision cannot be a substitute for good corporate governance and a continuous monitoring of the institutions by other market players.

As mentioned in section 2, the philosophy of banking supervision has been evolving in most developed countries from a strict and narrow approach focused on the monitoring of quantitative regulations to assessment of the banks' risk-management capacity and development of means to transfer more responsibility to other market players. This has required, among other things, efforts to improve the overall legal and institutional framework, clarify the duties and responsibilities of board members, improve disclosure, enhance the role of noninsured depositors, and strengthen the external audit function. The pension industry in some countries may face similar challenges.

Emerging countries implementing mandatory systems may conclude that it is inevitable to introduce proactive pension supervision policies in the first stages of reform implementation because these countries still do not have the legal and institutional structures required for a more decentralized but reliable supervision mode. However, as the long-run objective, the supervisor should ensure the strengthening of the regulatory framework and institutional mechanisms that would allow a more distributed burden of supervision in the future.

The need to start the reforms with more proactive supervision policies may imply the need to restrict entry initially and limit the number of institutions to a manageable size. However, the regulatory framework should not prevent the entry of employer-based schemes, but rather limit entry through the imposition of a minimum number of members and other professional requirements. Increasing the number of players raises many additional issues, particularly the issue of economies of scale and scope. It is sometimes argued that increasing the number of players may improve competition but also produce inefficiencies in scale. There is a misunderstanding in this area because small and medium-size funds in the OECD primarily outsource the administration and the management of their assets. The administration and asset management industries are more consolidated and may well be scale efficient.

At the same time, increasing the number of players does not mean aiming at a very fragmented structure, such as the one observed in most OECD countries (table 5.2). The target number should probably be on the order of dozens or hundreds, not tens and hundreds of thousands, as in most OECD countries. A very fragmented structure may indeed create problems in costs and compliance despite the outsourcing of tasks by smaller institutions. The total number of players and the minimum size required to obtain a license are important issues that require more empirical examination. Whitehouse (2000) shows that average administrative costs of externally managed funds in Australia decline very fast when the number of members increases from less than 100 to more than 500, but also that funds with 5,000–10,000 members may reap most scale economies.

These results suggest that a hybrid system that allows more employer-based funds and group contracts may succeed in curtailing marketing costs without simultaneously increasing other costs because of scale inefficiencies, provided that excessive fragmentation is avoided. They also

Table 5.2. Number of Banks, Pension Funds, and Asset Managers in Selected Countries

Country	Banks	Pension funds	Asset managers
Chile	28	8	8
Argentina	83	13	13
Hungary	43	32 in 2nd pillar 240 in 3rd pillar	45
Poland	83	19 in 2nd pillar 10 in 3rd pillar	29
Czech Republic	50	38	n.a.
United Kingdom	468	Hundreds of thousands	n.a.
United States	10,956	c.a. 700,000	n.a.
Australia	50	c.a. 150,000	n.a.
Switzerland	394	c.a. 11,000	Hundreds
Netherlands	99	c.a. 21,000	Several hundred
Ireland	71	c.a. 64,000	18

n.a Not applicable.
Sources: OECD (1999); Bank supervision agencies in several countries.

indicate the need for more empirical research on scale and scope economies in the pension industry and related industries through the estimation of well-specified cost functions, to provide useful inputs to pension regulators and to the design of pension reforms.[14]

Independence of Regulators. When faced with a crisis in the financial sector, policymakers have often brought pressure on bank regulators to engage in policies of forbearance or to delay interventions. The result has often been to ultimately make problems deeper or more costly when they finally are addressed. While this has clearly been an issue with banking regulators for some time, it is also of concern for the regulation of pension funds. Although pension funds are much less subject to systemic runs and failures, they may well be subject to political pressures to invest in government paper and other sectors favored by the government. The regulator may be induced to tailor the investment guidelines to these objectives, ignore the violation of existing regulations, and postpone intervention in pension funds subject to fraudulent practices. Insulating the regulator from these pressures is of paramount importance, and in many cases requires establishing an independent institution with clear board responsibilities and terms independent of the political cycle. Ensuring independence in pension supervision may be even more important, because it is more difficult to design "prompt corrective action" rules similar to those applied to bank supervisors, at least in the case of DC schemes.

The need to coordinate the activities of pension supervision with other supervision agencies is another issue that is on the agenda of regulators in many countries. Pension fund supervisors have to rely on the supervision of many other sectors of the financial system performed by different agencies. Although the need for coordination is clear, some legal systems restrict even the flow of information among supervisors, on the assumption that information sharing violates secrecy. At a minimum, the legal framework should allow supervisors to share information and even promote coordination by having the chief supervisors of different agencies participating on each other's boards or creating a commission of capital market supervision comprising the head of each supervision agency. A more structured solution would involve a fully integrated supervision agency, such as the one recently implemented in the United Kingdom.

Summary and Conclusions

This chapter has two major objectives: review of the regulation of the pension industry and identification of possible improvements in regulation, in light of developments in banking regulation in recent decades. In reviewing the literature on pension funds, we draw attention to the great variety of pension fund structures across countries but concentrate on the two most important and common structures: open funds operated by management companies and occupational-based trusts/foundations/mutuals. We identify prudential regulations that are applicable to both models while also stressing that the same regulation is frequently adapted to the specific model and that some regulations are entirely model-specific. Regulations common to both models include asset segregation rules, imposition of independent custodian and external audits, disclosure requirements, and portfolio diversification rules. There are some differences in disclosure requirements between the two models and marked differences between investment requirements between models and even between countries following the same model.

Some countries have introduced guarantees on second-pillar benefits that raise important issues related to viability, costs, and incentives. Relative guarantees are generally not very ambitious and do not seem to have caused financing problems or induced moral hazard. However, they are blamed for the intense herding behavior in the countries that adopt them. Absolute guarantees raise more substantive questions about sustainability and incentives. The few countries that have adopted them have not reported major problems, possibly because there are other, more informal channels linking the guarantee with the capital of the sponsors. However, a more explicit legal base is still lacking in these countries.

The chapter stresses the marked differences in the approach to supervision in the two models. Countries adopting the open fund model have introduced a very proactive supervision approach, which generally establishes strict entry criteria and closely monitors compliance with detailed disclosure requirements and investment regulations by a limited number of licensed funds. Countries that have historically adopted the occupational model follow a reactive supervision approach, largely because of the much larger number of institutions. The reactive model has proved functional, but requires a level of institutional and legal development that many emerging countries do not have at the present time.

The main section of the chapter examines whether there is scope for improvements in pension regulation. This section starts by examining worst case scenarios involving financial crisis while also pointing out the smoothing effects of long asset holding periods and the fact that multipillar constructions already contain an element of risk diversification. However, it also indicates that private funded systems will always be subject to market risk and looks at five possible solutions to deal with this risk, including DB schemes, absolute guarantees, multiple portfolios, pension deferrals, and the introduction of different annuity packages, including variable annuities and sequenced fixed annuities.

Most attempts to deal with market risk may introduce complications and negative side effects. In this regard, pension deferrals and the introduction of different annuity packages are probably the best options to deal with market risk, while absolute guarantees are the option that may cause the most damage. The chapter recommends that absolute guarantees be avoided while also providing more specific suggestions for design in the countries where they are introduced. These include keeping the guarantees low, putting private capital (of sponsors and asset managers) explicitly at risk before granting access to a central guarantee fund, and exploring the scope for introducing risk-based insurance premia.

We also identify other possible lessons from the banking industry. These include the need for more flexible rules aimed at enhancing portfolio diversification and the strengthening of governance rules in general, including the duties and responsibilities of boards and the scope and responsibilities of external auditors. The chapter stresses the need to achieve progress in these areas in order to spread the burden of supervision more evenly among a larger number of players. This is even more important in countries envisaging hybrid systems comprising both open and occupational funds, since hybrid systems would involve a larger number of institutions and would stretch the capacity of the supervisory agency.

Notes

1. The authors are grateful to the inputs and comments provided by Donald Duval of AON Consulting (United Kingdom); the former supervisor of pension funds in Australia, Rafael Rofman, of Nacion Pension Fund; and the former supervisor of pension funds in Argentina, Judit Spat, of the supervision department of the National Bank of Hungary.

2. A comprehensive survey of the literature on banking regulation is beyond the scope of this chapter. For in-depth analysis of financial regulations, see, for example, Benston and Kaufman (1988, 1996); Benston and others (1989); Bhattacharaya, Boot, and Thakor (1998); Calomiris (1998); Estrella (1998); Federal Reserve Bank of New York (1998); Goodhart and others (1998); Llewellyn (1999); and Randall (1993). This short list probably excludes important contributions to the literature.

3. A detailed review of these proposals and a description of the status of deposit insurance can be found in Benston (1993); FDIC (1998); Garcia (1998); Kopcke (1995); Kupiec and O'Brien (1998); Kuprianov and Mengle (1989); Rolnick (1993); Thomson (1990); and White (1989).

4. Briault (1999) provides a strong case for integrated supervision, and Taylor and Flemming (1999) provide a generally positive assessment of the experience with integrated supervision in Scandinavian countries. Goodhart and others (1998) propose a system with six different regulators

with clear mandates. Taylor (1995) proposes a simpler dual (twin peaks) model, comprising all prudential regulation in one agency and conduct of business rules in another.

5. There are probably other factors explaining the relatively low returns in these two countries during this period. For example, the guarantee of a minimum 4 percent return may have led Swiss funds to adopt conservative portfolio strategies. However, pressures for improved performance grew during the 1990s, resulting in increasing equity holdings and much higher returns among Swiss funds.

6. Srinivas, Whitehouse, and Yermo (2000) adopt the same classification. See also OECD (1998).

7. The OECD (1998 and 1999) provides an extensive and detailed comparison of investment regulations in OECD countries. Srinivas, Whitehouse and Yermo (2000) provide a similar comparison for Latin American countries.

8. Herding is stronger in Latin America, possibly because of the effect of guarantees (as discussed below), but is also observed in the OECD, even among countries following the prudent man rule.

9. Queisser (1998), Srinivas, Whitehouse and Yermo (2000), and Vittas (1995, 1995a, 1995b, 1998) provide a description of guarantees in Latin American countries and some Central and Eastern European countries.

10. The question is if herding is really a problem when portfolios are similar but well diversified.

11. The funds in Chile and Argentina also have a "profitability reserve" at the level of the pension fund itself (not the asset manager). This reserve is accumulated in periods of high returns and used in periods where returns fall below the minimum.

12. Palacios (1998) correlates wage growth (a proxy for PAYG returns) with equity returns (a proxy for second-pillar returns) for five OECD countries in the 1953–95 period and obtains very low or negative correlation coefficients.

13. Alier and Vittas (2000) show that a gradual switch into bonds five years before retirement would not significantly reduce differences in replacement ratios across cohorts.

14. There have been many studies of scale and scope economies in banking, but the authors are not aware of similar studies for the pension industry. The empirical literature on banks generally concludes that the average cost curve is relatively flat, with scale inefficiencies for both the smallest and largest banks. There is substantial disagreement on the minimum efficient scale of production, and the results seem to vary significantly according to the specific sample. There is no consensus on the existence of scope economies. Clark (1996) provides a brief survey of the literature.

References

Note: The word *processed* describes informally reproduced works that may not be commonly available through libraries.

Basle Committee on Banking Supervision. 1997. *Core Principles for Effective Banking Supervision.* Basle Committee on Banking Supervision.

Benston, George J. 1993. "Market Discipline: The Role of Uninsured Depositors and Other Market Participants." Paper presented at the conference "Safeguarding the Banking System in an Environment of Financial Cycles," November 18, Federal Reserve Bank of Boston.

Benston, George J., and George G. Kaufman. 1996. "The Appropriate Role of Bank Regulation." *The Economic Journal* 106 (May): 688–97.

_____. 1988. "Regulating Bank Safety and Performance." In William S. Haraf and Rose Marie Kushmeider, eds., *Restructuring Banking and Financial Services in America.* Washington, D.C.: American Enterprise Institute.

Benston, George J., R. Dan Brumbaugh, Jr., Jack M. Guttentag, Richard J. Herring, George G. Kaufman, Robert E. Litan, and Kenneth E. Scott. 1989. "Blueprint for Restructuring America's Financial Institutions: Report of a Task Force." Washington, D.C.: Brookings Institution.

Bhattacharya, Sudipto, Arnoud W. A. Boot, and Anjan V. Thakor. 1998. "The Economics of Bank Regulation." *Journal of Money, Credit and Banking* 30 (November): 745–70.

Briault, Clive. 1999. "The Rationale for a Single National Financial Services Regulator." Financial Services Authority, Occasional Paper No. 2 (May), London.

Calomiris, Charles. 1998. *The Postmodern Bank Safety Net.* Washington, D.C.: American Enterprise Institute.

Clark, Jeffrey. 1996. "Economic Cost, Scale Efficiency, and Competitive Viability in Banking." *Journal of Money, Credit and Banking* 28(3).

Davis, E. P. 1995. *Pension Funds, Retirement-Income Security, and Capital Markets—An International Perspective.* Oxford University Press.

Demarco, Gustavo, Rafael Rofman, and Edward Whitehouse. 1998. "Supervising Mandatory Funded Pension Systems: Issues and Challenges." Social Protection Discussion Paper No. 9817. World Bank, Washington, D.C.

Estrella, Arturo. 1998. "Formulas or Supervision? Remarks on the Future of Regulatory Capital." In *Financial Services at the Crossroads: Capital Regulation in the Twenty-First Century.* Federal Reserve Bank of New York, *Economic Policy Review*, vol. 4 (October): 191–200.

FDIC (Federal Deposit Insurance Corporation). 1998. "A Brief History of Deposit Insurance in the United States." Paper prepared for the

International Conference on Deposit Insurance, FDIC, Washington, D.C., September.

Federal Reserve Bank of New York. 1998. *Financial Services at the Crossroads: Capital Regulation in the Twenty-First Century, Economic Policy Review*, vol. 4, October.

Garcia, Gillian. 1998. "Comparative Analysis of Established Deposit Insurance Schemes." Paper presented at the FDIC's International Conference on Deposit Insurance, September, Washington, D.C.

Goodhart, Charles, P. Llewellyn, L. Rojas-Suarez, and S. Weisbrod. 1998. *Financial Regulation*. London and New York: Routledge.

Kopcke, Richard W. 1995. "Safety and Soundness of Financial Intermedaries: Capital Requirements, Deposit Insurance, and Monetary Policy." *New England Economic Review*, Federal Reserve Bank of Boston, December.

Krishnamurthi, Sudhir. 1999. "Applying Portfolio Theory to DB and DC Plans." Paper presented at a World Bank conference "Pension Systems in Eastern Europe and the Middle East: Achieving Effective Fund Management," Paris, March 22–24.

Kupiec, Paul H., and James M. O'Brien. 1998. "Deposit Insurance and the Design of Regulatory Policy." *Economic Policy Review*, vol. 4 (October), Federal Reserve Bank of New York: 201–11.

Kuprianov, Anatoli, and David L. Mengle. 1989. "The Future of Deposit Insurance: An Analysis of the Alternatives." *Federal Reserve Bank of Richmond Economic Review* 75(3): 3–15.

Llewellyn, D. 1999. "The Economic Rationale for Financial Regulation." Occasional Paper No. 1. Financial Services Authority, London.

OECD (Organization for Economic Cooperation and Development). 1997. "Ageing Populations and the Role of the Financial System in the Provision of Retirement Income in the OECD Area." Directorate for Financial, Fiscal, and Enterprise Affairs. OECD, Paris

_____. 1998. "Selected Principles for the Regulation of Investments by Insurance Companies and Pension Funds." Note by the Secretariat. OECD, Paris.

_____. 1999. "Comparative Tables on Regulation and Supervision of Pension Occupational Schemes." Note by the Secretariat. OECD, Paris.

Palacios, Robert. 1998. "A Note on Diversification Between Funded and PAYG Pension Schemes." World Bank, Washington D.C., December. Processed.

Queisser, Monika. 1998. "Regulation and Supervision of Pension Funds: Principles and Practices." *International Social Security Review* 51 (April–June): 1–21.

Randall, Richard E. 1993. "Safeguarding the Banking System from Financial Cycles: An Overview." Paper presented at the conference

"Safeguarding the Banking System in an Environment of Financial Cycles," November 18, Federal Reserve Bank of Boston.

Rolnick, Arthur J. 1993. "Market Discipline as a Regulator of Bank Risk." Paper presented at the conference "Safeguarding the Banking System in an Environment of Financial Cycles," November 18, Federal Reserve Bank of Boston.

Srinivas, S. P., Edward Whitehouse, and Juan Yermo. 2000. "Regulating Private Pension Funds' Structure, Performance and Investments: Cross-Country Evidence." Social Protection, Pension Primer Series. World Bank, Washington, D.C.

Taylor, Michael. 1995. "Twin Peaks: A Regulatory Structure for the New Century." Center for the Study of Financial Innovation, London.

Taylor, Michael, and Alex Flemming. 1999. "Integrated Financial Supervision: Lessons of Northern European Experience." International Monetary Fund and World Bank, Washington, D.C. Processed.

Thomson, James B. 1990. "Using Market Incentives to Reform Bank Regulation and Federal Deposit Insurance." *Federal Reserve Bank of Cleveland Economic Review* 26(1): 28–40.

Vittas, Dimitri. 1995a. "Strengths and Weaknesses of the Chilean Pension Reform." World Bank, Washington, D.C. Processed.

_____. 1995b. "The Argentine Pension Reform and Its Relevance for Eastern Europe." World Bank, Washington, D.C. Processed.

_____. 1998. "Regulatory Controversies of Private Pension Funds." World Bank, Washington, D.C. Processed.

Vittas, Dimitri, and Monika Queisser. 2000. "The Swiss Pension System: Triumph of Common Sense?" The World Bank and OECD. Processed.

White, Lawrence J. 1989. "The Reform of Federal Deposit Insurance." *The Journal of Economic Perspectives* 3 (Fall): 11–30.

Whitehouse, Edward. 2000. "Administrative Charges for Funded Pensions: An International Comparison and Assessment." Social Protection Discussion Paper No. 0016. World Bank, Washington, D.C.

6

Managing Public Pension Reserves: Evidence from the International Experience

Augusto Iglesias and Robert J. Palacios

MOST GOVERNMENTS FORCE THEIR CITIZENS to save for retirement.[1] In a pay-as-you-go pension scheme, contributions are immediately used to pay current pensions. Today, a majority of publicly mandated pension schemes are financed this way. In contrast, more than 50 countries have built up reserves to cover some (partially funded) or all (fully funded) of their pension liabilities. We estimate that the stock of pension assets, including voluntary pensions, is now as much as 50 percent of world gross domestic product (GDP).[2]

This percentage is likely to increase because more countries are choosing to prefund their pension obligations. For example, Canada and Ireland have recently decided to increase the funding levels of their partially funded public schemes. Meanwhile, a growing number of countries include privately managed and funded schemes as part of their mandatory system. Management of these reserves is of vital importance both to the pension systems and the economies involved.

Government mandate does not necessarily imply government management. Countries increasingly rely on private firms to manage the mandated contributions from workers. This does not mean government abdicates any role over investment policy. Rather, there are usually many restrictions on investment options.[3] In extreme situations regulations may be so heavy-handed as to effectively eliminate the discretion of private managers. Conversely, governments that directly control reserves may contract out management to the private sector or introduce some market-based, objective criteria to their internal investment policy. In other words, government interference is more usefully thought of as a continuum rather than as a simple distinction between public and private management.

The influence of government can be harmful when objectives unrelated to pension provision influence investment policies. Low investment returns compromise the underlying rationale for prefunding by threatening the solvency of a defined benefit scheme or, in the case of a defined contribution scheme, by reducing the risk-adjusted rate of return. Poor performance can also distort labor markets, as workers increasingly perceive their contributions to these schemes as a tax. Low risk-adjusted returns also signal an inefficient allocation of a country's savings. Meanwhile, good management can generate higher, more secure benefits for members and provide positive externalities to the economy.

Often, if the fund is large enough, there are important fiscal policy ramifications. Pension reserves are tempting sources of deficit financing, and methods of fiscal accounting encourage their use by government in this manner. This source of captive credit may lead to increased government consumption. It can also be addictive; once a government builds this source of borrowing into its budget process, it may be difficult to stop using it and make the necessary reforms underlying rationale for funding.

We observe that publicly managed funds almost always face serious political obstacles that hamper their ability to invest effectively. Their asset allocation is systematically biased toward targeted investments and lending to government at low yields. As a result, returns are much lower than those found in privately managed funds and mostly lower than bank deposit rates.

Using an index of governance as an explanatory variable, we find that normalized returns across countries are positively correlated with better government. Accounting for this factor, we also find that private management generates significantly better returns. These results should be considered preliminary. Data are not strictly comparable, and the sample is small. Nevertheless, the empirical analysis supports the anecdotal evidence: publicly managed pension funds have not been well managed.

In many countries, especially those with poor governance records, the best policy may be to use available resources to provide a safety net where traditional old age support systems have started to unravel. Most countries have already introduced forced savings schemes. If they are still running surpluses, they must find a way to manage these funds. A second-best policy would try to minimize problems by introducing competition and accountability into fund management. Competition should promote good investment policies, while accountability should protect members against fraud or abuse. Short of outright privatization, some improvement may be possible.

Despite the high stakes involved, little has been written on the international experience with managing public pension reserves, and this chapter only begins to fill the gap. The first section of the chapter distinguishes between types of prefunding, while the second section looks at public versus private management. The third section reviews the international evidence. In the last section, we draw some preliminary policy conclusions.

Types of Funding of Publicly Mandated Pensions

Publicly mandated pension schemes with some degree of prefunding fall roughly into three categories. The most common form is the partially funded, defined benefit scheme. Younger countries in which pension schemes are still immature, such as those in Francophone Africa or the Middle East, often have these types of systems.[4] A few older countries, such as Sweden and Japan, also fall into this category. The extent to which these defined benefit schemes are actually funded varies across countries and over time. However, to our knowledge, a fully funded defined benefit plan run by a national government does not exist.[5]

In contrast, the second type comprises the decentralized, defined contribution schemes that are fully funded in the sense that assets match liabilities at any given moment.[6] Decentralized and privately managed defined contribution schemes now operate in more than a dozen countries as part of multipillar pension systems. About half are in Latin America, but recently this model has spread to Hungary, Poland, and Hong Kong, among other countries. Australia, Switzerland, and the United Kingdom are examples in the Organization for Economic Cooperation and Development (OECD). This way of prefunding publicly mandated pension obligations has become more prevalent over the last two decades.

Finally, the third type of prefunded scheme, often called the provident fund model, constitutes defined contribution and is centrally managed. Fewer than a dozen countries—mainly former British colonies in Africa and Asia—use this model, and the number is shrinking. The largest one in terms of membership is the Employees' Provident Fund (EPF) in India, which has more than 20 million members. The Central Provident Fund of Singapore is the best known, however, with just over 1 million contributors. Most prescribe the yield to individual accounts every year and force investment in government bonds.

No single institution systematically collects international data on funded pension schemes. The figures in table 6.1 compare the ratio of accumulated reserves to national output for 55 countries using various sources documented in Palacios and Pallares-Miralles (2000). Data are derived from the late 1980s to mid-1990s, and are grouped according to the three categories

Table 6.1. Publicly Mandated Pension Fund Reserves in Selected Countries, by Type of Funding

Partially funded defined benefit		Centrally managed DC (Provident Funds)		Privately managed DC	
		Percent of GDP			
Egypt	33.1	Malaysia	55.7	Switzerland	117.0
Sweden	32.0	Singapore	55.6	Netherlands	87.3
Japan	25.0	Sri Lanka	15.2	United Kingdom	74.7
Jordan	16.9	Kenya	12.1	Australia	61.0
Mauritius	13.1	Tanzania	9.4	Chile	45.0
Philippines	11.2	Swaziland	6.6	Denmark	23.9
Gambia	11.1	India	4.5	Argentina	3.0
Canada	11.0	Nepal	4.0	Colombia	2.9
Belize	10.5	Indonesia	2.8	Peru	2.1
Ghana	9.4	Brunei	2.4	Poland	1.1
Morocco	8.7	Zambia	0.7	Uruguay	1.0
Switzerland	7.1	Uganda	0.6	Bolivia	1.0
Rep. of Korea	7.0			Mexico	0.5
Tunisia	6.9			Kazakhstan	0.5
Swaziland	6.6			Hungary	0.4
Jamaica	5.7			El Salvador	0.3
Costa Rica	5.4			Croatia	0.0
United States	5.0			Sweden	0.0
Yemen	4.0			Hong Kong	0.0
Honduras	3.5				
Senegal	1.6				
Ethiopia	1.4				
Algeria	1.2				
Chad	0.5				
Namibia	0.4				
Paraguay	0.4				

Notes: (i) The list does not include all countries known to have reserves; (ii) since 1995, India has had both a partially funded defined benefit scheme and a provident fund; (iii) India and Sri Lanka also have employer-managed funds; (iv) -privately managed assets in column three may include some voluntary retirement savings.
Source: Palacios and Pallares-Miralles (2000).

mentioned above. The first column shows the most common case—the partially funded, defined benefit plan. The Swedish and Egyptian schemes had accumulated assets worth almost one-third of GDP by the mid-1990s. Japan, Mauritius, Jordan, and the Philippines also had accumulated large funds relative to their respective economies. The smallest funds in countries like Paraguay and Yemen had assets equal to less than 1 percent of GDP.

The countries in bold are those for which this ratio is likely to grow significantly in the next few decades. For example, projections for the Republic of Korea suggest that the ratio of reserves to GDP will more than double in just the next 10 years. Recent reforms in Canada that raised contribution rates and aimed to increase returns should also lead to a much higher level of funding over the next two decades. In other countries, such as Japan, the funds will soon begin to dissipate as the schemes mature and populations age.

The largest provident funds relative to national income are those of Singapore and Malaysia. Their size is the result of four decades of accumulation, relatively high coverage and gradually rising contribution rates. Most of the other provident funds in the second column cover a minority of workers in each country, helping to explain why they are smaller by this measure. The fact that investment returns have trailed income growth is also partly to blame.

Among the privately managed schemes in the third column, those of Australia, the Netherlands, Switzerland, and the United Kingdom are the largest in terms of assets. These multipillar systems were built on preexisting, voluntary private pension sectors. Among the others, only Chile has the coverage levels and a long enough history to have accumulated significant assets. The rest of the Latin American countries in column three, along with the new schemes in Croatia, Hungary, Kazakhstan, Poland, and Sweden are projected to grow rapidly in the next two or three decades. For example, accumulated funds in Argentina, Hungary, and Poland are each expected to reach 40 percent of GDP by 2030.[7]

Public versus Private Management

The government influences the investment policies of all funded pension schemes. Private, voluntary pension funds rely on favorable tax treatment and are often subject to certain restrictions on investments and withdrawals.[8] Private managers in mandatory schemes sometimes face an intrusive regulatory regime and often must obey strict limits on the type of assets they hold. Taken to an extreme, portfolio limits can severely curtail competition or choice in the market, and government may even manipulate them to force private funds to invest exactly as it chooses.

At the same time, a centrally run government monopoly could use private managers and apply market-based criteria for their selection and compensation. Some countries are trying to build governance mechanisms that limit the direct role of politicians in the investment process. In principle, a centrally managed fund that incorporates market-based criteria could face a less restrictive environment than a privately managed scheme subject to onerous regulations.

Given the range of possibilities, it is more useful to express government's potential influence on the investment of publicly mandated pension funds along a continuum rather than as a sharp and simplistic distinction between public and private management. In figure 6.1, the possibilities range from the direct control exerted by a state monopoly to a lightly regulated, private system in which market forces operate freely. In Australia, for example, government regulation of investment of pension funds is very light. On the contrary, many countries fall closer to the left-hand side of the circle (nine o'clock), where direct public management involves a parastatal monopoly. There is no competition and government officials determine investment policy.

As we move from the laissez-faire point on the right towards direct control on the left, the level of government intervention rises. A clockwise shift represents stricter government regulation of the private sector. Movement counterclockwise signals an increase in the direct role of the government as manager of the funds. In either case, government influence on investment decisions increases.

A draconian regulatory regime gives government a large degree of control over private managers. For example, some of the countries in the third column of table 6.1 force private pension funds to invest a minimum share of their portfolios in government bonds.[9] In extreme cases in which

Figure 6.1. Role of Government in Management of Pension Reserves

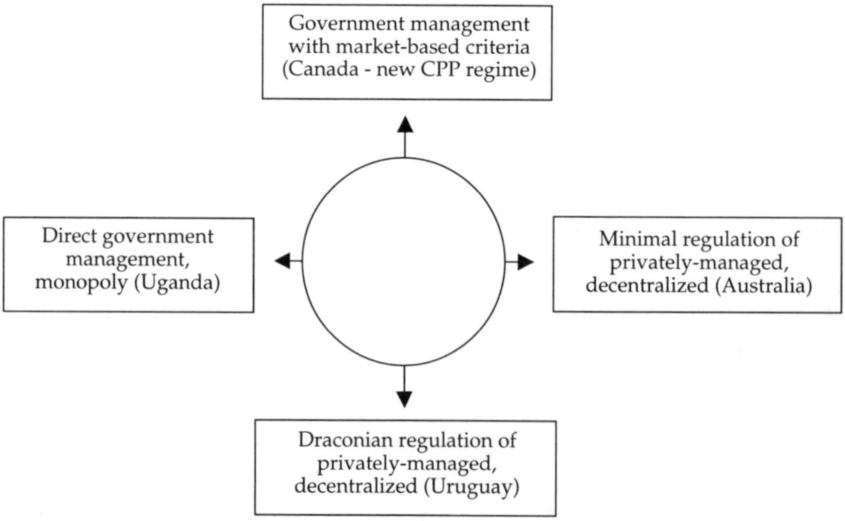

discretion is practically nonexistent, the difference between direct control of asset allocation and indirect control through regulations can disappear altogether. This is evident in the employer-based, "exempt funds" of India that are contracted out of the centrally managed EPF. Until recently, government has forced them to invest their entire portfolio in government guaranteed debt.

In contrast, even in a centralized structure, the government may set up mechanisms to limit political influence over investment decisions. It may, for example, create an objective benchmark based on some desired level of risk and target return and contract with private sector financial institutions to manage the assets. It may also subject the parastatal pension agency to the same standards applied to private sector pension managers.

Most of the multipillar schemes, including those in Latin America and Eastern Europe, are privately managed and heavily regulated. Here again, there are important differences in degree; in figure 6.1 Chile and Argentina would fall somewhere between Uruguay and Australia (say, at four o'clock) because they are less restricted than the former and more restricted than the latter. Most of the countries listed in the first two columns of table 6.1 lie closer to the left side of the circle. This may be changing; recently, for example, Singapore and Fiji have allowed some members to pick private managers and to determine how a portion of their Central Provident Fund balance will be invested.[10]

The case of Bolivia provides another classification challenge. There the government split the pension market into two regional monopolies and auctioned the management rights to private consortia. The exclusive concession will end eventually; new firms will be allowed to enter the market and workers permitted to switch between them. This is an example of introducing private sector management while tightly controlling the nature and degree of market competition. A similar outcome could have been achieved by tight regulation of the conditions for entry into the market (for example, minimum capital requirements, minimum membership, and so forth.).

These examples illustrate the point that all countries lie somewhere along a continuum of government involvement in managing pension reserves. Regulation can influence investment just as much as direct control. Put another way, decentralized management does not ensure more freedom of investment decision.

In practice, however, regulatory constraints are rarely so extreme as to eliminate the discretion of private managers, while most public pension monopolies are not insulated from political interference. The next section focuses on the experience to date with the defined benefit schemes and provident funds found in the first two columns of table 6.1.

International Experience with Public Management of Pension Reserves

This section looks at the experience of governments or parastatal institutions that manage pension reserves around the world. After a brief discussion of fund governance, we turn to investment policies and observed portfolios. We then highlight the implications of our findings.

Governance Structure

Provident funds and social insurance agencies typically have boards that set investment policy. These boards are almost always tripartite, with rep resentatives from labor unions, employers, and the government.[11] Sometimes pensioners are also represented. In 25 countries for which information was available, only three did not have tripartite boards.[12] The government typically appoints chairpersons who usually come from the Ministry of Finance (MOF) or the ministry responsible for pension policy. The treasury or central bank often plays a leading role.

While the board may determine overall investment policy (subject to the constraints described in the next section), an investment committee often holds responsibility for more detailed decisions and monitoring as well as evaluating the investments of the fund, trading, valuation, and so on.[13] Most schemes do everything in house. We found only four countries that had used external asset managers, and in these cases the proportion of the portfolio involved was minimal. In some partially funded, defined benefit schemes, an actuarial unit performs funding assessments. A few countries use external actuaries.

The composition of boards reflects domestic political circumstances. For example, the government changed the composition of the Committee for National Pension Fund Operation in Korea as part of a reform of the National Pension Scheme (NPS) in 1998. The minister of health replaced the minister of finance as chairman, and the number of members rose from 11 to 20. The members include the vice ministers of finance, agriculture, industry, and labor; the president of the National Pension Corporation (which administers the NPS); three employer and employee representatives, respectively; six representatives of farmers, fishermen, and the self-employed; and two pension experts.

The changes reflected two recent developments. First, the shift of ministerial power was due to broader decline of the standing of the MOF in the wake of the East Asian financial crisis. The addition of new representatives of the insured population and employers was a consequence of the expansion of coverage to new groups such as the self-employed in 1999.

It is not always clear how the composition of the board affects investment policy. In the case of Korea, the MOF had been able to tap the NPS surpluses for the last decade to finance projects and public works. After the "reforms," the Ministry of Health and the new worker representatives may have other uses for these funds.

Sometimes, the composition and operating procedures of the board are irrelevant. In Malaysia, for example, during the East Asian financial crisis the Mahathir government used the EPF to support certain government projects against the objections of the Board of Trustees.[14] Another example is found in Munnell and Ernsberger (1989), who note that the U.S. Secretary of the Treasury, when constrained by a debt ceiling in 1985, ordered the conversion "of 28 billion dollars in long-term bonds held by the trust funds into non-interest bearing cash balances without notifying the two public trustees." More often, however, government control is assured through political appointments and the direct representation of the executive branch on the board. There is usually little need to resort to extreme measures.

Restrictions and Mandates

Typically, a set of rules explicitly limits the governing boards' investment options. Restrictions on investment choices and mandates to invest in certain projects comprise the most common way that their discretion is curtailed. In Korea, for example, legal statutes automatically channeled two-thirds of the National Pension Fund to the MOF in the form of special loans. In the United States, all monies must be invested in nonmarketable government bonds.

Table 6.2 shows the portfolio restrictions of the EPF in India. These restrictions refer to new investments as opposed to limits on the actual portfolio held at any given time. Notably, the EPF must make 90 percent of investments in government or government-guaranteed debt, leaving only 10 percent to invest in private corporate bonds with investment-grade rating. Prior to 1998, the EPF could not invest in the private sector even on this limited basis. Interestingly, the EPF board has thus far decided not to invest in the corporate bonds despite higher potential returns. This decision was apparently due to the risk aversion of union representatives combined with the practice of stipulating the annual minimum yield in advance.[15]

But mandates and restrictions are not always so explicit. They can also take the form of investment principles or guidelines that steer the portfolio toward social and economic development objectives. Guidelines in Mauritius provide that 30 percent of the portfolio should be invested in areas with a "social dimension" and even specify the acceptable loss of return from this type of investment.[16] As one of its major principles, Jordan's public pension scheme aims at

> contributing to the development of the productive base of the national economy through participation in economically feasible projects that, at the same time, have an appropriate

Table 6.2. Prescribed Investment Limits for Employee Provident Fund in India, 1998.

Instrument	Percent of amount invested
(i) Central government bonds	25
(ii) (a) State government bonds (b) Government guaranteed bonds	15

(iii)   (a) Securities of public financial institutions,
      public sector enterprises, banks, and
      Infrastructure Development Finance Co.
      (b) CDs issued by public sector banks
	40

(iv) Above three categories as determined by board of trustees	20
(v) Private sector bonds with investment grade credit rating from two credit rating agencies *(from (iv) above)*	10

Source: Employee Provident Fund (EPF) Act, as amended, 1998.

> developmental dimension (Social Security Corporation Annual Report 1996).

The expression "developmental dimension" opens the door to a wide array of possibilities, which probably explains why politicians find this approach convenient. They can justify "social investments," for example, on the basis that they will improve the lives of members of the scheme in ways other than receiving a pension. Personal loans for housing and education, subsidies to mortgage loans and housing construction, and investment in social infrastructure (hospitals, clinics) are common examples.

Economic or development objectives give rise to another kind of mandate—"economically-targeted investments," or ETIs. Some proponents of this type of investment claim that inefficiencies in the capital markets leave worthwhile projects without financing and that there are externalities to some projects that can produce quantifiable benefits for members. However, such claims are difficult to substantiate.[17] More often, the motives for ETIs relate to the popularity of the projects being financed. We are not aware of any countries that apply rigorous and objective criteria to the selection of these targeted investments. Anecdotally, the selection of projects appears to be based mostly on the priorities of the government in power. In this case, the lower returns that typically accompany ETIs are a tax on at least some members of the scheme.

There are examples of economically targeted investments involving pension funds in every region of the world and in countries of every income level. They are often sanctioned at a very broad policy level. Public pension funds in five African countries responded positively when asked if there was a formal link between the government's economic development plan and the use of pension reserves (ISSA 1997). Mahdi (1990) reports that in Turkey the State Planning Board can directly intervene in investment policy. In Jordan the board that manages investments tries to "meet criteria, which include those established within the framework of the National Development Plan."

Infrastructure projects and state enterprises often benefit from pension fund investment. In Venezuela, for example, a substantial portion of the pension fund portfolio during the 1980s consisted of state enterprise bonds. In Tunisia the government required investment in "equipment bonds."[18] Development banks invest the Egyptian and Moroccan reserves. Since 1987 Iran has used its reserves to provide "financial facilities to industrial units of the country, to buy raw materials and machinery and [to] improv[e] business activities (SSRI 1997, p. 76). Whatever the social returns of these investments, all appear to have generated returns below market rates.

In East Asia publicly managed pension funds have used ETIs extensively. In Japan, for example, the Trust Fund Bureau receives a portion of the surpluses that it in turn makes available to the Fiscal Investment Loan Program. Under the direction of the Ministry of Finance, this agency invests in hospitals, housing, infrastructure projects, resorts, and welfare facilities. Korea has followed the Japanese model closely. The Ministry of Finance in Korea invests a substantial portion of the reserves, which it takes on loan, in various public projects. This portion has grown to more than two-thirds of the total portfolio. These funds also make social investments. In Korea and Japan, investments in the category labeled "welfare" had risen from 0 to about 3 percent and 17 percent of the portfolio, respectively, by 1995.[19]

Government mandates are most popular for the purpose of providing housing. Investments by pension funds in this sector can take many forms. A government might force the pension fund to purchase mortgage bonds in an effort to create a market for such instruments. Alternatively, the pension fund could provide loans directly to members for construction or purchase of housing. It could also invest in public housing projects through special bonds or loans to developers.

Sweden offers an example. In the 1960s and 1970s, the Swedish government was interested in expanding housing opportunities. Growing public pension reserves presented a convenient source of long-term financing. This match was made when the central bank effectively forced the public pension funds, or AP funds, to purchase low-interest housing bonds. As a result, note Munnell and Ernsberger (1989), "the priorities of the AP managers were often at odds with the goals of the Central Bank." The pension fund managers lost the battle, and the AP funds earned lower returns in order to meet the government's housing policy objectives.

Housing and medical facilities comprise the main social investments in Algeria, Iran, Jordan, Morocco, and Tunisia (see World Bank 1994, 1996). Jordan favors housing projects that "meet the needs of medium- and low-income families" and charges interest rates on these loans that "are below prevailing interest rates on normal deposits." Vittas (1993) reports that Tunisia was phasing out social housing investments in the early 1990s but was replacing them with housing and personal loans at below-market interest rates. In Iran the social insurance agency made housing loans to cooperatives and individuals between 1987 and 1993 (SSRI 1997). Algeria invested its pension funds in social infrastructure projects yielding negative returns (Börsch-Supan, Palacios, and Tumbarello 1999).

A recent study of a dozen Anglophone African countries also found that housing was the most popular social investment. ISSA (1997) reports that the public pension funds in Gambia, Ghana, Kenya, Mauritius, Nigeria, Swaziland, Tanzania, Uganda, and Zambia played a role in housing finance and/or construction (see ILO 1994, 1996; National Provident Fund 1996, 1997; National Social Security Fund of Kenya 1998). In Tanzania and Zambia, for example, the fund itself constructs housing that it then rents to individuals. Sometimes these loans are not directed at the average worker. In Nigeria, for example, housing investments "are restricted to the provision of commercial housing largely for high net worth individuals," although the fund was "considering the development of mass housing for middle- and low-income persons in urban areas" (ISSA 1997).

The government can also use restrictions and mandates to force pension funds to lend it money. Governments prefer to borrow from public pension funds for at least three reasons: (i) the flow of pension fund surpluses is usually predictable, making it easier to finance anticipated deficits in comparison to issuing bonds in the market; (ii) by forcing the pension funds to purchase nontradable bonds with no transparent market pricing mechanism, the government may be able to reduce its borrowing costs; and (iii) fiscal accounting practices may reward this form of borrowing, since purchase of government securities by a public pension fund reduces net government debt.[20] Many countries apply rules that explicitly or implicitly force public pension fund managers to purchase government bonds. In some cases, such as the United States, this is the only investment allowed. Figure 6.2 summarizes the type of mandates and restrictions found in a sample of more than 30 countries. Some portion of the portfolio in all countries was composed of ETIs, social investments, or the purchase of government or state enterprise debt. Housing was the most popular type of directed investment.

Figure 6.2. Directed Investment of Publicly Managed Pension Funds
(percentage of funds with these practices)

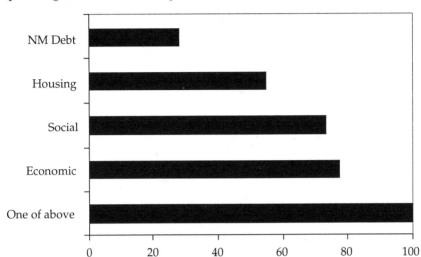

Note: NM Debt = nonmarketable government debt.
Source: Authors' calculations based on various country sources.

Limited Domestic Investment Options

In addition to the constraints imposed by governments, underdeveloped capital markets and shallow financial sectors can be major obstacles for pension fund managers, whether they are public or private. While allowing for investment abroad would ease this constraint (and is generally to be recommended), it is often not an option because of exchange controls, high transaction costs, and, perhaps most importantly, political pressure to keep scarce investment funds at home.

Figures 6.3 and 6.4 use stock market capitalization and commercial bank credit as a percentage of GDP to highlight the wide variation in the depth of financial sectors across countries.[21] Not surprisingly, the countries with the lowest ratios are found in Sub-Saharan Africa and the poorer parts of the former Soviet Union. Pension fund managers in these countries would encounter few options for investment in domestic markets. These countries also have the weakest legal and regulatory structures, thinnest market for

Figure 6.3. Distribution of Countries by Financial Sector Depth
(stock market capitalization as percentage of GDP)

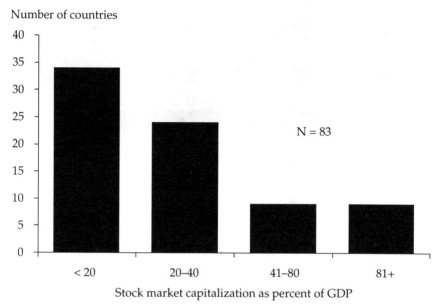

Number of countries

N = 83

Stock market capitalization as percent of GDP

Source: World Development Indicators 1997, Table 5.10.

government bonds, and the most limited human resources for operation and supervision of funded pension schemes.

Clearly, public pension fund managers in different countries face very different constraints. Sometimes options in the domestic market are practically nonexistent. In some countries, the rule of law, definition of property rights, and basic financial infrastructure do not meet minimum standards. In such a situation, the riskless benchmark does not exist since the government may default on its bonds or fail to ensure the solvency of the banking system. Cameroon, unfortunately, is not a unique case (see box 6.1).

But even in countries where domestic capital markets do provide potential investment outlets for large public pension funds, at least three obvious problems emerge: (i) ownership of a large proportion of the shares by the government would effectively nationalize the industries involved. At the very least, it would raise important questions regarding corporate governance; (ii) the government may be tempted to use the pension fund to support the stock market or specific firms with political influence;[22] and (iii) the government may find itself in the awkward position of regulator and

Figure 6.4. Distribution of Countries by Financial Sector Depth
(commercial bank credit as percentage of GDP)

Number of countries

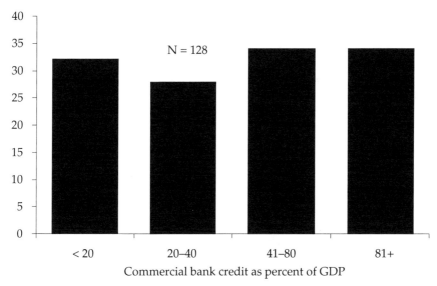

N = 128

Commercial bank credit as percent of GDP

Source: World Development Indicators 1997, Table 5.10.

owner of certain industries, creating other possible conflicts of interest. These are among the major challenges facing supporters of the idea of investing public funds in private markets.[23]

OBSERVED PORTFOLIOS

Table 6.3 reports broad portfolio allocations for public pension schemes in more than 30 countries from every region of the world. The data come from various sources, and the original categories were reclassified into four broad asset classes. The share in each category is rounded. Clearly, there is a bias in most countries toward holding large shares in bank deposits and government securities. For the sample as a whole, the simple average of holdings in this category is 75 percent of total assets. In most of these cases, there is little or no secondary market for the government bonds held by the pension fund. Most of the bank deposits are in state-owned banks.

Only five countries invest less than half of the portfolio in bank deposits or government bonds. These countries—Ecuador, Philippines, Sudan, Sweden, and Tunisia—have above average holdings of loans for housing

---

Box 6.1. Cameroon: No Safe Haven for Public Pension Funds

In the 1980s the public pension fund in Cameroon (CNPS) had a difficult time finding safe places to invest its growing funds. There were few private securities available domestically. It was forced to purchase medium-term, low-interest bonds from the National Investment Company and invested some more in the Bank for Trade and Industry, but all of this accounted for only a small part of the overall portfolio.

Bank deposits were the second largest item in the portfolio, but these deposits turned out to be quite risky. The accounts were frozen when several banks were closed in the 1980s. A small part of the portfolio was in real estate. This provided rental income and appeared to have maintained its real value over time.

But the largest part of the portfolio was held in the form of government bonds. Naturally, it would be safe there. Or would it? In the mid-1980s, the government of Cameroon covered part of its burgeoning deficit by borrowing large sums from the CNPS. More loans were mandated to state enterprises like the Cameroon Sugar Corporation and the Cameroon Banana Organization. Social housing was financed through loans to the Cameroon Housing Company. These loans were made upon the instruction of the President of the Republic or the Minister of Finance, while the CNPS management was restricted to carrying out instructions. The duration of the loans was 10 or 20 years, and the interest rates were often lower than those given on bank deposits. Some state companies were unable to repay the loans, while others simply chose not to repay. One official expressed his dismay, "The managers of the CNPS have no real means of exerting pressure on the government since the Fund is a public establishment. . . . This situation justifies the fears of those who worry that the temptation of the abundant reserves accumulated by social security schemes will be too strong for public authorities, which will draw on them for more dubious purposes."

Frustrated managers at the CNPS even advocated depositing some of the pension fund money abroad, but government rejected this idea. In the end, there seems to be no safe haven for the savings of Cameroon's workers.

Source: This material is drawn from Mounbaga (1995).

---

and other purposes. This is the second most popular category for investments. Loans represented a significant share of the portfolio in 19 of the countries, and there is no obvious pattern by income level or region. Most of these loans involve implicit subsidies.

The last column includes property such as hotels, commercial office space, and land, along with some other items not easily classified. Nineteen countries had some investments in these items, but, with the exception of four countries, none held more than one-fifth of their portfolio in this type of asset. Typically, these transactions involve long-term ownership in an

Table 6.3. Publicly Managed Pension Fund Portfolios in 34 Countries, 1980s and 1990s

Country	Year	Gov't. bonds/ fixed deposits	Loans/ mortgages/ housing bonds	Shares/ equity	Real estate/ other	Total
		Percentages				
Canada (CPP)	1991	100	0	0	0	100
Egypt	1995	100	0	0	0	100
Pakistan	1981	100	0	0	0	100
Sri Lanka	1997	100	0	0	0	100
Switzerland	1997	100	0	0	0	100
United States	1997	100	0	0	0	100
Yemen	1996	100	0	0	0	100
Colombia	1982	100	0	0	0	100
India	1995	100	0	0	0	100
Venezuela	1981	100	0	0	0	100
Niger	1980	96	3	1	0	100
Senegal	1980	93	6	1	0	100
Jamaica	1987	91	9	0	0	100
Tanzania	1996	90	0	0	10	100
Korea	1997	89	3	3	6	100
Rwanda	1980	82	4	5	8	100
Ethiopia	1996	80	0	0	20	100
Costa Rica	1987	79	15	0	6	100
Burundi	1981	78	9	6	8	100
Peru	1988	76	7	0	17	100
Kenya	1994	73	0	11	16	100
Uganda	1994	68	8	1	23	100
Japan	1995	63	17	19	0	100
Malaysia	1996	63	21	15	1	100
Togo	1981	59	1	3	37	100
Morocco	1994	58	32	7	3	100
Cameroon	1989	57	40	2	1	100
Mauritius	1996	56	0	2	42	100
Jordan	1995	52	25	17	6	100
Philippines	1995	44	38	10	8	100
Tunisia	1990	43	30	0	27	100
Sweden	1996	42	40	0	18	100
Sudan	1982	26	58	0	16	100
Ecuador	1986	10	83	3	3	100
Mean		75	14	3	8	100

Note: Provident funds appear in bold.
Source: Palacios and Pallares-Miralles (2000).

illiquid real estate market, making valuation extremely difficult. Again, there was no clear pattern with regard to the proportions of real estate held.

Table 6.3 illustrates the very limited use of private capital markets by public pension funds. The least popular investment is in equities. Only about one-third of the countries had any investment in this category. On average only 3 percent of the portfolios in the sample are invested in shares. The size and liquidity of the stock market is not necessarily the constraint, for low equity holdings are not correlated with capital market depth or liquidity. For example, Korea had a relatively large and liquid stock market, but less than 3 percent of pension reserves were invested in equities. Similarly, the absence of shares in U.S. and Canadian portfolios has nothing to do with the domestic capital market conditions. Certainly, thin local capital markets in many countries could discourage pension fund managers, especially if foreign investment were prohibited. It is doubtful, however, that it has been a binding constraint in most cases.

Private pension portfolios looked much different during the same period. A recent study of 10 OECD countries found that the unweighted average proportion of private pension portfolios invested in equity in 1996 was around 32 percent. Weighted by assets, the figure rises to almost 50 percent.[24] Investments in equities in Latin America's new private pension schemes also tend to be significantly higher than what is observed in table 6.3. Private pension funds in Peru and Argentina, for example, held 22 and 35 percent of their respective assets in equities in mid-1997. Since restrictions on equity investments were lifted in the mid-1980s, Chilean AFPs increased investments in shares, reaching about 30 percent by mid-1997. Around three-fourths of Hong Kong's private pension assets were in the form of equities between 1990–95. We also find no evidence of mandates for social investment or ETIs in private pension systems.

As already noted, investment abroad by public pension funds is rare. We found only a few countries where public pension funds held foreign securities, including Japan (less than 1 percent), Mauritius (5 percent), and Sweden (2 percent). A 1997 legislative change allowed the main public scheme in the Philippines to invest up to 7.5 percent abroad, but this had not occurred by 1999.[25] This is poor policy in light of the limited investment options available in most countries, especially when the funds are large relative to domestic capital markets. Nevertheless, the political pressure to keep workers' savings at home is a common theme in the policy debates of rich and poor countries alike.[26]

In contrast, data for seven OECD countries (including voluntary schemes) show that private pension funds have increased the average share of their portfolio in foreign assets from 12 to 17 percent between 1990 and 1996.[27] This trend will likely continue, and many OECD countries have already relaxed restrictions on cross-border investments by pension funds.

Investment Returns and Volatility

The rate of return perhaps represents the most important single indicator of how public pension reserves are being managed. This measure provides an important signal as to whether investment decisions allocate capital efficiently in the economy. It also measures the extent to which prefunding is actually offsetting defined benefit liabilities or generating retirement wealth in defined contribution accounts. It does not, of course, describe social returns just as measures of enterprise efficiency (for example, factor productivity, profits, etc.) do not incorporate externalities to society. An attempt to measure these indirect effects, while interesting, is beyond the scope of this chapter.

Unfortunately, data are not readily available for most countries and, when they are available, are not strictly comparable. For example, valuation methods vary, with most countries using book values rather than marking to market. In other countries, returns are simply not published. The dearth of good information in this area is itself symptomatic of a lack of accountability and transparency in this area.

With these caveats in mind, this subsection looks at two types of returns for a small sample of countries. The first type is the return credited to the accounts of provident fund members. The second refers to the reported return on investments of partially funded, defined benefit schemes. The sample includes countries with data for at least eight consecutive years (see annex).

Figure 6.5 plots the annual compounded rates of return for a sample of 22 countries for different time periods against the standard deviations of annual returns. About half of the sample, or 10 countries, failed to generate positive real returns. For those that did, returns were low, mostly between 1–2 percent. Only members of provident funds in Malaysia and the partially funded defined benefit scheme in Korea earned real returns in excess of 3 percent. The Korean performance was the best at 5.4 percent per annum. Uganda (-50.5 percent), Peru (-46.6 percent), and Zambia (-30.5 percent) had the worst returns.

A striking feature of figure 6.5 is that volatility, as measured by the standard deviation of annual returns, is inversely related with the average compounded return. Given that the data are from different countries and years, they do not represent a comparable set of points along a risk-return frontier. Nevertheless, we would expect that cross-country results would be roughly consistent with the idea that higher returns reward higher risk. This is not the case. Instead, half of the sample holds risky portfolios and gets dismal returns. The other half gets low but stable returns. We also include the returns in Chile for the private pension industry between 1982 and 1997 as reported in Srinivas and Yermo (1999).

Figure 6.5 is difficult to interpret. The domestic risk/return profiles of the investments available to public pension fund managers vary greatly

Figure 6.5. Annual Compounded Real Returns and Volatility in 22 Publicly Managed Pension Funds

Standard deviation, percent

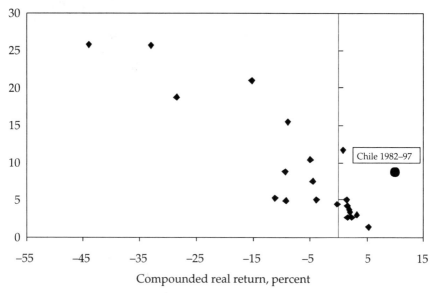

Compounded real return, percent

Source: Author's calculations based on data in Palacios and Pallares-Miralles (2000).

across countries. Public pension managers in each country had to deal with the available investment universe in their respective economies. Recent evidence suggests that these may be low even in capital-scarce countries.[28] The mandates and restrictions described above further constrain the opportunity set. Finally, country-specific factors affecting particular economies during the period covered here could skew the cross-country results. In short, while figure 6.5 confirms low or negative returns for all of the publicly managed schemes, it does not reveal whether the returns were reasonable given prevailing conditions or domestic benchmarks.

In order to get a clearer picture, we looked at the returns relative to bank deposit rates in the same countries during the same periods. Normalizing in this way should help control for some of the country-specific factors and provide a crude benchmark for investment alternatives. Figure 6.6 shows the difference between pension fund returns and short-term bank deposit rates for 20 countries. There was a very high correlation between the rates of return on pension funds and the bank deposit rate. This is not surprising given the high shares of the portfolio that are invested in bank deposits

Figure 6.6. Difference between Annual Compounded Real Publicly Managed Pension Fund Returns and Bank Deposit Rates in 20 Countries
(from worst to best)

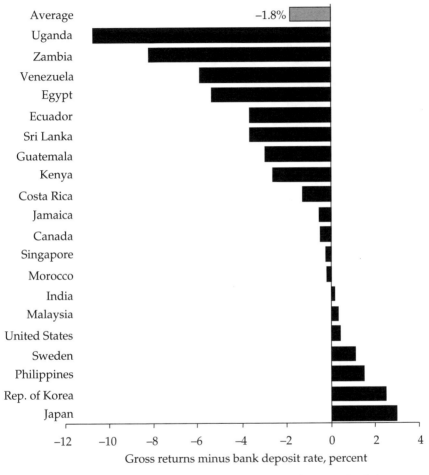

Gross returns minus bank deposit rate, percent

Sources: International Monetary Fund (IMF), *International Finance Statistics Yearbook*, various years; figure 6.4; authors' calculations.

and/or short-term government bonds and the effect of sudden bouts of inflation on both.

There is significant variation across the sample. Using a simple average, returns are 180 basis points lower than bank deposit rates. However, four countries—Korea, Japan, Philippines, and Sweden—show returns that are more than 100 basis points higher than deposit rates. Japan and Korea stand out with returns exceeding deposit rates by 300 and 250 basis points, respectively. We should note, however, that this differential disappears if the yield on t-bills is used instead of bank deposit rates.

Most of the sample posted returns well below the short-term interest rate. In the worst cases, the funds would have earned 400–1000 basis points more per annum by keeping all of their money in bank deposits. Worse yet, lower risk did not compensate these poor returns for workers in these countries; the volatility of bank deposit interest rates was the same as or lower than the volatility of pension fund returns (see annex). By contrast, compounded real returns for Chile's private pension funds outpaced bank deposit rates by 370 basis points between 1982–97 according to Srinivas and Ycrmo (1999).

Figure 6.6 suggests that returns in most of our sample are not even as high as the short-term returns that can be obtained in banks by individual savers. In some cases, the returns are much worse. But pension funds handle long-term savings that should be able to earn higher returns in exchange for lower liquidity. Rather than the riskless rate of return on liquid assets, they should be able to earn something closer to the economy's long-run return on capital. This could only be achieved of course, if investments were made in the private capital markets. We have already seen that this is uncommon for publicly managed funds.

In assessing the gap between actual and potential returns, we can look to the growth of incomes as a rough benchmark. In a dynamically efficient economy, returns to capital are higher than the growth in incomes over long time horizons. As shown by Abel and others (1989), this can be the case even when the riskless rate of return (for example, interest on t-bills) is below GDP growth. Thus, with other factors remaining constant, the returns available to publicly managed pension funds from a diversified portfolio should be greater than income growth. This relationship is also important if the pension scheme is to generate reasonable replacement rates.

Figure 6.7 shows that only two publicly managed pension schemes (Philippines and Morocco) earned returns that were greater, by a small margin, than the growth of income per capita during the periods in question.[29] In most countries returns trailed income growth. In half the sample, the differential in favor of income growth was greater than 300 basis points.

The results for Singapore and Malaysia merit further discussion. Both provident funds exhibit low but positive real rates of returns. However, incomes in both countries were among the fastest growing in the world over the last three decades. Another similarity is that prescribed yields to members have been based on short-term interest rate, while actual investment returns are believed to have been much higher. For example, Asher (1998) suggests that the actual investment return in Singapore may have been more

Figure 6.7. Difference between Real Annual Compounded Publicly Managed Pension Fund Returns and Real Income Per Capita Growth in Selected Countries

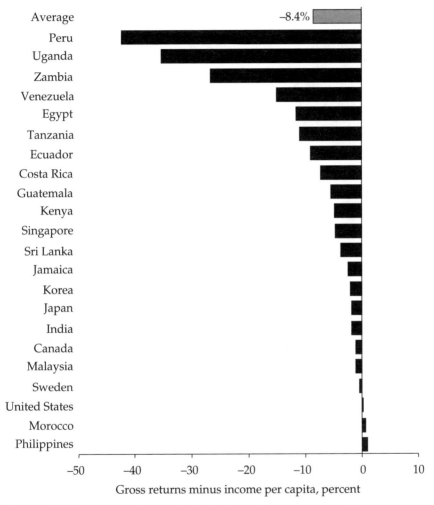

Gross returns minus income per capita, percent

Sources: IMF *International Finance Statistics Yearbook;* authors' calculations

than 3 percentage points higher than what has been credited to members' accounts. In other words, part of the effect being observed here is an implicit taxation of returns rather than poor investment performance.[30]

From the worker's perspective, the result of this implicit taxation is a low replacement rate. Assuming that average wages and income per capita moved in tandem in both countries, a worker who began his or her career in 1960 would have seen his or her wage grow eightfold in Singapore and almost tenfold in Malaysia by 1995. Meanwhile, the contribution this worker made in 1960 would only have doubled in Singapore and tripled in Malaysia. Not surprisingly, criticism of these schemes has increased as retiring workers, having contributed their entire working lives, find that low balances are insufficient to maintain preretirement living standards.[31]

Private pension fund returns, in contrast, almost always exceed the growth of incomes over the long run. Figure 6.8 shows that this difference is usually at least 200 basis points. Although the time periods considered here are different, public and private pension returns over long periods of time can also be compared for a few countries. For example, privately managed funds in Sweden and Japan earned returns that were, respectively, 300 and 500 basis points higher than their public sector counterparts.

Underlying Causes of Low Returns in Publicly Managed Schemes

In Figures 6.5 and 6.6, we ranked publicly managed pension funds in our sample based on the difference between investment returns and bank deposits or income per capita growth. The first measure served to crudely control for broader policies and shocks that would affect most investments. It also provided a benchmark return that was presumably available to all investors in the same country during the same time period. The second measure focused on the gap between actual returns and the return that should be available in the private markets, specifically, a return exceeding the growth of incomes. In both cases we found that public pension fund returns fared badly; in some cases they were disastrous. We also noted that where data are available, private pension fund returns are almost always greater than income growth.

The direct causes for underperformance have already been mentioned. They include government interference in investment, ranging from the imposition of social or development objectives on the pension fund to forcing pension funds to finance deficits or state enterprise losses, often at interest rates lower than what is available on the market. The common prohibition on investment abroad posed another major challenge to public pension fund managers trying to diversify their (often significant) country-specific risk. While we noted that thin and/or badly regulated capital markets might not provide the investment opportunities required by large funds, this constraint did not seem to be binding in most countries. It certainly could not explain why returns were lower than bank deposit rates.

We also noted that normalized returns vary widely across publicly managed pension funds. This suggests that additional factors are either exacerbating or mitigating the general deficiencies that affect public management. The obvious question is why do some countries perform better than others.

Figure 6.8. Difference between Real Annual Private Pension Fund Returns and the Real Income Per Capita Growth in Selected Countries

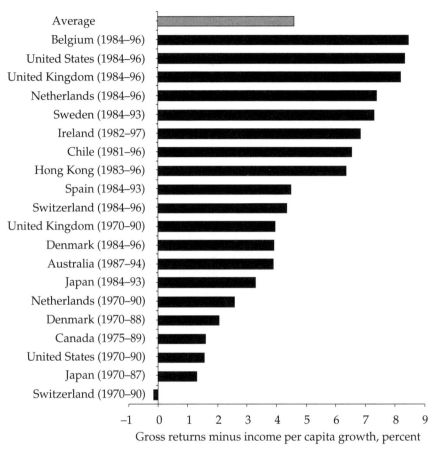

Gross returns minus income per capita growth, percent

Sources: Davis 1993; OECD 1998; Wyatt 1998; Superintendencia de AFP, Chile 2000; Piggott 1999; IMF, *International Finance Statistics Yearbook*, various years.

Explaining private pension fund performance has focused on strategic asset allocation. These decisions have been found to explain more than 90 percent of the variation in risk-adjusted returns across private pension funds (Brinson, Hood, and Beebower 1986; Brinson, Singer, and Beebower 1991). In public pension funds we have shown that the mandates and restrictions imposed on public pension fund managers largely determine asset allocation. These decisions are largely political and have little to do with any application of portfolio theory. Furthermore, given that public managers tend to use criteria that ignore the concept of risk-adjusted return and typically invest very little in private capital markets, performance is not likely to depend very much on the skill of managers.

In short, the problem is that political motives drive investment policy. This means that performance differentials observed across countries are most likely correlated with lack of transparency that allows the fund to be used for nonpension purposes. Other characteristics would also reflect the quality of governance. Some governments may be less dependent on cheap borrowing from pension reserves while others may be more resistant to lobbies from special interests for social investments. Some may be even be more susceptible to corruption.

Recently, Kaufmann, Kraay, and Zoldo-Lobaton (1999) demonstrated the association between good government and a wide array of positive development outcomes across many countries. Conversely, after accounting for other factors, the countries that rank poorly in terms of bureaucratic efficiency and corruption have worse living standards.

In the case of public pension fund management, the link may be even more straightforward. The evidence motivated us to test the following hypotheses: (i) the level of governance in a country affects performance across countries, and (ii) there is a general "public management effect" that itself reduce returns. We tested these hypotheses in a multivariate regression analysis using gross returns minus bank deposit rates as the dependent variable. We used an index of governance and a dummy variable for private management as independent variables. The governance measure is an average of three indices covering surveyed perceptions of (i) the efficiency of the judiciary system, (ii) the amount of bureaucratic red tape and (iii) corruption as found in appendix 3 of Mauro (1995). The specific proposition here is that poor governance leads to conditions—corruption, politicized investments, the need for captive financing for deficits, etc.— that in turn lead to poor returns.

We attempted several specifications. The sample included 16 of the multiyear country observations of gross returns minus bank deposit rates from figure 6.5. The governance index was not available for the other countries.[32] The sample also included observations of the same indicator from 14 countries for which private pension returns were available. Observations of both public and private management were used from Canada, Japan, Sweden, and the United States. We included an intercept dummy for private management.

The functional form yielding the best fit was quadratic, suggesting that the impact of governance on performance is greater in the lower part of the range and gradually levels off. Using this specification, the adjusted R^2 was 0.58. Both variables were statistically significant (at the 5 percent level) and had the expected signs. Better country governance rankings were associated with higher returns; public management was associated with lower returns.

In figure 6.9 we plot the fitted lines for publicly and privately managed returns against different values of the governance index, showing the extent of these two effects. The effect of governance is strong: on a scale of 1–10, with 10 being the best governance, an increase from 4–5 to 8–10 increases returns relative to bank deposits by 5–7 percentage points. Most of the gains come at the lower part of this range and begin to disappear after a country achieves a governance rating of approximately 8.

The difference between the top and the bottom lines in figure 6.9 is due to the significant and positive coefficient of the private management dummy. This is an intercept dummy—a slope dummy was insignificant. According to our results, private management produces returns that are about 430 basis points higher than publicly managed schemes, after taking

Figure 6.9. Predicted Normalized Returns for Different Levels of Governance for Privately and Publicly Managed Schemes Based on Regression Results

Returns above bank deposits, percent

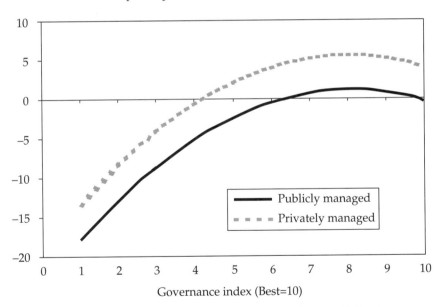

Note: Regression results used to generate the figure are from the following equation:

$$-2.36 + .06151 * GOVINDEX - .0038 * GOVINDEX^2 + .0437 * PRIVATEDUM$$
$$(2.14) \quad (1.96) \qquad\qquad (-1.83) \qquad\qquad\quad (3.83)$$

t-stats in parentheses; adjusted R^2 = .58; number of observation = 30.
An interactive term was tested and found not to be significant.
Sources: Figure 6.6; Mauro 1995.

into account differences in the governance index. In other words, as expected, the "public management effect" is strongly negative.

Several tentative conclusions emerge from the observation of the two effects shown in figure 6.9. First, based on the experience to date, publicly managed schemes are likely to perform very badly in countries with low governance ratings. Countries with good governments fare better but are unlikely to outperform short-term interest rates. This presents a major policy dilemma for countries that choose to partially fund their defined benefit obligations in the hope of improving sustainability and stabilizing payroll taxes in the face of population aging. It is an even greater problem for countries that choose to run centrally managed, defined contribution schemes in which benefits depend directly on the investment return.

Second, figure 6.9 shows that privately managed schemes are likely to outperform short-term interest rates in countries with medium or high governance ratings. In countries rated 7 or better, private returns exceed bank deposit rates by more than 400 basis points. On the other hand, countries with the worst governance ratings, say, below 4, would not produce reasonable returns even with private management. The difference between the normalized returns predicted for a privately managed scheme in a country with good government and a publicly managed scheme in a poorly governed country would be on the order of 10 percentage points.

The policy implications can be stated as follows: (i) unless public management can be improved or replaced by private management, prefunding is not likely to be effective in achieving the objectives of either a partially funded defined benefit or a funded defined contribution scheme; (ii) poor performance of publicly managed schemes is likely to signal misallocation of savings with important macroeconomic implications if the fund itself is large; and (iii) privately managed schemes tend to produce gross returns that are consistent with the objectives of pension policy but only where a certain level of governance has been attained. This implies that countries with low governance rankings probably should avoid altogether funding their mandatory pension systems.[33]

There are, however, several important caveats. First, this analysis ignores risk. This would not affect countries in the low governance category where poor returns are also very volatile (see figure 6.5). However, in the well-governed countries, adjusting the publicly managed scheme returns for risk would reduce the advantage to private management and increase the importance of good governance in our regression. At the same time, it is not clear that annual volatility is the appropriate measure of risk for these long-term savings vehicles. Considering longer periods favors private management.

The data set used suffers from certain problems of quality and comparability already highlighted. The sample is also quite small despite the fact that the 30 country observations for the dependent variable represent more than 400 country/year data points in the form of compounded averages.

Unfortunately, time series data on governance is not readily available. The cross-section regression implicitly assumes that relative governance capacity has not changed over the time periods analyzed.

Our results are also likely to be skewed by the fact that the privately managed schemes in our sample are from countries with better governance. In future work we hope to expand the overall sample, especially the available information on private pension funds in low-governance countries. Finally, the privately managed returns are sectoral averages hiding potentially significant variation across funds within a country. Despite these caveats, preliminary conclusions are quite robust and are consistent with anecdotal evidence.

Effect of Poor Management of Public Pension Reserves

The portfolios of publicly managed pension funds tend to fall into two categories—high proportions of government or government-guaranteed debt and bank deposits or a combination of these with socially and economically targeted investments. With a few exceptions, there is very little investment in private securities and almost no foreign investment. These practices produce several problems for members of the pension funds and for the economies as a whole.

The most visible consequence for the members of the fund is the low rate of return. For partially funded, defined benefit schemes, low returns hasten the day when benefits must be cut or contributions raised. This has already happened in many developing countries in which deficits have arisen or contribution rate increases have been forced after just one or two decades of operation, largely due to poor investment returns. In other words, poor investment policy leads to a lower internal rate of return to participation in the scheme. Low returns over long periods of time can gradually erode the credibility of the system. To the extent that workers increasingly perceive the lost returns as a tax, they will be encouraged to evade the scheme and hide their income from the government. An extreme case of this phenomenon occurred recently in the small island nation of Vanuatu. In February 1999, workers voted with their feet. The Australian press reported the following:

> Over two thousand members of the National Provident Fund have received their contribution payments totaling just over two million dollars. The fund's acting general manager, Joses Kenneth, says the fund is processing a daily payment of forty thousand dollars to some 500 members. The decision to pay out the money was reached after riots broke out in Port Vila last month when worried depositors stormed the fund's head office, which the Ombudsman said gave preferential loans to politicians and their supporters.[34]

Public Management of Pension Reserves and Savings

A vast literature exists on the complexity of the relationship between public pension systems and national savings. One specific question that is directly relevant to public management of pension reserves is how fiscal policy is affected by the presence of pension surpluses. There is some evidence, for example, that forced purchase of government debt may lead to increased government consumption. Cogan (1998) provides econometric evidence of such an effect in the United States, and Von Furstenberg (1979) finds that spending at the provincial level in Canada increased due to the subsidized credit provided by the Canadian Pension Plan.

Unfortunately, evidence is scarce, but the idea that easy access to these funds increases the government's appetite for spending seems a reasonable hypothesis. The effect is made more likely by the fiscal accounting methods that consider public pension fund government bond holdings as repurchase of government debt, as is the case in the current framework of the International Monetary Fund's Government Finance Statistics. If such an effect does exist, the rationale for prefunding will be seriously undermined. In the extreme case where borrowing increases exactly in step with the surpluses, the "funded" scheme would have the same intertemporal economic impact as a pure pay-as-you-go scheme. Maintaining pay-as-you-go financing but simply reporting the liabilities as part of the fiscal accounts could obtain a similar result.[35]

How likely is it that nonpension government spending increases (or nonpension taxes are reduced) in such a way as to completely offset pension surpluses? The answer depends to some extent on the government's target budget deficit concept. Most governments focus on a deficit concept that includes the central budget as well as pension spending and revenues.[36] These "headline" deficits may not accurately reflect the intertemporal fiscal stance of the government but are nevertheless often at the center of the annual budget discussions.

This important point was made by a number of prominent economists analyzing the emerging surpluses of the U.S. Social Security program in the late 1980s (Weaver 1990). The question addressed was whether these surpluses were likely to add to national savings, a key underlying assumption of the commission that raised contribution rates in the early 1980s in order to generate surpluses. One of the analysts, James Buchanan, described the scenario in which a comprehensive deficit target is used but the public pension program is running surpluses as follows:

> [S]uppose that the comprehensive budget was in deficit . . . but that medium range legislative targets were established to reduce and then eliminate the comprehensive budget deficit. . . . In this case, surpluses in the social security account allow the deficit reduction targets to be satisfied, while still allowing for increases

in the non-social security deficit. Much the same results emerge under any scheme for deficit control that uses balance or imbalance in the comprehensive budget as a criterion for policy achievement. As a final example, suppose that a decision is made to keep the relationship between the measured comprehensive budget deficit and the gross national product constant. Again, satisfaction of this norm would allow non-social-security deficits to increase during the period of trust fund accumulation. (Buchanan 1990)

The consequences are straightforward. If the additional spending induced by the availability of these surpluses takes the form of government consumption, "there will be no induced increase in the rate of private capital formation in the economy. There will be no direct or indirect funding of the future pension obligations" (Buchanan 1990). In other words, as long as governments focus on targets based on the standard definition of its budget deficit, the intergenerational fiscal burden does not improve through this type of prefunding.

Summary and Conclusions

This chapter reviewed some of the available information on how publicly managed pension funds invest and how their returns compare to relevant benchmarks. The general finding is that public pension funds are subject to a series of restrictions and mandates that produce poor returns. The nonpension objectives of the government often lead to social and economically targeted investments and forced loans to the government to finance its deficits. These investments yield returns that are often below bank deposit rates and almost always below the growth of incomes. This contrasts with privately managed pension fund returns, which generally exceed income growth. Public management in countries with poor governance records produces the worst returns.

The low rates of return found in many publicly managed schemes over the last few decades have negative consequences for the finances of the pension scheme as well as for the output of the overall economy. The members are affected because partially funded schemes must charge higher contributions or pay lower benefits. Provident fund members receive lower returns (or prescribed yields), which directly reduces their balances and makes it impossible to maintain preretirement consumption levels.

Meanwhile, the presence of these reserves may lead to higher nonpension government deficits if target deficit levels are based on the consolidated budget. Additionally, the diversion of an important pool of long-term savings to projects with low returns or for higher government consumption implies an important opportunity cost for the economy. Private capital markets are robbed of liquidity, and good projects do not find financing. The larger the fund is, relative to the capital markets, the greater this cost.

There is considerable evidence that public management of pension funds should be avoided despite a number of caveats and the need for further research. Moreover, the discussion ignores recent policy initiatives in some countries that seek to address historical problems with public management. Faced with demographic aging and scheme maturation, some publicly managed funds are starting to invest more of their portfolio in the private capital markets. This trend is likely to continue, raising a new set of policy issues. In particular, as public pension funds become shareholders in private industry, the government faces a potential conflict between its role as regulator and its role in corporate governance.

Notes

1. Robert Holzmann, Estelle James, Olivia Mitchell, Sylvester Schieber, Yvonne Sin, and Juan Yermo provided useful comments for this chapter, which is a condensed version of a longer paper of the same title published as part of the World Bank's Pension Reform Primer series. Electronic copies are available at www.worldbank.org/pensions.

2. These are rough estimates based on available country data (see Palacios and Pallares-Miralles 2000).

3. See Srinivas, Whitehouse, and Yermo (2000).

4. The International Labor Office recommended the concept of the "scaled premium," which involves the accumulation of reserves in order to smooth out contribution rates over time, and many developing countries adopted it in the 1950s and 1960s (ILO 1983). Much of North Africa and Francophone Sub-Saharan Africa adopted the scaled premium approach. Mesa-Lago (1991) reports nine scaled premium countries in Latin America.

5. There is no standard methodology for calculating unfunded public pension liabilities across countries. Nevertheless, we believe this statement to be true under any reasonable definition of full funding currently applied to private sector defined benefit schemes.

6. Some of these schemes include guarantees or prescribed yields that are not funded.

7. See Rofman, Stirparo, and Lattes (1998) for Argentina; Palacios and Rocha (1998) for Hungary; and Chlon, Gora, and Rutkowski (1999) for Poland.

8. See Whitehouse (1999) on tax treatment of funded pension schemes.

9. Srinivas, Whitehouse, and Yermo (2000) discuss the effect of government regulation on the countries in column three of table 1.

10. See Asher (1999) on Singapore and http://fiji.gov.fj for information on Fiji.

11. Privately managed, employer-based schemes in many countries include representatives of employees and employers. In Australia and Switzerland half of the membership of the boards constitutes employees.

12. The number of board members varies by country: India (42), Jordan (15), Korea (20), Malaysia (20) and Sweden (9), Tanzania (12), and Kenya (10) (compiled from national sources).

13. The number of staff handling investments also varies among countries: Ghana (11), Kenya (62), Malaysia (6), Nigeria (12), Sudan (62), Uganda (6), and Zambia (21) (compiled from national sources).

14. See *Far Eastern Economic Review*. "Savings at Risk: Malaysia Is Being Criticized for Using Its National Pension Fund to Funnel Cash to Companies." *Far Eastern Economic Review*, April 30, 1998.

15. Discussions with EPF officials in November 1998.

16. "The yield to investments with a social dimension is expected to be 2.5 percent above the bank rate, and commercial bank loans are expected to yield 4.5 percent above the Bank rate" (Government's Actuary Department, United Kingdom, 1998).

17. For examples of the debate over ETIs in the United States, see Watson (1994) and Nofsinger (1998). Munnell and Sunden (1999) provide a long list of examples from the U.S. experience.

18. Vittas (1993) states that the government was lifting these restrictions in the early 1990s.

19. The Employees' Pension Insurance and the National Pension System have 63 percent of their funds in national financial investments and loan programs, 17 percent in welfare operations, and 20 percent in market-based investments (24 trillion yen in 1998).

20. The International Monetary Fund's Government Finance Statistics (GFS) methodology treats the purchase of government bonds by public pension funds as repurchase of government debt.

21. Other indicators such as M3/GDP, stock market capitalization and liquidity, etc., produce a similar distribution across countries.

22. A recent example is the use of Taiwan's state-controlled pension fund to prop up the stock market (see *Wall Street Journal*, "Taipei Signals Willingness to Discuss Unification If Beijing Accepts Taiwan as Diplomatic Equal," July 19, 1999, p. A10).

23. See Angelis (1998) for a good review of the issues in the U.S. context.

24. See table V.5, OECD (1998). This average includes Australia, Belgium, Canada, France, Italy, Japan, Germany, Netherlands, Switzerland, the United Kingdom, and the United States.

25. In fact, the finance minister recently announced that no foreign investments would be allowed.

26. For example, Canadian unions have hotly contested proposals by the new Investment Board to allow the Canadian Pension Plan to invest as much abroad as private pension funds (20 percent).

27. The sample did not include Australia, where pension funds tend to hold more than 15 percent in foreign assets.

28. Easterly (1999), for example, finds very low returns to capital in Sub-Saharan Africa.

29. It should be noted that, as in all of the countries, our data refer to the main public scheme for private employees—in the case of the Philippines, the social security system. However, returns to a fund of similar magnitude for civil servants during this period appear to have been much lower.

30. As noted above, we do not consider the social returns that are generated from the use of these funds; for example, investment in urban housing in Singapore. This would be a difficult exercise in the case of Singapore, where the government owns the land upon which the housing is built, and it represents a substantial portion of the value of the housing. In any case, we are not aware of any study that attempts to estimate net social returns to public pension fund investments in Singapore or elsewhere.

31. See, for example, Asher (1999) and Leong and Das-Gupta (1998) on Singapore.

32. We ran a separate set of regressions with estimated values for four countries based on the correlation between Mauro's index and the corruption index produced by Transparency International. The regression was more robust with these observations included.

33. A possible criterion would be the governance level at which the regression would predict that returns would be greater than bank deposit rates. Based on the indices shown in Mauro (1995) and the estimated relationship between governance and returns, a number of countries such as Haiti, Bangladesh, Nigeria, and Liberia would not be likely to succeed with a prefunding strategy.

34. There was a similar reaction recently among provident fund members in Papua, New Guinea, when they learned that their balance of the fund was to be written down by one-half to recognize losses.

35. See Kane and Palacios (1996) for a discussion of reporting the implicit pension debt.

36. Munnell and Ernsberger (1989) claim that the Swedish government is an exception in that its targets exclude the AP fund surpluses.

References

Note: The word *processed* describes informally reproduced works that may not be commonly available through libraries.

Abel, A. B., N. G. Mankiw, L. H. Summers, and R. J. Zeckhauser. 1989. "Assessing Dynamic Efficiency: Theory and Evidence." *Review of Economic Studies* 56: 1–20.

Angelis, Theodore J. 1998. "Investing Public Money in Private Markets: What Are the Right Questions?" Presentation at the 1998 National Academy of Social Insurance Conference, January. Processed.

Asher, Mukul. 1998. "Investment Policies and Performance of Provident Funds in Southeast Asia." Paper prepared for the Economic Development Institute of the World Bank workshop in China, January. Processed.

_____. 1999. "The Pension System in Singapore." Social Protection Discussion Paper No. 9919. World Bank, Washington, D.C.

Börsch-Supan, Axel, Robert Palacios, and Patrizia Tumbarello. 1999. "Pension Systems in the Middle East and North Africa: A Window of Opportunity." Processed.

Brinson, Gary, L., Randolph Hood, and Gilbert L. Beebower. 1986. "Determinants of Portfolio Performance." *Financial Analysts Journal*, July–August.

Brinson, Gary, Brian Singer, and Gilbert Beebower. 1991. "Determinants of Portfolio Performance II: An Update." *Financial Analysts Journal*, May/June.

Buchanan, James. 1990. "The Budgetary Politics of Social Security." In Carolyn L. Weaver, ed., *Social Security's Looming Surpluses: Prospects and Implications*. Washington, D.C.: American Enterprise Institute.

Chlon, A., M. Gora, and M. Rutkowski. 1999. "Shaping Pension Reform in Poland: Security Through Diversity." Social Protection Discussion Paper No. 9923. World Bank, Washington, D.C.

Cogan, John F. 1998. "The Congressional Response to Social Security Surpluses, 1935–1994." Hoover Institution, Stanford University, Palo Alto, Calif. Processed.

Davis, E.P. 1993. "The Structure, Regulation and Performance of Pension Funds in Nine Industrial Countries." World Bank, Financial Sector Development Department, Washington, D.C.

Easterly, W. 1999. "Are African Savings Too Low?" World Bank, Washington, D.C. Processed.

Government's Actuary Department, United Kingdom. 1998. "Mauritius National Pensions Fund, Actuarial Review as at June 30, 1995." London.

ILO (International Labour Office). 1983. "Methods of Financing Social Security Schemes in Developing Countries with Particular Reference to the Accumulation of Reserve Funds." Paper presented at the Meeting of Experts on the Investment of Social Security Funds in Developing Countries, Geneva. Processed.

_____. 1994. "United Republic of Tanzania: The Investment Policy and Financial Management of the National Provident Fund of Tanzania, Project Findings and Recommendations." Geneva.

_____. 1996. "Uganda: Rehabilitation and Development of the National Social Security Fund, Actuarial Study of Proposals for Reform." Geneva, UNDP programme.

IMF (International Monetary Fund). Various years. *International Finance Statistics Yearbook*. Washington, D.C.

ISSA (International Social Security Association). 1997. "Investment of Social Security Funds by Social Security Organizations in English-Speaking Africa." Paper presented at Meeting of Directors of Member Organizations in English-Speaking Africa, Kampala, Uganda. Processed.

Kane, C., and R. Palacios. 1996. "The Implicit Pension Debt." *Finance and Development* 33: 36–38.

Kaufmann, D., Aart Kraay, and Pablo Zoldo-Lobaton. 1999. "Governance Matters." World Bank, Washington, D.C. Processed.

Leong, Lun Yee, and Arindam Das-Gupta. 1998. "Returns to Social Security in Singapore: A Life-Cycle Evaluation." Nanyang Business School, Nanyang Technological University, Singapore. Processed.

Mahdi El Farhan, Mohammad. 1990. "Investment of Social Security Funds: Comparative Report on Pension Schemes in Asia and the Pacific." In Proceedings to Meeting of Experts on Investment of Social Security Funds in Developing Countries, ISSA. Processed.

Mauro, Paolo. 1995. "Corruption and Growth." *The Quarterly Journal of Economics* 110 (August): 681–712.

Mesa-Lago, Carmelo. 1991. "Portfolio Performance of Selected Social Security Institutes in Latin America." World Bank Discussion Paper No. 139, Washington, D.C.

Mounbaga, Emmanuel. 1995. "The Investment of Social Security Reserves During Periods of Crisis: The Experience of Cameroon." *International Social Security Review* 48(2): 95.

Munnell, Alicia, and C. Nicole Ernsberger. 1989. "Public Pension Surpluses and National Saving: Foreign Experience." *New England Economic Review*, March/April: 16–38.

Munnell, Alicia, and Annika Sunden, 1999. "Investment Practices of State and Local Pension Funds." Paper presented at the 1999 Pension Research Council Symposium, April.

National Provident Fund. 1996. "Annual Report for the Financial Year 1995/96." Head Office, Bibi Titi Mohammed/Morogoro Road, Dar es Salaam, Tanzania.

_____. 1997. "Annual Report for the Financial Year 1996/97." Head Office, Bibi Titi Mohammed/Morogoro Road, Dar es Salaam, Tanzania.

National Social Security Fund of Kenya. 1998. "Annual Report for 1996/97."

Nofsinger, John. 1998. "Why Targeted Investing Does Not Make Sense." *Financial Management* 27(3): 87–96.

OECD (Organization for Economic Cooperation and Development). 1998. "Private Pension Systems: Regulatory Policies." Working Paper AWP 2.2. Paris.

Palacios, R., and M. Pallares-Miralles. 2000. "International Patterns of Pension Provision." Social Protection Discussion Paper No. 0009. World Bank, Washington, D.C.

Palacios, R., and R. Rocha. 1998. "The Hungarian Pension System in Transition." Social Protection Discussion Paper No. 9805. World Bank, Washington, D.C.

Piggott, John, and Geoffrey Kingston. 1999. "The Geometry of Life Annuities." *Manchester School* (United Kingdom) 67: 187–91.

Rofman, Rafael, Gustavo Stirparo, and Pablo Lattes. 1998. "Proyecciones del Sistema Integrado de Jubilaciones y Pensiones, 1995–2050." Serie Estudios Especiales 12, SAFJP, Buenos Aires.

Social Security Corporation. 1996. *Annual Report*. Kingdom of Jordan.

SSRI (Social Security Research Institute). 1997. "Social Security in Iran." Tehran, Iran.

Srinivas, S. P., and J. Yermo. 1999. "Do Investment Regulations Compromise Pension Fund Performance?" World Bank Latin American and Caribbean Studies, Discussion Paper Series. Washington, D.C.

Srinivas, S. P., E. Whitehouse, and J. Yermo. 2000. "Portfolio Limits in Mandatory Pension Schemes, Human Development Network, Social Protection Working Paper Series, World Bank, Washington, D.C.

Superintendencia de Administradoras de Fondes de Pensiones. 2000. Evolución del Sistema Chileno de Pensiones. Santiago de Chile, Gobierno de Chile.

Vittas, Dimitri. 1993. "Options for Pension Reform in Tunisia." World Bank Policy Research Working Paper Series, WPS 1154. Washington, D.C.

Von Furstenberg, George. 1979. *Social Security versus Private Saving*. Cambridge, Mass.: Ballinger Press.

Watson, Ronald. 1994. "Does Targeted Investing Make Sense?" *Financial Management* 24(4): 69–74.

Weaver, C. 1990. *Social Security's Looming Surpluses*. Washington, D.C.: American Enterprise Institute.

Whitehouse, Edward. 1999. "The Tax Treatment of Funded Pensions." Social Protection Discussion Paper No. 9910. World Bank, Washington, D.C.

World Bank. 1994. "The Democratic and Popular Republic of Algeria: Country Economic Memorandum: The Transition to a Market Economy." World Bank Report No. 12048-AL, Middle East and North Africa Region. Washington, D.C.

———. 1996. "Report on Social Security Corporation of Jordan." Processed.

———. 1997. *World Development Indicators 1997*. Washington, D.C.

Annex

Summary Tables for Data Used in Figures 6.5–6.9

Table A.6.1. Compounded Real Annual Pension Fund Returns, Standard Deviation and Sharpe Ratio
(Ranked from highest to lowest average return)

Country	Period	Compounded return (%)	Standard deviation (%)	Sharpe ratio
Rep. of Korea	1988–97	5.4	1.4	3.83
Malaysia	1958–96	3.2	3.1	1.05
Morocco	1985–96	2.3	2.7	0.85
Sweden	1961–95	2.1	3.4	0.60
United States	1955–96	2.0	3.4	0.58
Canada	1971–89	1.8	3.8	0.48
India	1977–97	1.6	2.7	0.57
Singapore	1961–95	1.5	4.2	0.36
Japan	1970–94	1.4	5.0	0.27
Philippines	1978–91	0.8	11.7	0.07
Sri Lanka	1960–97	–0.3	4.5	–0.08
Kenya	1978–90	–3.9	5.1	–0.76
Jamaica	1979–86	–4.5	7.5	–0.60
Guatemala	1985–95	–4.9	10.4	–0.47
Costa Rica	1980–96	–5.0	15.5	–0.32
Egypt	1981–95	–9.1	4.9	–1.85
Ecuador	1980–87	–9.3	8.8	–1.06
Tanzania	1986–96	–11.2	5.2	–2.14
Venezuela	1979–89	–15.3	21.0	–0.73
Zambia	1980–91	–28.5	18.7	–1.52
Uganda	1986–94	–33.1	25.6	–1.29
Peru	1981–87	–44.0	25.7	–1.71
Unweighted average		–6.7%	8.8%	–17.5%
Maximum		5.4%	25.7%	
Minimum		–44.0%	1.4%	
Total observations (country x years)		325		

Table A.6.2. Compounded Real Annual Bank Deposit Rates and Standard Deviation

Country	Period	Compounded return (%)	Standard deviation
Canada	1975–89	2.6	2.5
Costa Rica	1982–96	–2.3	11.7
Ecuador	1980–87	–5.6	6.7
Egypt	1981–95	–3.7	3.5
Guatemala	1985–95	–1.9	5.2
India	1977–97	1.3	3.3
Jamaica	1979–86	–4.3	7.5
Japan	1970–94	–1.6	4.3
Kenya	1978–90	–1.3	5.0
Rep. of Korea	1988–97	2.9	1.2
Malaysia	1958–96	3.0	2.8
Morocco	1985–96	2.5	2.1
Peru	n.a.	n.a.	n.a.
Philippines	1978–91	–0.4	7.1
Singapore	1972–95	1.1	3.6
Sri Lanka	1978–97	2.8	5.1
Sweden	1962–95	0.9	2.5
Tanzania	n.a.	n.a.	n.a.
Uganda	1986–94	–22.7	27.3
United States	1960–96	1.7	2.4
Venezuela	1982–89	–8.6	13.1
Zambia	1980–90	–18.4	15.4
Unweighted average		-2.6%	6.2%
Maximum		3.0%	27.3%
Minimum		-22.7%	1.2%

n.a. Not available.

Table A.6.3. Compounded Real Annual Income Per Capita Growth and Standard Deviation

Country	Period	Compounded return (%)	Standard deviation (%)
Canada	1971–89	2.9	2.6
Costa Rica	1980–96	2.2	5.8
Ecuador	1980–87	–0.3	3.8
Egypt	1981–95	2.3	2.9
Guatemala	1985–95	0.5	1.6
India	1977–97	3.3	3.2
Jamaica	1979–86	–2.1	4.7
Japan	1970–94	3.2	3.6
Kenya	1978–90	1.0	5.1
Rep. of Korea	1988–97	7.4	3.3
Malaysia	1961–96	4.3	2.7
Morocco	1985–96	1.7	4.7
Peru	1981–87	–1.6	3.3
Philippines	1978–91	–0.2	3.2
Singapore	1961–95	6.2	3.8
Sri Lanka	1960–97	3.4	4.5
Sweden	1961–95	2.5	2.2
Tanzania	1986–96	–0.4	4.5
Uganda	1986–94	2.3	3.4
United States	1955–96	1.8	2.1
Venezuela	1979–89	–0.4	4.0
Zambia	1980–91	–1.9	4.8

Table A.6.4. Governance Index for Sample of Countries

Sample	Governance index[a]
Japan	9.08
Rep. of Korea	6.08
Philippines	4.75
Sweden	9.25
United States	9.75
Malaysia	7
India	5.5
Morocco	5.88
Singapore	10
Canada	9.58
Jamaica	5.44
Kenya	5.08
Sri Lanka	6.67
Ecuador	5.58
Egypt	4.25
Venezuela	5.42
Switzerland	10
Hong Kong	9.25
United Kingdom	9
Australia	9.75
Denmark	9.58
Spain	6.42
Chile	8.58
Netherlands	10
Belgium	9.08
Ireland	8.67
Extended sample[b]	
Zambia	5.3
Uganda	4.5
Costa RIca	6.4
Guatemala	4.2

a. Taken from Appendix 3, Mauro (1995).
b. Based on Transparency International Corruption Index.
Description of governance index: There are a wide variety of governance indicators available (see Kaufmann, Kraay, and Zoldo-Lobaton 1999). The index used here is constructed on the basis of nine indicators collected by the Economist Intelligence Unit for the period 1980–83, which Mauro (1995) used to generate three composite indices. These three indices measure (i) the efficiency of the judiciary system, (ii) the cost of dealing with bureaucracy ("red tape"), and (iii) corruption. In this chapter, the average of these three indices (referred to as "bureaucratic efficiency" by Mauro) is used as a measure of governance. For more details, see Mauro (1995). The extended sample figures shown in table A6.3 were based on a simple regression of this governance indicator with the one published by Transparency International. The major conclusions of the analysis presented here were borne out when these observations were included, but the results reported here exclude these four countries.

7

Administrative Costs and the Organization of Individual Account Systems: A Comparative Perspective

Estelle James, James Smalhout, and Dimitri Vittas

PREFUNDING IS NOW SEEN AS A desirable characteristic of old age security systems because it can help increase national saving, makes the financial sustainability of the systems less sensitive to demographic shocks, and reduce the need to increase taxes as populations age.[1] With prefunding comes the need to determine how the funds will be managed. Those who fear political manipulation of publicly managed funds see defined contribution individual accounts (IAs) as a way to decentralize control and, thereby, achieve a better allocation of the funds. But IAs have been criticized on other grounds, especially for having high administrative costs. Many countries now in the process of establishing their IA systems are concerned about these costs and seek ways to keep them low.

This chapter investigates the cost-effectiveness of two alternative methods for organizing mandatory IAs: (i) investing through the retail market, in which workers choose their own pension fund, open entry is subject to regulations, and the fund sets prices, and (ii) investing through the institutional market under conditions in which entry and price are negotiated for a larger group or for the entire covered labor force and group choice constrains worker choice. In a competitive bidding process, which is a recommended way of determining group choice, primary competition takes place at the point of entry to the market, and a more limited secondary competition for individual workers occurs among the winners of the primary competition. In both the retail and institutional cases, government "organizes" the markets, but in the former it uses regulations while in the latter it uses competitive bidding or other group mechanisms. Additionally, in both cases most countries will end up with a relatively concentrated market due to scale economies, but the paths as well as the equilibrium costs and fees, differ. We pose the question of what is the most cost-effective way to organize a mandatory IA system.

In the first section we start with a simple, stylized illustration of retail and institutional markets that decomposes total costs into investment, record-keeping, marketing, and start-up components. In the second section, to analyze actual costs in the retail market, we use data from mandatory schemes in Chile and other Latin American countries. In the third section we complement these data with data on U.S. mutual funds, which offer an example of a relatively well-run, voluntary retail financial industry that has much in common with decentralized IA systems. To analyze costs in the institutional market, in the fourth section we use data from large centralized pension funds in the United States as well as from mandatory and voluntary IA systems in various countries. The fifth section of the chapter analyzes these IA systems that operate in the institutional market in Bolivia, Sweden, and in the U.S. Thrift Saving Plan (TSP). These systems operate by aggregating small contributions into large blocks of money, constraining choice regarding investment portfolios and managers, and negotiating fees on a group or centralized basis. In Bolivia and the TSP entry has been limited and fees set in a competitive bidding process; in Sweden price ceilings attempt to mimic the marginal cost function and the sliding fee scale in the institutional market.

Empirical evidence in this chapter and elsewhere finds substantial economies of scale and scope in asset management. Both the retail and institutional markets exploit these economies, but in different ways. The retail market pools funds from many individual investors, enabling them to benefit from scale economies but at the cost of high marketing expenses—about half of total costs—that are needed to attract and aggregate small investments into large pools. In the Chilean Administradores de Fondos de Pensiones (AFP) and U.S. mutual fund industries, most annual fees range from 0.8–1.5 percent of assets, and marketing is the largest cost component. Slightly larger numbers obtain in retail personal pension plans in the United Kingdom and master trusts in Australia (Bateman 1999; Bateman and Piggott 1999; Blake 2000; Murthi, Orszag, and Orszag 2000). A 1 percent annual fee reduces retirement accumulations by 20 percent for a lifetime contributor, so administrative costs in the retail market reduce pensions by 15–30 percent.

The institutional market, which caters to large investors, benefits from scale economies without large marketing costs; hence, its total costs are much lower. We investigate whether and how mandatory IA systems that consist of many small investors could be set up to capture these same advantages. We find that use of the institutional market in IA systems in Bolivia, Sweden, and the United States has reduced fees to less than 0.6 percent and in some cases to less than 0.2 percent of assets. These lower fees stemming from lower administrative costs in the institutional market reduce pensions by only 10 percent or less, a potential saving of 10–20 percent relative to the retail market.

Costs must always be weighed against benefits. Potential pitfalls inherent in the institutional approach include the increased probability of corruption, collusion, regulatory capture, decreased performance incentives, rebidding problems, and inflexibility in the face of unforeseen contingencies (see sections 5 and 6). If these problems can be surmounted, the institutional approach is worth serious consideration, especially for countries with small asset bases and at the start-up phase of a new IA system.

How Administrative Costs Vary across Time and Systems and How to Compare Them

We start by setting forth a small model of the components of administrative costs that can be used to understand differences in costs across time and systems:

$$\text{TOTADMINCOST}^i_t = \text{STARTUPCOST} + \text{R\&C} + \text{INV} + \text{MARKETING}$$

where TOTADMINCOST^i_t = total administrative cost for pension fund or system i in year t; STARTUPCOST = capital costs incurred in the early years of a new system or fund; R&C = record-keeping and communication costs, INV = investment cost; and MARKETING = marketing cost.

Each of these cost components is determined quite differently. R&C costs tend to be technologically determined and standardized, depending on quality of service and number of accounts. Passive investment costs are also technologically determined, depending on volume and allocation of assets. Active investment costs are market-determined, stemming from the premium that a manager who is deemed to be superior can command in a market for differentiated investment skills. Marketing expenses usually go together with active management, since they are used to sell the skills of a particular asset manager and depend on profit-maximizing calculations about costs versus returns of incremental marketing activities.

In comparing costs across funds or systems and trying to ascertain how these are likely to change in the future, it is necessary to take into account the main arguments of the fund's production function—the volume of assets and the number of accounts that determine costs. Looking simply at current costs can be misleading as an indicator of efficiency or long-run costs in comparing systems of different sizes or stages of development.

Table 7.1 illustrates the total administrative cost and its breakdown between R&C and INV in two hypothetical systems as they evolve through time. Two cost measures are used—*dollars per account* and *basis points per unit of assets* (1 basis point = .01 percent). The first measure is useful because it tells us how much it costs to operate an account for an average worker, while the second measure tells us by how much administrative costs are whittling away gross returns. While economies of scale are probable (see James and Palacios 1995; Mitchell 1998), in this section, for expositional purposes, we assume that R&C cost per account and INV cost per unit of assets are constant, and that start-up costs are incurred in the first three years.

Panel A illustrates a stylized cost profile for an IA system that uses the institutional approach, with passive investing costs of 0.1 percent of assets annually and R&C costs of US$20 per account. Panel B does the same but increases the gross annual contribution from US$520 to US$2,020. Panel C illustrates the retail approach, with marketing plus active investment expenses of 1.1 percent of assets and R&C costs of US$30 per account. We see that costs per account and per unit of assets change over time, and in a given year differences appear among these systems, even if they are equally efficient:

- *Start-up costs* greatly accentuate total cost in the early years.
- *Cost per account* starts relatively low and rises through time as average account size grows, due to increased investment and/or marketing costs.
- *Cost as a percentage of assets* starts high and falls as average account size grows, due to constant R&C costs per account. Scale economies in asset management would accentuate this effect.
- *R&C costs* dominate at the beginning, but their impact on net returns becomes much smaller in the long run, when investment and marketing costs dominate.
- A *higher contribution rate* leads to a faster buildup of assets, and a lower cost as percentage of assets, even if two systems are equally efficient (panel A versus B).
- An *expensive investment and marketing strategy*, as in the retail market, increases cost per unit of assets and leads to faster growth in cost per account and per unit of assets, while the institutional approach keeps these costs low, both in the short and long run (panel B versus C).

If we apply this production function approach across countries, in attempting to evaluate the cost-effectiveness of different systems, additional problems arise because wages, infrastructure, and productivity vary widely. If the relevant technologies tend to be capital-intensive, then capital-rich

Table 7.1. Administrative Costs over Time as a Percentage of Assets and Dollars per Account (Hypothetical System)

Panel A. Low Costs, Small Contribution Base

Year	Year-end accumulation of individual (in \$000s)[a]	Average account size in system (in \$000s)[b]	Costs as percentage of assets		Costs as dollars per account		R&C/ total exp.
			R&C	R&C + Inv	Inv per account	R&C + Inv per account	
1	0.5	0.5	4.00	4.10	0.5	20.5	0.98
2	1.0	1.0	2.20	2.30	1.0	21.0	0.96
3	1.6	1.6	1.28	1.38	1.6	21.6	0.93
4	2.2	2.1	0.95	1.05	2.1	22.1	0.90
5	2.8	2.7	0.76	0.86	2.7	22.7	0.88
10	6.4	5.6	0.36	0.46	5.6	25.6	0.78
15	10.9	8.8	0.23	0.33	8.8	28.8	0.70
20	16.7	12.1	0.17	0.27	12.1	32.1	0.63
25	24.1	15.4	0.13	0.23	15.4	35.4	0.57
30	33.6	18.5	0.11	0.21	18.5	38.5	0.52
35	45.6	20.8	0.10	0.20	20.8	40.8	0.50
40	61.0	22.0	0.09	0.19	22.0	42.0	0.47

Panel B. Low Costs, High Contribution Base

Year	Year-end accumulation of individual (in \$000s)[a]	Average account size in system (in \$000s)[b]	Costs as percentage of assets		Costs as dollars per account		R&C/ total exp.
			R&C	R&C + Inv	Inv per account	R&C + Inv per account	
1	2.0	2.0	1.00	1.10	2.0	22.0	0.91
2	4.0	4.0	0.50	0.60	4.0	24.0	0.83
3	6.4	6.4	0.31	0.41	6.4	26.4	0.76
4	8.8	8.4	0.24	0.34	8.4	28.4	0.70
5	11.2	10.8	0.19	0.29	10.8	30.8	0.65
10	25.6	22.4	0.09	0.19	22.4	42.4	0.47
15	43.6	35.2	0.06	0.16	35.2	55.2	0.36
20	66.8	48.4	0.04	0.14	48.4	68.4	0.29
25	96.4	61.6	0.03	0.13	61.6	81.6	0.25
30	134.4	74.0	0.03	0.13	74.0	94.0	0.21
35	182.4	83.2	0.02	0.12	83.2	103.2	0.19
40	244.0	88.0	0.02	0.12	88.0	108.0	0.19

(Table continued on next page)

Table 7.1 continued

Panel C. High costs, high contribution base

Year	Year-end accumulation of individual (in $000s)[a]	Average account size in system (in $000s)[b]	Costs as percentage of assets		Costs as dollars per account		R&C/ total exp.
			R&C	R&C + Inv	Inv per account	R&C + Inv per account	
1	2.0	2.0	1.50	2.10	2.60	12.0	52.0	0.58
2	4.1	4.1	0.74	1.34	1.84	24.3	74.5	0.40
3	6.2	6.0	0.50	1.10	1.60	36.3	96.5	0.31
4	8.5	8.2	0.37	0.97	1.57	49.0	119.9	0.25
5	10.8	10.2	0.29	0.89	1.39	61.4	142.6	0.21
10	23.9	21.0	0.14	0.74	1.24	126.1	261.2	0.11
15	39.8	32.1	0.09	0.69	1.19	192.7	383.3	0.08
20	59.3	43.3	0.07	0.67	1.17	259.8	506.2	0.06
25	82.9	53.9	0.06	0.66	1.16	323.2	622.5	0.05
30	111.6	63.1	0.05	0.65	1.15	378.8	724.5	0.04
35	146.6	70.1	0.04	0.64	1.14	420.4	800.8	0.04
40	189.1	73.2	0.04	0.64	1.14	439.0	834.9	0.04

Note:
Panel A: US$520 is contributed each year, R&C costs = US$20 per account, net contribution (NC) = US$500, gross rate of return = 5.1 percent, investment costs = 0.1 percent of assets, net return (NR) = 5.0 percent.
Panel B: annual contribution = US$2,020, R&C costs = US$20 per account, net contribution = US$2,000, gross rate of return = 5.1 percent, investment costs = 0.1 percent of assets, net return = 5.0 percent.
Panel C: annual contribution = US$2,020, R&C costs = US$30 per account, net contribution = US$1,990, gross rate of return = 5.1 percent, investment costs = 0.6 percent, marketing cost = 0.5 percent of assets, net return = 4 percent.

a. Individual's account accumulates at the following rate: $AA_t = AA_{t-1} (1 + NR) + NC$.

b. Account size increases at specified rates for individuals who stay in system. Withdrawals by high account individuals who retire and their replacement by incoming workers with small new accounts cause a decrease in average account size in system relative to individual's account.
Source: Authors' calculations.

countries with relatively cheap capital will have lower costs per account and asset unit, while the opposite is true if the feasible technology set uses labor intensively, especially unskilled labor. Funds that operate in countries with a facilitating legal and physical infrastructure, including, for example, enforceable contract rights and telephone lines that work, will be able to use their own labor and capital more productively. Regulations that vary across countries also influence the feasible production function. Data gaps do not allow us to control for differences in types and quality of service, which, therefore, become part of the "random" variation.

While we have been defining costs to the fund and the system, costs (fees) to consumers may vary from this. In the short run, at the start-up of a new system, funds may run temporary losses, in the expectation that they will increase their market share and recoup their capital expenses later on. In the medium term, they may earn profits that offset the earlier losses. Thus fees over time might be smoother than costs over time.

We would expect that in the long run competition would eliminate pure profits, so fees will just cover fund costs. But the existence of marketing competition, as well as potential skill and wage differentials across asset managers, makes it difficult to predict the cost and fee level at which this zero-profit equilibrium will occur. New computerized technologies may reduce variable costs in the long run but raise fixed costs in the short run. New financial instruments may increase benefits but also transaction costs and cost differentials across managers and funds. And oligopolistic profits may remain if scale economies are large relative to the size of the market. Moreover, price discrimination, used to recover fixed costs when heterogeneous consumers have different price elasticities, means that cost may have different relationships to price for different groups of investors. In this chapter we presume that in the long run fees will bear a close relationship to real costs, and costs depend on how the system is organized.

The retail market for IAs incurs R&C costs for many small accounts, expensive investment strategies may be chosen, and marketing costs are often high (as in panel C). Proponents of centralized funds point to the cost advantages that stem from lower R&C, investment and marketing expenses. We provide evidence that by operating in the institutional market an IA system may achieve most of the cost advantages of centralized funds but with greater political insulation and responsiveness to workers' preferences. The institutional approach aggregates many small accounts into large blocs of money and negotiates investment fees on a group basis, thereby keeping costs and fees low by (i) cutting STARTUPCOST by avoiding excess capacity, (ii) minimizing MARKETING cost, (iii) constraining worker choice to portfolios and strategies with low INV costs, and (iv) using increased bargaining power to shift costs and reduce oligopoly profits. R&C expenditures may also be organized to cut costs and facilitate compliance, although we have less evidence of this.

When these strategies are utilized, the cost to workers of an IA system are in the same neighborhood as a centralized system but with greater competition and choice, which are the key elements of a privately managed funded pillar.

How High Are Administrative Fees in Latin America and How Are They Spent?

In this section we examine costs and fees charged by individual account systems in Chile and other Latin American countries. These fees have been subject to great criticism by opponents of IA systems. AFP fees do not necessarily represent real costs nor do they represent a long-term commitment. AFPs in Chile (and other Latin American countries) suffered losses in the early years of the new system because of large fixed and start-up costs that exceeded their revenues, but the industry has been quite profitable in recent years. We might expect competition to eliminate these profits, but price insensitivity among investors may prevent this from happening quickly. In the future deregulation and increasing oligopoly may alter costs and their relationship to fees, in ways difficult to predict. For example, in an industry characterized by differentiated competition, marketing costs play a large role, and we do not know whether they will increase or decrease as the industry grows more concentrated. As regulations are liberalized, portfolio diversification increases and managerial skill is deemed increasingly important, which may raise managerial wages, marketing costs, and fees. Despite this uncertainty about the future, the current fee structure poses costs to investors that reduce their net returns, so we take them as given, and in this section we examine their implications.

Costs and Fees in Latin America across Time, Countries, and AFPs

Tables 7.2 and 7.3 present information about aggregate fees, costs, and their impact on member accounts for AFP systems in a variety of Latin American countries in 1998. Table 7.4 presents a longer time series on Chile, for which we have data since 1982.

Most Latin American countries have adopted the Chilean method of charging fees: they impose a fee when the contribution first enters the system and charge no management fees on that contribution thereafter. In Chile the fee started at more than 20 percent of contributions but has now fallen to an average level of 15.6 percent (and possibly less for the many workers who are said to get unofficial rebates). Table 7.2 shows that in other Latin American countries, such as Argentina and Mexico, fees are still 20 percent of contributions or even higher. In Bolivia, which is experimenting with an institutional approach to administrative costs, they are lower. Table 7.3 shows that in systems that are still in their early years, these fees do not even cover full cost.

Besides the problems inherent in cost comparisons across countries that were listed in section 1, additional problems appear in Latin American, where the allocation of fees and expenses among administration, insurance,

Table 7.2. Administrative Fees in Latin American IA Systems, 1999

Country[a]		Gross fee as % of wages[b]	Net fee as % of wages	Net fee as % of total contribution	Net fee as % of current assets, 1998	Net fee as % of lifetime annual assets[g]	% Reduction in final capital and pension
Argentina[c]	(10.0)	3.25	2.30	23.0	7.66	1.13	23.0
Bolivia[d]	(10.6)	4.60	0.60	5.5	3.0	.54	11.1
Colombia[c]	(11.6)	3.50	1.64	14.1	4.0	0.69	14.1
Chile[e]	(11.8)	2.47	1.84	15.6	1.36	0.76	15.6
El Salvador	(12.1)	3.18	2.13	17.6	—	0.86	17.6
Peru	(12.4)	3.74	2.36	19.0	7.31	0.93	19.0
Mexico[f]	(8.7)	4.42	1.92	22.1	9.19	1.08	22.1
Uruguay	(14.4)	2.68	2.06	14.3	—	0.70	14.3

— Not available.

a. Total contribution rate = contribution to IA system + net fee, as a percentage of wages. This number is given in parentheses after each country. In Argentina, Mexico, and Uruguay, the fee is taken out of the worker's account, unlike other countries where the fee is added on.

b. Gross fee includes premium for disability and survivors insurance. Net fee excludes this premium.

c. Some AFPs in Argentina also charge a fixed fee. The split between administrative fee, insurance, and other fees and costs is difficult to disentangle in Argentina and Colombia.

d. This includes a fee of 0.5 percent of wages plus 0.235 of assets that is charged by the AFP's, plus 0.2 percent of assets to the custodian. The asset-based part will increase over time as assets grow, so total fee as a percent of wages and contributions will also grow and will be higher than numbers given in columns 1, 2, and 3 in the future. Gross fee includes 2 percent of wages for disability and survivors benefits.

e. Most Chilean AFPs also charge a small flat fee per month, increasing the net fee. Anecdotal evidence indicates that part of the fee is rebated when workers switch AFPs, decreasing the net fee.

f. In Mexico the government contributes 5.5 percent of the minimum wage, which is estimated to be 2.2 percent of the average wage, to each account. This is included in the total contribution rate given above. Source for Mexico: CONSAR tabulations (1997).

g. This is based on a simulation of a full-career worker who works 40 years with an annual wage growth of 2 percent and an annual interest rate of 5 percent.

Sources: Iglesias, personal communication; PrimAmerica Consultores.

and other AFP activities is not always apparent. In Argentina the division between insurance and administrative costs may be arbitrary, and in Colombia the management of unemployment insurance and voluntary insurance provides additional revenues. Generally only contributors pay fees, although noncontributing affiliates also generate costs. The ratio of contributors to affiliates varies across countries. Nevertheless, some effects are striking. While initially the differences among countries may appear to be random, upon closer examination clear patterns emerge:

Table 7.3. Assets, Accounts, and Costs in Latin America, 1998
(US$)

Panel A. Using 1998 Exchange Rate

Country	No. of contributors (millions)	No. of affiliates (millions)	Exchange rate	Assets (mill. US$)	Total assets/ contributors (US$)	Total assets/ affiliates (US$)
Mexico	11.38	13.83	0.100600	5,484.43	482	397
Bolivia		0.46	0.177900	238.39		518
Colombia	1.39	2.91	0.000654	2,127.57	1,531	731
Peru	0.90	1.98	0.319600	1,745.38	1,939	882
Argentina	3.46	7.07	1.000200	11,528.70	3,332	1,631
Chile	3.15	5.97	0.002111	31,056.17	9,859	5,202

Country	Fee/ contributor (US$)	Expenses/ contributor (US$)	Fee/ affiliate (US$)	Expenses/ affiliate (US$)	Fee/unit of asset (%)	Expenses/ unit of assets (%)
Mexico	43	44	35	36	8.82	9.19
Bolivia		16	21	3.00	4.04	
Colombia	61	101	29	48	4.00	6.63
Peru	142	158	64	59	7.31	6.74
Argentina	261	200	128	98	7.66	6.80
Chile	134	111	71	59	1.36	1.13

Panel B. Using 1997 PPP

Country	No. of contributors (millions)	No. of affiliates (millions)	Exchange rate	Assets (mill. US$)	Total assets/ contributors (US$)	Total assets/ affiliates (US$)
Mexico	11.38	13.83	0.25	13,629.30	1198	986
Bolivia		0.46	0.5263	705.26		1,533
Colombia	1.39	2.91	0.0025	8,132.92	5851	2,795
Peru	0.90	1.98	0.6667	3,640.93	4045	1,839
Argentina	3.46	7.07	1.1111	12,806.98	3701	1,811
Chile	3.15	5.97	0.0058	85,338.19	27,091	14,295

Country	Fee/ contributor (US$)	Expenses/ contributor (US$)	Fee/ affiliate (US$)	Expenses/ affiliate (US$)	Fee/unit of asset (%)	Expenses/ unit of assets (%)
Mexico	106	110	87	91	8.82	9.19
Bolivia		46	62	3.00	4.04	
Colombia	234	388	112	185	4.00	6.63
Peru	296	273	134	124	7.31	6.74
Argentina	290	222	142	109	7.66	6.80
Chile	368	307	196	162	1.36	1.13

Note: Countries are arranged in order of total assets/affiliates at 1998 exchange rate.
In Colombia and Argentina AFPs engage in other insurance activities whose fees and costs are difficult to disentangle from pension administration. In Bolivia an additional 0.2 percent of assets is paid to the custodian.
Source: PrimAmerica Consultores, taken from reports of Superintendencias.

Table 7.4. Assets, Fees, and Expenditures in Chile through Time

Year	No. of affiliates (millions)	Contributors/ affiliates	Assets (1998 US$ million)	Total assets/ contributors (1998 US$)	Total assets/ affiliates (1998 US$)	Marketing costs as % of total expend.
1982	1.44	0.74	1277.74	1205	887	46
1983	1.62	0.76	2212.50	1799	1366	40
1984	1.93	0.70	2842.46	2090	1473	36
1985	2.28	0.68	2290.61	1470	1003	30
1986	2.59	0.68	3112.55	1779	1201	24
1987	2.89	0.70	3812.46	1884	1319	21
1988	3.18	0.68	4868.26	2246	1529	23
1989	3.47	0.65	5844.70	2577	1684	22
1990	3.74	0.61	8144.61	3558	2178	24
1991	4.11	0.61	11999.98	4825	2920	26
1992	4.43	0.61	14265.43	5292	3217	30
1993	4.71	0.59	17839.38	6389	3788	35
1994	5.01	0.57	24206.33	8406	4827	38
1995	5.32	0.56	27039.54	9129	5082	43
1996	5.57	0.56	28366.44	9088	5091	49
1997	5.78	0.57	31133.98	9445	5386	52
1998	5.97	0.53	31060.16	9861	5206	46

Year	Fee per contributor (1998 US$)	Expenses per contributor (1998 US$)	Fee per affiliate (1998 US$)	Expenses per affiliate (1998 US$)	Fee per unit of assets (%)	Expenses per unit of assets (%)
1982	113	145	83	106	9.39	12.00
1983	101	102	77	77	5.63	5.65
1984	102	97	72	68	4.90	4.65
1985	52	50	36	34	3.54	3.41
1986	52	46	35	31	2.93	2.57
1987	49	42	34	29	2.60	2.22
1988	58	50	39	34	2.57	2.23
1989	64	51	42	33	2.49	1.97
1990	71	63	43	39	2.00	1.77
1991	81	68	49	41	1.68	1.41
1992	95	74	58	45	1.79	1.39
1993	103	92	61	54	1.61	1.43
1994	123	114	71	65	1.47	1.35
1995	143	124	79	69	1.56	1.35
1996	145	128	81	72	1.59	1.41
1997	148	131	84	75	1.56	1.38
1998	134	112	71	59	1.36	1.13

Note:
Exchange Rates: 1982—0.017103, 1983—0.013734, 1984—0.011233, 1985—0.005445, 1986—0.004878, 1987—0.004200, 1988—0.004041, 1989—0.003372, 1990—0.002969, 1991—0.002668, 1992—0.002616, 1993—0.002320, 1994—0.002475, 1995—0.002456, 1996—0.002353, 1997—0.002274, 1998—0.002111.
Sources: PrimAmerica Consultores, based on reports of Superintendencias; authors' calculations.

- High start-up costs characterize new systems until a sharp drop occurs around year four. This helps account for the higher expenses outside of Chile in 1998.
- Thereafter, cost per account climbs gradually due to the increased investment costs associated with larger assets, while cost per unit of assets falls as the constant R&C costs per account are spread over a larger asset base. Figures 7.1 and 7.2 demonstrate the negative relationship between cost per unit of assets and average account size implied by these tables, with the exception of Bolivia, which has a much lower expense ratio than would be expected. In contrast, Mexico, which is one of the newest systems with the smallest account size, has the highest expense ratio relative to assets in the region. As Mexico's system matures, we would expect its cost per account to rise but its cost per unit of assets to fall.

Costs and Fees in Chile

Chile, which has by far the largest account size due to its age and contribution rate, has the smallest expense ratio per unit of assets. In Chile in 1998, using the official exchange rate for conversion, the average account size was US$5,000 per affiliate and US$10,000 per contributor; cost per affiliate and

Figure 7.1. Costs of Chilean AFP System, 1982–1998: Relation between Fee as a Percentage of Assets and Average Account Size

Fee per unit of assets, percent

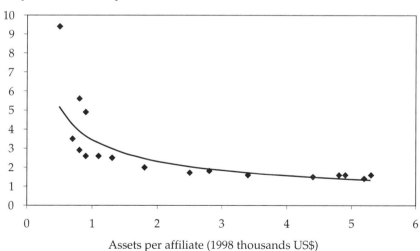

Assets per affiliate (1998 thousands US$)

Source: Authors' calculations.

Figure 7.2. Costs of Latin American AFP Systems, 1998: Relation between Cost as a Percentage of Assets and Average Account Size

Expenses per unit of assets, percent

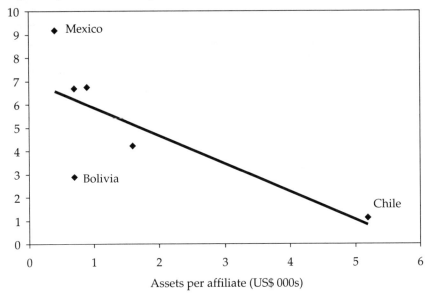

Assets per affiliate (US$ 000s)

Source: Authors' calculations.

contributor was US$59 and US$112, respectively; and fees were somewhat higher.[2] While fees per account have been rising, as a percentage of assets they have fallen sharply, from over 9 percent in 1982 (much like Mexico today) to 1.36 percent in 1998 (much like the U.S. mutual fund industry today).

Table 7.5a presents the results of a simple regression analysis that sums up this relationship between aggregate assets, costs, and fees for the Chilean system over time. Start-up costs and assets alone explain 96–98 percent of the variance in costs and fees across time. Very high correlations among assets, affiliates, and contributors, together with small sample size, preclude including more than one variable in this analysis of aggregate costs.

However, disaggregation by AFP as well as by year introduces larger sample size and greater variation that allows us to decompose total costs and fees into their major determinants—assets and affiliates—and to explore potential scale economies. Table 7.5b presents the results of a panel data (fixed effects) analysis of Chilean AFP costs, 1982–98, using these independent variables, and shows how the system has evolved through time. In Chile we found the following:

Table 7.5a. Regression Analysis: Determinants of Costs and Fees, Chile, 1982–98: Aggregate Analysis

Independent variables	Dependent variables					
	Total admin. cost	Total cost/ assets	Total cost/ affiliates	Total fee revenues	Total fee/ assets	Total fees/ affiliates
Assets	0.012	-0.00004	0.001	0.013	-0.00005	0.002
	(24.38)a	(4.14)a	(12.00)a	(30.47)a	(5.39)a	(16.48)a
Dummy, start-up year = 82	92.781	9.581	77.936	47.948	6.629	50.182
	(4.74)a	(20.16)a	(14.91)a	(2.54)c	(16.14)a	(11.61)a
Dummy, start-up years =83-4	53.611	2.787	42.486	43.532	2.567	39.383
	(3.44)a	(7.81)a	(10.83)a	(3.07)b	(8.33)a	(12.14)a
Constant	45.780	2.476	26.704	55.269	2.826	31.078
	(5.18)a	(12.22)a	(2.23)c	(6.87)a	(16.14)a	(16.87)a
R2	0.976	0.974	0.951	0.985	0.967	0.956
N	17	17	17	17	17	17

Note: t-statistics are in parentheses.
Units of measurement: costs, fees, and assets are 1998 US dollars in millions; no. of contributors and affiliates are in millions; cost/assets and fees/assets are in percentages; cost/affiliates, fees/affiliates, and assets/affiliates are in 1998 US dollars.
a. Significant at 0.1% level; b. Significant at 1% level; c. Significant at 5% level.
Source: Authors' calculations.

- Start-up fees and, even more, start-up costs in the first three years of operations were high.
- As the number of affiliates grows (R&C), costs and fees grow en toto and relative to assets.
- As assets grow, (investment) costs and fees grow, en toto and per account, but costs and fees as a percentage of assets, which ultimately determine net return, decrease due to scale economies.
- The fact that affiliates and assets both have a coefficient of less than 1, singly and summed, in the logged regressions on total costs further demonstrates scale economies, but the negative term (although insignificant) in the quadratic implies that these scale economies may eventually come to an end. Calculations using these coefficients suggest that this occurs when the AFP has about 3 million affiliates and US$15 billion—half of the current Chilean market.

Table 7.5b. Fixed Effects Regression for Chile: Disaggregated by AFP and Year

Independent variable	Cost		Cost/affiliate			Cost/asset	
	Quadratic	Logs	Quadratic	Logs	No logs	Quadratic	Logs
Affiliate	3.711	0.350	−78.510	−0.650	11.712	13.587	0.350
	(0.65)	(5.54)[a]	(−0.79)	(−10.31)[a]	(0.49)	(3.71)[a]	(5.54)[a]
Affiliate square	−2.211		28.336			−3.651	
	(−0.95)		(0.70)			(−2.47)[c]	
Asset	0.011	0.535	0.046	0.535		−0.002	−0.465
	(11.95)[a]	(14.53)[a]	(2.76)[b]	(1.248)		(−2.82)[b]	(−12.61)[a]
Asset square	−1.5e−07		−5.5e−06			1.3e−07	
	(−1.01)		(−2.10)[c]			(1.33)	
Asset/affiliate					0.009		
					(4.56)[a]		
Dummy, start-up year = 82	6.692	1.248	89.603	1.248	96.328	15.121	1.248
	(5.38)[a]	(16.45)[a]	(4.14)[a]	(16.45)[a]	(4.89)[a]	(19.06)[a]	(16.45)[a]
Dummy, start-up year = 83, 84	3.384	0.655	44.172	0.655	47.804	4.316	0.655
	(3.50)[a]	(11.53)[a]	(2.63)[b]	(11.53)[a]	(3.15)[b]	(7.00)[a]	(11.53)[a]
Constant	3.556	−0.339	84.942	−0.339	51.181	0.695	4.266
	(3.94)[a]	(−0.98)	(5.42)[a]	(−0.98)	(4.57)[a]	(1.21)	(12.33)[a]
R-sq:							
Within	0.923	0.917	0.134	0.703	0.173	0.681	0.868
Between	0.938	0.931	0.137	0.775	0.036	0.110	0.533
Overall	0.916	0.935	0.0003	0.817	0.210	0.335	0.753
N	234	232	234	232	234	234	232

(Table continued on next page)

Mergers have indeed been occurring. We can expect that Chile, Mexico, and other Latin American countries will benefit further from maturation and scale economies in the future, so their future costs will be lower than present costs for that reason.

Implications of Front-Loaded Fees: How to Convert Them into Annualized Fees

Charging fees based on new contributions is an extremely front-loaded method as compared with the customary practice in mutual funds of charging an annual fee based on assets. Such a fee basis has a different impact on returns depending on how long the worker will keep his or her money in the system, which in turn depends on the age and career pattern of the worker. For comparability, we have converted the 15.6 percent front-loaded fee in Chile into an equivalent annual fee based on assets that will yield the same final-year accumulation (table 7.6). This tells us how much, effectively, gross investment returns are being reduced each year, and it

Table 7.5b continued

Independent variable	Fee		Fee/affiliate			Fee/asset	
	Quadratic	Logs	Quadratic	Logs	No logs	Quadratic	Logs
Affiliate	16.266	0.803	−146.971	−0.197	−3.719	3.865	0.803
	(2.66)[b]	(9.99)[a]	(−2.94)[b]	(−2.45)[c]	(−0.36)	(2.28)[c]	(9.99)[a]
Affiliate square	−9.792		27.307			−1.631	
	(−.97)[a]		(1.36)			(−2.39)[c]	
Asset	0.010	0.389	0.047	0.389		−0.002	−0.611
	(10.27)[a]	(8.17)[a]	(5.64)[a]	(8.17)[a]		(−5.37)[a]	(−12.86)[a]
Asset square	5.5e–7		−3.8e–06			1.9e–07	
	(3.45)[a]		(−.90)[b]			(4.36)[a]	
Asset/affiliate					0.010		
					(12.81)a		
Dummy, start-up year = 82	4.433	0.828	16.121	0.828	32.772	5.401	0.828
	(3.35)[a]	(8.41)[a]	(1.49)	(8.41)[a]	(3.87)[a]	(14.72)[a]	(8.41)[a]
Dummy, start-up year = 83, 84	3.992	0.814	33.096	0.814	44.289	2.969	0.814
	(3.88)[a]	(11.07)[a]	(3.94)[a]	(11.07)[a]	(6.81)[a]	(10.41)[a]	(11.07)[a]
Constant	2.569	1.439	85.478	1.439	33.238	2.428	6.044
	(2.68)b	(3.23)b	(10.91)[a]	(3.23)b	(6.92)[a]	(9.13)[a]	(13.56)[a]
R-sq:							
Within	0.946	0.903	0.285	0.552	0.495	0.699	0.715
Between	0.947	0.946	0.138	0.179	0.882	0.850	0.697
Overall	0.956	0.915	0.278	0.275	0.832	0.702	0.566
N	234	234	234	234	234	234	234

Note: t–statistics are in parenthesis. See table 7. 5a for units of measurement. Similar results were obtained in a random effects analysis.
a. Significance level: 0.1%; b. Significance level: 1%; Significance level: 5%.
Source: Authors' calculations.

enables us to compare it with fees charged by mutual funds and other financial institutions. This simulation assumes that the same fee schedule remains in effect over the worker's lifetime, although, of course, there is no guarantee that this will be the case. If a worker contributes only for her first 20 years of employment, the equivalent average annual fee for all her contributions is 0.57 percent. If contributions are made only in the last 20 years, however, the equivalent average annual fee is 1.65 percent (column 2). For a worker who contributes every year for 40 years, paying a fee on each new contribution, the annual equivalent of all these front-loaded fees is 0.76 percent (column 3). Suppose that one-half of all workers contribute for 40 years, and one-quarter each for their first and last 20 years. The systemwide annual expense ratio that is equivalent to the 15.6 percent fee on contributions would then be 0.94 percent, almost 1 percent of assets per year.

Table 7.6. Annual Asset-Based Fee Equivalent to 15.6 Percent Fee on New Contributions in Chile
(as percentage of assets)

Starting age	Contribution made for one year only at given age 1	Contributions made for 20 years only, starting at given age 2	Contributions made every year until age 65, starting at given age 3
25	0.45	0.57	0.76
35	0.60	0.85	1.05
45	0.91	1.65	1.65
55	1.86	—	3.50
64	33.37	—	33.37

— Not applicable.

Note: Assumptions: This table shows the annual fee based on assets that will yield the same capital accumulation at age 65 as would a 15.6 percent front-loaded fee on incoming contributions. In column 1 a single year of contributions is assumed at the starting age. The annual fee for age 64 is 33.37 percent because contributions and fees are assumed to be paid monthly, including the last month. In column 2 the worker continues contributing a fixed percentage of wage for 20 years. In column 3 the worker continues investing a fixed percentage of wage from starting age until age 65. A rate of return of 5 percent is assumed. For columns 2 and 3, annual wage growth of 2 percent is assumed. Similar results were obtained for 3 percent rate of return and 1 percent rate of wage growth. The average contributor pays US$134 today in Chile. The fee would increase 2 percent per year under these assumptions.

Source: Authors' calculations.

A front-loaded fee means that workers with different employment histories will end up paying different annual equivalents as a subtraction from their gross returns, even if they impose the same real cost on the fund. Frontloading of fees may induce evasion among workers in their later years, since they can avoid all investment costs on accumulated assets if they simply stop making new contributions. It may induce AFPs to reject transfers from older workers with larger assets and investment costs. Thus, front loads may not be desirable in the start-up phase of a mandatory system because of their distributional impact and may not be sustainable in the long run if AFPs are permitted to change their fee structure, but they are frequently used, perhaps as a device to help AFPs cover their costs, which are also front-loaded.

Comparison between Chilean AFP Fees and Mutual Fund Fees

Annualized Chilean fees are similar to fees of mutual funds that operate in the U.S. domestic market (section 3). American mutual funds, because they are voluntary, cater to a higher socioeconomic group and provide much greater diversification and service than Chilean AFPs, which would make their costs higher. But they also benefit from much greater economies of scale and better infrastructure, which would make their costs lower. AFP costs are much lower than costs of U.S. mutual funds that operate in emerging markets. They are much lower than mutual fund fees for voluntary saving in Chile, which during the early 1990s averaged around 6 percent per year for equity funds and 2 percent for bond funds, plus entrance and exit charges (Maturana and Walker 1999). AFP fees are also lower than those of mutual funds in most other countries, where the combination of front loads and annual fees exceeds levels in the United States. Chilean AFPs are therefore relatively inexpensive if the standard of comparison is fees in other diversified mutual funds that invest individuals' savings. However, they are more expensive than savings accounts in commercial banks, either in Chile or elsewhere (Valdes 1999b).

The breakdown of costs among AFPs shows that over 45 percent of total expenditures were for marketing costs, especially sales commissions. This proportion is similar to marketing expenses in the retail financial markets in the United States and other countries. In both countries the number would probably exceed 50 percent if we included staff salaries involved in marketing. These similarities suggest that a study of U.S. mutual fund data will yield insights into how costs might evolve in IA systems and how these costs might be reduced—for example, by reducing marketing costs.

Finally, AFP fees are much higher than fees paid by institutional investors, and they have a substantial impact on ultimate pension amounts, raising the question of whether it is possible to organize a mandatory system so that it captures the lower costs and higher benefits of the institutional market, and, if so, what trade-offs are involved.

Costs in the Retail Market of American Mutual Funds

The mutual fund in the United States has been a hugely successful retail financial institution. Assets have grown from less than US$1 billion in 1949 to almost US$140 billion in 1980 to over US$4 trillion by the end of 1997. They now exceed the combined total of savings bank deposits and life insurance assets (Pozen 1998). Each mutual fund investor has an individual account that can be transferred from fund to fund, so this might provide information on how an IA system would operate in a competitive retail market. An earlier paper analyzed the determinants of these fees and the cost structure that underlies them. We used regression analysis and frontier analysis based on a large data set of mutual funds (4,254 funds in 1997 and 1,300–2,000 each year for 1992–96), as well as information culled from annual reports, surveys conducted by mutual fund associations, and discussions with fund officials. In this section we summarize these results and consider the policy implications for a reformed social security system that includes individual accounts (for a fuller account and numerous references, see James and others 1999).

Costs and Fees in the Mutual Fund Industry

In the U.S. mutual fund industry, the fund pays annual fees to its investment adviser and distributor (which is usually the same group or "sponsor" that originally set up the fund), and much smaller fees to lawyers, auditors, transfer agents, and others. The charges are allocated among shareholders proportional to their assets and determine the fund's reported "expense ratio" that it subtracts from its gross return to obtain the net return passed on to shareholders. In addition, for many funds individual investors pay front-loaded and back-loaded commissions directly to brokers or other sales agents upon purchase or sale. These entry and exit fees are part of the price to relevant shareholders, although the fund does not receive them. The expense ratio also does not incorporate brokerage fees paid by the fund for securities transactions, but these are costs to shareholders, netted out of the fund's reported gross returns.

We have constructed a "total investor cost ratio" that equals the reported expense ratio plus average brokerage (trading) costs and annualized front-loaded sales commissions (table 7.7).[3] In 1997 the total investor cost was 1.85 percent of assets, compared to the reported expense ratio of 1.28 percent. Weighted by assets, the total and reported numbers fall to 1.43 percent and 0.91 percent (or US$360 and US$228 per account), respectively. Asset-weighted numbers are more relevant for our purposes.[4]

Most funds are members of a mutual fund complex (for example, Fidelity and Vanguard). A common investment adviser supplies certain activities, such as advertising, research, and new product development, to all members of the complex. Estimates of where the expenses can be absorbed with smallest loss of clients may influence the allocation of these expenses among the funds. Thus the relative fees paid by members of a fund complex do not necessarily reflect the real cost of producing them. For example, small and new funds that are expensive to run may be allocated only a small share of costs to attract new customers, and index funds that are marketed to cost-conscious consumers may similarly be allocated a small share. Business strategy concerning joint cost allocation may be different in a mandatory IA system. These caveats should be kept in mind as we analyze fund costs below.

We conducted a regression analysis designed to explain the "expense ratio"—reported expenses (excluding trading fees and loads) as a percentage of assets.[5] We sought to discover the extent to which cost variation is random or systematic, to identify the factors that determined the

Table 7.7. Composition of Mutual Fund Expenses, 1997
(as percentage of assets and dollars per account)

	Simple Average	Average	Asset-weighted Active	Passive
Expenses included in expense ratio				
Investment advisor	0.56	0.49	0.52	0.08
Distributor for 12b1 fees[a]	0.35	0.21	0.22	0.02
Transfer agent (R&C)	0.13	0.12	0.12	0.05
Other (legal, audit, etc.)	0.23	0.09	0.08	0.13
Reported expense ratio	1.27	0.91	0.95	0.28
Dollars per account[b]	320	228	238	70
Other investor costs				
Brokerage fees (trading costs)	0.26	0.12	0.12	0.03
Annualized front-loaded sales charge paid by shareholder[b]	0.31	0.40	0.43	0.01
Total investor costs as percentage of assets	1.85	1.43	1.50	0.32
Dollars per account[b]	463	360	375	80

a. The 12b1 fee is a fee paid annually by the fund, primarily for distribution of new shares and related service. It is financed by a charge paid by all shareholders, whether or not they have purchased their shares through a broker. It is part of the fund's expense ratio and is based on assets. The front-loaded sales charge is paid directly to the distributor by investors who purchase through brokers, as a percentage of their new investment. It is not included in the fund's expense ratio. The average front-loaded fee is 4.48 percent. It is charged by about one-third of all funds. In this table, this one-time fee has been annualized according to the procedure described in endnote 1. These numbers are averaged over all funds, ignoring the big distinction in costs to shareholders between funds that impose sales charges and those that do not.
b. For average account size = US$25,000
Source: Authors' calculations and estimates (see endnote 3).

systematic variation, and to assess the implications for IA systems. We ran the OLS regressions separately for each year between 1992 and 1997 and also conducted a frontier (envelope) analysis for 1992–97. Table 7.8 reports results from the OLS regression for 1997, and table 7.9 reports the frontier analysis for 1992–97. The regressions in table 7.8 explain 64 percent of the variance when all the above variables are included. Most of the variance in costs is, therefore, systematic rather than random. Costs faced by

Table 7.8. Determinants of Expense Ratios of Mutual Funds in the United States, 1997

(dependent variable is total expenses/total assets, in basis points)[a]

	1		2		3		4		5	
Core group										
Intercept	113.7	$(59.63)^c$	112.1	$(55.35)^c$	111.0	$(22.22)^c$	83.4	$(22.03)^c$	125.0	$(26.09)^c$
Assets in US$ billions	−9.2	$(−9.55)^c$	−7.9	$(−10.03)^c$	−9.1	$(−9.61)^c$	−3.9	$(−5.65)^c$	−5.2	$(−5.67)^c$
Asset[b]	0.1	$(5.22)^c$	0.1	$(7.20)^c$	0.1	$(5.48)^c$	0.1	$(−6.17)^c$	0.1	$(4.51)^c$
No. shareholders in 000s	0.1	$(3.14)^c$			0.1	$(3.02)^c$	0.0	$(−1.48)$	0.0	(0.89)
Assets/shareholders			−0.4	$(−4.9)^c$						
Assets in fund complex	−0.1	$(−7.99)^c$	−0.1	$(−7.61)^c$	−0.1	$(−8.66)^c$	−0.1	$(−7.31)^c$	−0.1	$(−10.07)^c$
3–year net return[b]	−1.5	$(−13.73)^c$			−0.9	$(−6.26)^c$	−0.7	$(−6.37)^c$	−0.7	$(−4.84)^c$
No. year gross return			−1.1	$(−9.73)^c$						
3 Year Standard Deviation	4.6	$(29.56)^c$	4.4	$(27.93)^c$	3.5	$(14.24)^c$	3.1	$(17.94)^c$	3.3	$(14.32)^c$
Asset allocation										
Bond					−1.9	$(−0.52)$	−9.6	$(−3.71)^c$	−8.0	$(−2.35)^d$
Small cap					3.2	(0.76)	11.6	$(3.98)^c$	−0.2	(0.05)
Specialty					23.0	$(6.01)^c$	11.7	$(4.33)^c$	16.4	$(4.61)^c$
International					28.9	$(7.61)^c$	24.1	$(8.96)^c$	24.5	$(6.89)^c$
Emerging market					37.6	$(5.25)^c$	37.5	$(7.43)^c$	39.9	$(5.53)^c$
Investment and marketing strategy										
Institutional							−15.4	$(−4.23)^c$	−52.8	$(−11.45)^c$
Initial investment							−0.4	$(−3.22)^c$	−0.4	$(−1.9)^d$
Index							−38.5	$(−8.72)^c$	−51.7	$(−8.86)^c$
12b1 fee < 1, > 0							18.4	$(9.73)^c$		
12b1 fee = 1							43.5	$(14.19)^c$		
Front load							2.7	$(−1.43)$		
Deferred load							47.3	$(16.86)^c$		
Turnover							4.3	$(8.21)^c$	6.0	$(8.65)^*$
Bank advised							−8.1	$(−4.44)^c$	−18.7	$(−7.88)^*$
Fundage							−0.2	$(−3.26)^c$	−1.1	$(−12.37)^*$
Adjusted R2	23.8		22.2		26.9		64.2		38.0	
Dep mean	127.6		127.6		127.6		127.6		127.6	
N	3610		3610		3610		3610		3610	

a. Brokerage fees and front and deferred loads are not included in expense ratios. For each equation, first column gives coefficient and second column gives t statistics. 1 basis point = 0.01 percent; b. Three–year net returns are gross returns adjusted for expense ratio and loads; c. Significant at 0.2 percent level; d. Significant at 5 percent level.
Source: Authors. calculations.

investors vary in large part because of business choices made by fund managers, and these same costs could be substantially influenced by policy choices in a mandatory IA system. Our major empirical findings and their implications for IA systems follow.

Considerable Evidence of Economies of Scale and Scope

Expense ratios fall when total assets in fund, assets in the entire fund complex, and assets per shareholder increase. A simple cross-tabulation shows

Table 7.9. Determinants of Expense Ratios of Mutual Funds, United States, 1992–97

(dependent variable is total expenses/total assets, in basis points)[a]

	1		2		3		4		5	
Core group										
Intercept	22.6	(12.73)c	23.0	(12.31)c	26.4	(9.17)c	65.0	(31.91)c	125.0	(26.09)c
Assets in US$ billions	−3.5	(−5.97)c	−2.2	(−5.97)c	−2.7	(−7.05)c	−2.3	(4.64)c	−5.2	(−5.67)c
Asset[b]	0.1	(5.77)c	1.0	(5.33)c	0.1	(6.18)c	0.1	(6.21)c	0.1	(4.51)c
No. shareholders in 000s	0.03	(2.68)d					0.0	(1.3)	0.0	(0.89)
Assets/shareholders			−1.0	(−3.11)c	−0.1	(−3.17)c				
Assets in fund complex	−0.1	(−6.27)c	−0.1	(−8.47)c	−0.1	(−8.23)c	−0.1	(−12.94)c	−0.1	(−10.07)c
3-year net return[b]			−0.6	(−16.25)c	−0.5	(−13.5)c			−0.7	(−4.84)c
No. year gross return	−0.4	(−11.31)c					−0.3	(−8.89)c		
3-year standard deviation	0.13	(16.79)c	1.5	(19.2)c	1.0	(−11.59)c	1.0	(12.82)c	3.3	(14.32)c
Asset allocation										
Bond					−12.6	(−7.57)c	−23.8	(−19.25)c	−8.0	(−2.35)d
Small cap					14.9	(5.12)c	11.5	(6.25)c	−0.2	(0.05)
Specialty					15.7	(5.59)c	6.8	(3.96)c	16.4	(4.61)c
International					18.5	(7.65)c	21.7	(13.72)c	24.5	(6.89)c
Emerging market					59.9	(12.92)c	48.2	(15.64)c	39.9	(5.53)c
Investment and marketing strategy										
Institutional							−15.4	(−8.09)c	−52.8	(−11.45)c
Initial investment							−0.3	(−2.48)d	−0.4	(−1.9)d
Index							−38.6	(−14.18)c	−51.7	(−8.86)c
12b1 fee < 1, > 0							17.7	(13.84)c		
12b1 fee = 1							49.9	(23.16)c		
Front load							6.2	(4.71)c		
Deferred load							49.7	(25.3)c		
Turnover							2.0	(7.46)c	6.0	(8.65)c
Bank advised							−2.4	(−1.92)d	−18.7	(−7.88)c
Fundage							−0.4	(−8.95)c	−1.1	(−12.37)c
Time	2.3	(11.17)c	2.3	(10.66)c	2.3	(10.96)c	1.2	(6.41)c	38.0	

a. Brokerage fees and front and deferred loads are not included in expense ratios. For each equation, first column gives coefficient and second column gives t statistics. 1 basis point = 0.01 percent.;
b. Three–year net returns are gross returns adjusted for expense ratio and loads; c. Significant at 0.2 percent level; d. Significant at 5 percent level.
Source: Authors' calculations.

the average expense ratio for funds with assets of less than US$10 million is 1.6 percent, while for those with assets of US$1 to US$10 billion and more than US$20 billion, it is 0.96 percent and 0.6 percent, respectively. While all funds need industry analysts, portfolio managers, computers, and access to electronic trading facilities, large funds can be managed with a relatively small increase in total resources. But these economies from asset aggregation do not continue indefinitely. The positive sign on the coefficient of Asset^2 in the regressions eventually halts the fall in the expense ratio. Thus aggregation brings economies that lead to industry concentration, but the limit to these economies nevertheless leaves space for multiple mutual funds (and pension funds), the exact number of which depends on the total market size of each country.

Significant Fixed Costs per Account

Holding aggregate assets constant, the expense ratio increases with the number of shareholders and decreases as average account size rises. The basic reason, as discussed in section 1, is that funds incur a fixed cost per account for record-keeping and shareholder communication (R&C), and the larger each account, the smaller this cost will be, as a percentage of assets. According to these regressions and corroborating evidence from periodic surveys of transfer agents (the organizations that provide these services for mutual funds), average R&C costs per account are US$20–$25. Fixed costs of R&C pose a potential problem for IA systems if the accounts are small. These fixed costs help explain the high expense ratios of new AFPs in developing countries. This raises the question of whether an investment option with lower R&C costs should be used or whether R&C costs should be amortized over a long time period, to avoid imposing a heavy burden on early cohorts when new IA systems are started.

High Marketing Costs

Using brokers, other sales persons and mass advertising methods, the industry has successfully alerted potential shareholders to the advantages of equity investing, using mutual funds as the vehicle. The major marketing expense to shareholders consists of sales commissions. Two-thirds of all funds are sold through third parties (brokers, insurance agents, and financial planners) who receive some kind of commission (through front or deferred loads or annual 12b1 fees). And most of these sales commissions are passed on to consumers. If we define the "total annual marketing cost" paid by the shareholder as the 12b1 fee plus annualized front load, it is 0.61 percent—around 43 percent of all fund expenses (table 7.10). This is very similar to the marketing proportions in Chile's AFP system. From a social point of view, marketing probably provides a mixture of useful information, misleading information, an impetus to good performance, and zero-sum game raiding. Other studies have shown that the funds that have gained the most are those that combine vigorous marketing with good performance (Sirri and Tufano 1997). The possibility of spreading favorable information by marketing probably acts as a spur to good performance and product innovation. But most methods to keep IA costs low involve a reduction in marketing expenses, under the assumption that much of it is zero-sum and not the most efficient way to provide useful information to new investors.

Table 7.10. Marketing Expenses in U.S. Mutual Funds

	Unweighted		Weighted	
	1992	1997	1992	1997
Prevalence of commissions				
(% of total funds)				
Funds with 12b1 fees	55.00	61.00	49.00	46.00
Funds with Fload	50.00	35.00	52.00	42.00
Funds with Dload	9.00	27.00	9.00	12.00
Funds with no load or 12b1 fee	34.00	32.00	36.00	44.00
Expenses as % of assets – all funds				
Average 12b1 fee	0.21	0.35	0.18	0.21
Average annualized Fload	0.46	0.31	0.50	0.40
Reported expense ratio	1.16	1.28	0.87	0.91
Brokerage fees (trading costs)	0.27	0.26	0.15	0.12
Total expenses	1.89	1.85	1.52	1.43
Marketing expenses as	*35.00*	*36.00*	*45.00*	*43.00*
% of total expenses				
Expenses as % of assets—				
funds with either 12b1 or Fload				
Average 12b1 fee	0.38	0.52	0.36	0.37
Average Fload	0.65	0.46	0.75	0.72
Reported expense ratio	1.27	1.46	0.98	1.09
Brokerage fees	0.28	0.28	0.15	0.11
Total investor cost ratio	2.20	2.20	1.88	1.92
Marketing expenses as	*46.82*	*44.55*	*59.04*	*56.77*
% of total expenses				
Expenses as % of assets—				
funds without 12b1 or Fload				
Average 12b1 fee	0	0	0	0
Average Fload	0	0	0	0
Reported expense ratio	0.94	0.89	0.68	0.68
Brokerage fees	0.29	0.23	0.17	0.12
Total investor cost ratio	1.23	1.12	0.85	0.80

Note: For 12b1 fee, Fload, and total expenses, see table 7 and endnotes.
Source: Authors' calculations and estimates.

Lower Expense Ratios for Institutional Funds

A small number of mutual funds are limited to institutional investors (that is, bank trust departments, corporations, and small foundations). These funds have a significantly lower expense ratio compared to funds for individual investors. The same assets can be amassed with much lower

distribution, communication, and record-keeping expenses from one large
institution than from numerous small individuals. Institutions are much less
likely to pay sales commissions to brokers because they have more efficient
ways of gathering information. On the rare occasions when they pay these
fees, they obtain lower rates. As a result, the expense ratio of institutional
funds is 0.6 percent lower than that of other funds in the regressions, and
the total investor cost for institutional funds is less than half those of retail
funds (table 7.11). This led us to investigate the institutional market in
greater detail, to determine whether IAs were doomed to have high expense
ratios due to their small account size or could benefit from low expenses
due to the large aggregate amounts in the mandatory system.

Lower Costs of Passive Management—for Some Assets

Also important is the large significant negative sign on passively managed
funds, known as index funds, which do not have to pay the high fees that

**Table 7.11. Institutional Versus Retail, Passive versus Active Mutual
Funds**
(average expense ratios and investor costs as percentage of assets, 1997)

		All		Active		Passive	
	All	Retail	Institutional	Retail	Institutional	Retail	Institutional
A. Expense ratio—unweighted							
Domestic stock funds	1.43	1.47	0.91	1.50	0.98	0.71	0.37
Domestic bond funds	1.08	1.12	0.62	1.12	0.62	0.65	0.35
International stock funds	1.69	1.75	1.09	1.77	1.15	0.95	0.66
Emerging market funds	2.12	2.19	1.39	2.21	1.39	0.57	
All funds in universe	1.28	1.31	0.79	1.33	0.81	0.72	0.42
B. Expense ratio—weighted by assets							
Domestic stock funds	0.93	0.94	0.51	0.99	0.85	0.31	0.19
Domestic bond funds	0.80	0.82	0.53	0.82	0.54	0.25	0.31
International stock funds	1.18	1.19	0.96	1.20	0.97	0.42	0.68
Emerging market funds	1.75	1.77	1.25	1.81	1.25	0.57	0.00
All funds in universe	0.91	0.93	0.56	0.96	0.69	0.31	0.20
C. Total investor costs, including							
Annualized floads and brokerage							
Fees—weighted by assets							
Domestic stock funds	1.44	1.47	0.60	1.55	0.97	0.37	0.21
Domestic bond funds	1.30	1.35	0.62	1.36	0.65	0.31	0.33
International stock funds	1.83	1.87	1.05	1.89	1.09	0.48	0.70
Emerging market funds	2.29	2.33	1.34	2.38	1.37	0.63	
All funds in universe	1.44	1.48	0.65	1.52	0.81	0.37	0.22

Note: For 12b1 fee, Fload, and total expenses, see table 7 and endnote 1.
Source: Authors' calculations and estimates.

popular active managers command. Passively managed funds mimic or replicate a stated benchmark, such as the Standard & Poor 500 or the Russell 2000. The manager does not engage in discretionary stock selection or market timing and, therefore, cannot claim a fee for superior information or judgement. Index funds generally benefit from low turnover, which reduces the expense ratio as well as brokerage fees. Their high correlation with the market (low nonsystematic risk) means that they are less likely to engage in heavy marketing and more likely to rely on price (cost) competition. Controlling only for asset allocation, fees of passive funds are less than one-third those of actively managed funds in the retail market (table 7.11).

The low cost of index funds should be interpreted with some caution, however. It could mean that fund complexes view these funds as the products that are designed to capture price-sensitive consumers, and for this reason they may allocate much of their joint expenses (advertising, new product development) to the other members of their complex. R&C charges also tend to be less for passively than for actively managed funds, and this may be a business strategy decision rather than a reflection of real cost differentials. Our regression results may, therefore, overstate the real cost savings to the economy from index funds, although real cost savings to individual investors remain. If index funds become a larger share of the total market, opportunities for cost shifting may decline. Finally, the lower costs of index funds are not statistically significant for small cap and emerging market funds. IA systems in large cap stock and bond markets in industrialized countries can keep their costs down and increase their net returns by using index funds, but this may be less true of developing and transitional countries where emerging markets and small cap stocks dominate.

Asset Allocation: International Funds

Asset allocation has a major impact on costs. Bond funds have lower costs and small cap funds have higher costs. Expenses are highest in international funds, especially emerging market funds—as a result of their smaller size, the greater difficulty in obtaining information in these countries, their high bid-ask spreads, transactions and custodial costs, currency hedging costs, and the relative paucity of effective cost-saving passive investment opportunities. These factors would also apply to local funds operating in emerging markets, although institutions based in a country need not hedge against currency risk and may have an information advantage over those that are based in a foreign country. It follows that IA systems in industrialized countries can economize on costs if they concentrate investments in large liquid domestic instruments; international diversification comes at a cost. In contrast, international diversification, including the use of foreign index funds, could mitigate the higher costs in developing countries.

Net and Gross Returns

Of course, the investor ultimately cares about net returns, not the expense incurred in earning them. If higher costs led to higher returns, they would be worth incurring. However, a large literature indicates that this is not the case (Elton and others 1993; Malkiel 1995; Malhotra and McLeod 1997). In fact, some of the same factors that increased costs actually reduced returns during this period. Most importantly, in our sample larger assets increase gross and net returns, but this effect stops after a point. Funds with front-loaded sales commissions do not earn higher gross returns, so their load-adjusted net returns are lower than for no-loads. Index funds earn significantly more overall than actively managed funds, particularly in the large cap stock and bond markets, but this effect is absent in small cap, international, and emerging market funds (see also Muralidhar and Weary 1998 and chapter 9 of this volume). Institutional funds have higher net returns. These results from separate equations are consistent with the negative sign on gross and net returns as control variables in our expense ratio equations. Cost and net returns appear to be negatively correlated. Thus strategies involving high administrative costs do not seem justified on grounds that they raise returns.

Changes over Time: Will Price Competition Reduce Investor Costs?

The question of whether expenses have been going up or down over time has been hotly debated (see Lipper 1994). This is an important question because it tells us whether policymakers can rely on market forces to reduce costs. Between 1992 and 1997, a shift of investors toward no-loads and a decrease in the size of front loads led to a small fall in the total investor cost ratio, despite the rise in the reported expense ratio (table 7.10). Over a longer time period (1980–97), the average investor cost ratio has fallen more substantially (by about one-third) for the same reasons (Rea and Reid 1998). But the picture remains mixed because total expenses per account (expense ratio times average assets per account) have gone up dramatically over the same period, primarily as a result of asset growth and, secondarily, as a result of the rise in nonmarketing expenses. More recently, investors have been shifting into cheaper, passively managed funds, but in 1997 these still held only 6 percent of all assets.

The movement to lower cost and higher performing funds generally occurs through the flow of new money to the funds rather than the reallocation of old money. The process, therefore, has been very gradual, and some poorly informed investors have not participated in it (Gruber 1996; Ippolito 1992; Patel, Zeckhauser, and Hendricks 1994; Sirri and Tufano 1997). It appears that in the short run we cannot count on competition to bring price down for many investors. Why is this the case? We hypothesize that competition through marketing rather than through price cuts may be a consequence of high volatility and the resulting high noise-to-signal ratio that makes it difficult for investors to distinguish between random luck versus systematic skill and low costs until many years of observations have elapsed (for a mathematical example, see James and others 1999). Funds spend on marketing, pointing to their lucky returns, rather than cutting costs and price. This poses a problem for IA systems, as an entire generation of workers may pass through the system before low-cost, high-performing funds are identified. The difficulty new investors have in processing financial information exacerbates this situation. An IA system that constrains investments to funds with low nonsystematic risk will encourage price competition relative to marketing competition, because such funds will be able to demonstrate their cost-based superiority more quickly than funds with greater fund-specific volatility. Reduced differentiation and fund-specific volatility may help explain why, on average, fees in Chilean AFPs are somewhat lower than fees in U.S. mutual funds.

Costs in the Institutional Market

Although small institutions invest through special low-cost institutional mutual funds, large institutions (for example, defined benefit plans of major corporations) do not invest through mutual funds that must treat all shareholders equally. They can get better asset management rates elsewhere.

How Much Do Institutional Investors Pay for Asset Management?

Table 7.12 presents illustrative cost data on costs of money management provided by a large manager of institutional funds operating outside the mutual fund framework. It also shows median costs for 167 large and 10 of the largest U.S. pension funds. These rates supply clear evidence of scale economies and the cost efficiency of passive management.

Fees as a percentage of assets decline over large ranges with volume of assets managed. Marginal fees are as low as 1 basis point for passive management of large cap stocks and 2.5 basis points for small and mid-caps, once assets in an account reach US$200 million. Fees for active management are higher but still far less than mutual fund rates. For large cap domestic equity exceeding US$25 million, investors pay 35–50 basis points. Not surprisingly, fees for emerging market investments are much higher than for domestic investments, but advantages to large institutional investors remain. Despite the sliding fee scale, most funds use multiple money managers and allocate less than a US$1 billion on average to each active manager, evidence that diversification benefits eventually outweigh scale economies. There appears to be no strong cost reason for aggregating assets per manager beyond a billion dollars.

Table 7.12. Marginal and Average Asset Management Fees for Institutional Investors: How they Vary with Amount of Investment
(basis points)

Passive domestic equity	Large cap.	Small & mid cap.
< US$5 million	20.0	25.0
US$5–10 million	10.0	15.0
US$10–25 million	8.0	10.0
US$25–100 million	6.0	7.5
US$100–200 million	3.0	5.0
Balance	1.0	2.5
Average fee for US$100 million	7.2	9.1
Average fee for US$500 million	2.6	4.3
Median cost-large U.S. pens. funds[a]	4.0	7.0
Median cost-largest U.S. pens. funds[b]	1.0	6.0

Active domestic equity	Value	Growth	Small cap.
< US$5 million	65.0	80.0	100.0
US$5–25 million	35.0	80.0	100.0
Balance	35.0	50.0	100.0
Average fee for US$100 million	36.5	57.5	100.0
Average fee for US$500 million	35.3	51.5	100.0
Median cost—large pension funds	37.0		69.0
Median cost—largest pension funds	25.0		55.0

International equity	Index	Active
< US$10 million	25.00	90.0
US$10–25 million	25.00	70.0
US$25–40 million	20.00	70.0
US$40–50 million	20.00	60.0
US$50–100 million	15.00	60.0
Balance	10.00	60.0
Average fee for US$100 million	18.75	66.0
Average fee for US$500 million	11.75	61.2
Median cost—large pension funds	12.00	54.0
Median cost—largest pension funds	8.00	34.0

Emerging market	Index	Active
< US$50 million	40	100
Balance	40	80
Average fee for US$100 million	40	90
Average fee for US$500 million	40	82
Median cost—large pension funds	23	77
Median cost—largest pension funds	12	70

(Table continued on next page)

Table 7.12 continued

Fixed income	Index	Active
< US$25 million	12.0	30
25-50 million	8.0	24
50-100 million	5.0	17
Balance	3.0	12
Average fee for US$100 million	7.5	22
Average fee for US$500 million	3.9	14
Median cost—large pension funds	6.0	24
Median cost—largest pension funds	5.0	25

Other asset management costs for institutional investors[c]	
Internal administrative costs	
- Median cost—large pension funds	6
- Median cost—largest pension funds	2
Brokerage costs (trading costs)	
- Median cost—large pension funds	10
- Median cost—largest pension funds	7

a. These are median costs of external money management for given type of assets, reported by 167 large U.S. pension funds ranging in size from less than US$100 million to more than US$100 billion. Median fund = US$1.5 billion. Average of 14 external money managers per fund, managing US$194 million each, median amount managed per manager = US$113 million.

b. These are median costs for the 10 largest U.S. pension funds, excluding CALPERS, ranging in size from US$29–$65 billion. Average of 34 external money managers per fund managing US$646 million each (US$543 million median).

c. This includes brokerage (trading costs) plus internal administrative costs of money management, such as executive pay, consultants, performance measurement, custodial arrangements, trustees, and audits. The breakdown by passive and active is not available, but brokerage costs are estimated to be much lower for passive.

Sources: Sliding scale fees for institutional commingled funds, the BT Pyramid funds, were supplied by Bankers Trust, a large money manager of indexed and actively managed institutional funds. For data on large U.S. pension funds, see "Cost-Effectiveness Pension Fund Report," prepared by Cost-Effective Management, Inc. (1997) for CALPERS.

Adding to these asset management costs another 3–10 basis points for brokerage fees and internal administrative costs that large institutions incur brings the total cost to 0.04–0.65 percent, depending on investment strategy. These numbers from large U.S. pension funds are roughly consistent with numbers from occupational pension plans in the United Kingdom, Switzerland, and South Africa, and from "industry funds" in Australia, all of which cost between 0.4 and 0.6 percent of assets for large defined benefit and defined contribution plans in which workers have no choice of investment manager.[6]

Why Do Institutions Get Better Rates?

In an imperfectly competitive market, large investors have greater reasons and resources to seek out asset managers who will provide good performance at low cost. They are better able to separate noise from signal, to evaluate whether a particular fee is warranted by the expected returns, and, therefore, to respond sensibly to price differentials. They are more likely to use passive investment strategies. They also have the credible threat of managing their money in house if they do not get good terms from an external manager. An all-or-nothing bargaining strategy for a large money bloc enables them to capture potential oligopoly profits or a fee that approaches marginal cost if this is less than average because of fixed costs.

Besides the greater information and bargaining power of institutional investors, they also require lower R&C and marketing costs by the asset manager. It is easier and less labor consuming for the asset manager to deal with the financial staff at a few large institutions than with numerous small, uninformed households. To reach the individual retail investor, asset management services must incur advertising expenses, send numerous brochures and statements to households, and often maintain commissioned salespersons. In contrast, marketing in the institutional marketplace is likely to consume fewer resources because of the concentration of investors, their greater financial expertise, and price sensitivity. Commissions are rarely paid. And, once the contract is secured, only one investor need be served in the institutional market. Even if the billion dollar investor gets better service than the thousand dollar investor (as is likely the case), total marketing and R&C demands relative to assets are much smaller for one institution than for a million small investors. These factors lead to costs for institutional investors as low as 0.04–0.65 percent of assets, depending upon the chosen asset category and investment strategy. This is much lower than retail costs ranging from 0.3 percent to 1.5 percent for the average passively and actively managed mutual funds, respectively.

Capturing Institutional Rates for a
Mandatory IA System: Constrained Choice

By operating through the institutional market, mandatory IA systems can also be structured to obtain scale economies in asset management without high marketing costs. In other words, they can offer workers an opportunity to invest at much lower cost than would be possible on a voluntary basis. To accomplish this requires aggregating numerous small accounts of a mandatory system into large blocks of money and negotiating fees for the investment function on a group or centralized basis. Competition takes place in two stages. In the first stage, a competitive bidding process might be used to limit entry to asset managers charging the lowest fees subject to performance specifications.[7] Limited entry avoids high start-up costs in the early years of a new system. Low fees create a disincentive for high marketing expenses. In the second stage workers choose from among funds that won the primary competition. The lowest fees are obtained when worker choice is constrained to low-cost investment portfolios and strategies, such as passive investment. Still, enough choice could be retained to satisfy individual preferences and avoid political control. With R&C costs of 0.1 percent of assets (as in the average mutual fund in table 7.7 and as calculated for an IA system with small contributions in table 7.1), and with investment costs as given above for institutions, an "institutional" IA system would cost 0.14–0.75 percent of assets in the long run (James and others 1999).

Several countries are now experimenting with variants of this approach. The three institutional IA systems described below all operate within this fee range and imply some trade-off of political insulation and individual freedom for the cost reduction. We start with the most constrained system, in Bolivia, that is appropriate for a small developing country, and conclude with the Swedish system, that offers considerable choice among existing funds, mimics the institutional market through a sliding scale of price ceilings, and is more appropriate for countries with advanced financial markets. We describe the cost savings that seem achievable, as well as the pitfalls of these schemes.

Auction off Entry Rights to a Single Portfolio: Bolivia

In 1997, in a widely publicized international bidding process, Bolivia auctioned off the asset management rights in its new defined contribution pillar to two investment companies. The new system was initially expected to have 300,000 participants, each contributing 10 percent of wages into their retirement accounts, bringing total annual contributions to US$300 per account or almost US$90 million en toto. Initially, to help finance the transition almost all of the assets had to be invested in government bonds, but over time the funds were expected to diversify.

The bidding process for management rights consisted of two stages that began with notices in the *Wall Street Journal*, *Financial Times*, and *Pensions and Investments* and proceeded through extensive Internet communications, which facilitated international competition. A Web site was established to exchange documents such as draft law and regulations, proposed contracts, and other data. Initial selection criteria included experience in asset management (at least 10 years of global asset management, at least US$10 billion in assets under management), experience in pension fund administration and record keeping (at least 100,000 accounts), and experience in establishing new systems. Reacting to this publicity, 73 asset managers expressed interest, and 12 consortia (including 25 separate companies) applied, of which nine were selected to bid. At the bidding stage, the managers competed with respect to asset management fees, and conditions regarding guarantees and regulations were added. Concerns about possible guarantees that might be required and the government's insistence that in the early years the AFPs must invest most incoming revenues in Treasury bonds led only three managers to submit bids at this stage.

The bidding process specified that a uniform fee of 0.5 percent of salary (5 percent of net contributions) would be imposed, and companies bid on the size of their additional asset-based fee. In the end the lowest bidder offered to charge 22.85 basis points of the first US$1 billion under management, 1.4 basis points on the next US$0.2 billion, 0.67 basis points on the next US$.3 billion and no management fee on assets above US$1.5 billion—strong evidence of the scale economies in asset management noted above. The second bidder quickly adopted this schedule, thereby ending the bidding process.[8]

Both winner consortia consisted of international consortia that included foreign and domestic partners: Invesco-Argentaria and Banco Bilbao Vizcaya S.A.-Prevision. Their contracts run for five years. Initially workers were assigned to a company and no switching was permitted. Starting in the year 2000, urban workers will be allowed to switch and new workers will be permitted to choose. After the five-year contractual period, additional companies will be allowed to enter and the price caps will be lifted (Von Gersdorff 1997; Guerard and Kelly 1997).

Why were international companies so interested in a small pension fund in a small country? The same companies that run the new defined contribution pillar will also manage the US$1.65 billion proceeds of a privatization program (an amount that is equal to 22 percent of Bolivia's gross national product). Bolivia undertook pension reform and state enterprise reform simultaneously and auctioned off management rights to the two sets of assets jointly. In addition to the fees paid by workers, the companies will receive a fee of 0.2285 percent of privatization assets, which will roughly double their revenues in the early years. Given that 5 percent of pension contributions equals US$15 per year, which would barely cover R&C costs, cross-subsidies from the management of privatization assets could well be involved. It is likely that bidders would have been less interested, and initial costs paid by workers in the IA system would have been higher without the presence of large privatization assets. But they probably would have been lower if the same scenario were repeated in a country with better financial markets and infrastructure. In other countries, bidders might be attracted because of complementarity with desired insurance and banking markets.

The Bolivian system is designed to keep average costs and fees low in the early years by reducing fixed costs and excess capacity, since only two companies are operating; decreasing marketing and record-keeping costs, since each company is given an initial monopoly for a group of workers and transfers are not allowed; amortizing infrastructure costs over several years, during which each company has an assured market share; and increasing information and bargaining power, since the government bargains on behalf of the entire system when fees are established in the contract. Was this accomplished? Initially fees in Bolivia were only 0.5 percent of wages (5 percent of incoming contributions) plus 0.23 percent of assets and 0.2 percent of assets for the custodian. This produced a fee that was less than one-third of that in Chile in the first year (3 percent of assets for Bolivia in 1998 compared with 9.4 percent in Chile in 1982; see tables 7.3 and 7.4). For workers who will only be in the system for 20 years or less, Bolivia is clearly much cheaper than Chile.

However, the differential is expected to narrow over time as the asset-based component grows. Under the current fee structure, a full-career worker who enters the system today would pay the equivalent of 0.56 percent of assets per year over his or her lifetime, as compared with 0.76 percent in Chile. Thus, in the long run, given the present pricing structure, the difference between the two countries is about 20 basis points. In the absence of cost-saving measures, we would have expected Bolivia to be more expensive than Chile due to its smaller accounts and less developed infrastructure and financial markets, so these numbers understate the true saving.

Restricted entry has other pros and cons besides the impact on costs. One advantage of a bidding process with only two or three winners, especially in small countries, is that for some period it provides a guaranteed market share that may entice international companies with financial expertise to enter the market. The established standards and practices of these firms may, to some extent, substitute for regulatory capacity in countries where this is weak. At the same time, the extreme concentration opens the door to corruption in the award of the initial contracts, collusion between the two firms, and possibly control of the contract monitors by the firms that they are supposed to regulate. In return for favorable regulatory treatment, the firms may agree to buy government debt at low rates rather than investing more broadly. The regulators may have weak power relative to the power of two large investment companies that control the market. The two companies may also constitute a controlling share of the securities market in Bolivia, once this begins to develop and they are permitted to diversify, and this is particularly a threat if international investments are not allowed. Thus this system is not as well insulated from political objectives and monopolistic distortions as would be a less concentrated system.

Another problem stems from the lack of incentives for service and from slow adaptability to unforeseen contingencies because of the incomplete nature of contracts. While certain service targets were set, the contract cannot specify every element of service that might be desired, and companies are likely to cut back on services that are not specified in order to maximize their profits while living within the contract. The fact that workers cannot switch companies initially removes competitive pressures to perform well for those circumstances and services that are not enumerated. Of course, the possibility of switches after three years, as well as the entry of new firms after five years, means that long-run contestability may prevent abuses of monopoly power. But it is also possible that political pressures from the first two companies may lead to a continuation of the restrictions on entry and switching. Moreover, competition in Bolivia has been dampened by an unexpected development—the merger of the parent companies of the two winning bidders, which in effect have become one. Thus the Bolivian approach keeps costs low at start-up, but the impact on costs and performance in the long run is uncertain.

One way to mitigate these problems is to maintain an auction process for the long run, but with rebidding every 3–5 years on the basis of performance as well as fees. However, the incumbent may have a big competitive advantage over potential newcomers, since it already has affiliates and R&C files. To facilitate contestability, it may be desirable to separate the fixed cost component of the operation (such as the R&C database) from the investment function, and to permit investment abroad, which will make the environment more inviting to asset managers from abroad.

With these caveats in mind, the limited entry-by-bidding approach is worth serious consideration, especially as a way to avoid excess capacity at the start-up of new systems and in the longer run for countries that have modest contribution and asset bases.

Competitive Bidding with Portfolio Choice: TSP

In Bolivia both funds offer the same portfolio (government bonds and bank deposits). A less constrained variation on this theme uses a competitive bidding process to select a limited number of varied portfolios and investment companies offering them, among which workers can choose. The federal Thrift Saving Plan (TSP), a voluntary plan for civil service workers in the United States, employs this approach. It has been proposed as one possible model that might be followed if the U.S. Social Security system were reformed to include IAs. In the TSP, the employer—the federal government—matches worker contributions up to a combined limit of 16 percent. Beginning with barely a million participants and US$3 billion in assets in 1987, the TSP had grown to 2.3 million participants and US$65 billion by 1998, with average annual contributions of US$2,600 and an average account size of US$27,400 that far exceeds the size of other plans analyzed in this chapter.

In the TSP model, several benchmarks are selected, and the right to run a fund through passive management based on the benchmarks is auctioned off periodically in a competitive bidding process. Initially only three portfolios were authorized: a money market fund that holds short-term government securities, a fixed-income fund that holds medium- and long-term government and corporate bonds, and a common stock fund indexed to the Standard & Poor 500. It is now in the process of adding a small cap fund and an international stock fund (the voluntary market provided these options many years ago). A bidding process is held every 2–4 years, with prospective managers evaluated on the basis of tracking ability, trading costs, fiduciary record, and fees. Workers have a choice among these funds and limited switching is permitted. However, the same investment company has been selected to run the stock and bond funds so workers do not have a choice among investment companies. Moreover, the contract holder has not changed over the lifetime of TSP, consistent with the "first mover" advantage mentioned above.

The TSP essentially operates as an institutional investor, passing the savings along to its investors. As a result of its information and bargaining power as well as its use of passive management, investment costs (including trading fees) are only a few basis points. The largest cost component, about US$20 per account, is for R&C, which a separate public agency executes. An alternative model might auction off the R&C function as well. While R&C costs have been quite constant over time in dollar terms, investment costs have been rising with assets, so total administrative costs are now US$30 per account. As a percentage of assets, administrative costs have fallen from 0.7 percent at the start-up of the system to 0.11 percent in 1998 (table 7.13).

The fee is less than 10 percent of what workers would pay, on average, if they were given a broad choice of portfolios and chose the same mix as retail mutual fund investors (who pay 1.43 percent of assets, on average). It is about half of what they would have to pay in the retail industry in the United States for similar funds (Standard & Poor index mutual funds are available for 21 basis points, including trading costs). This cost is exceptionally low partly because contributions are passed on by a single employer, the government, which also covers some additional communications costs. But the biggest cost saving in TSP (a saving of 1.2 percent of assets per year compared with the average mutual fund investment) comes from constraining the choice of investment strategy to domestic passive management; countries that did not have such deep financial markets could not achieve such large savings. Small additional savings (of 0.1 percent per year) accrue to TSP from using a competitive bidding process to enhance bargaining power, secure better rates, and eliminate marketing expenses.

Table 7.13. Administrative Costs of Thrift Saving Plan, 1988–98

Year	Expense ratio as % of assets	Average size account (in 000$'s)	Administrative cost per account (in $'s)	Administrative cost per account (in 1998 $'s)	Investment cost per account ($'s)	R&C cost per account (in $'s)	R&C cost per account (in 1998 $'s)
1988	.70	2.4	16.8	(22.7)	1.0	15.8	(21.4)
1989	.46	3.7	17.1	(22.21)	1.5	15.5	(20.2)
1990	.29	5.1	14.81	(18.00)	2.0	12.8	(15.6)
1991	.26	6.7	17.4	(20.71)	2.7	14.7	(17.6)
1992	.23	8.5	19.6	(22.53)	3.4	16.2	(18.6)
1993	.19	10.7	20.3	(22.81)	4.3	16.1	(18.0)
1994	.16	12.8	20.6	(22.39)	5.1	15.4	(16.7)
1995	.14	16.5	23.1	(24.57)	6.6	16.5	(17.6)
1996	.13	20.1	26.2	(27.01)	8.0	18.1	(18.7)
1997	.12	25.3	30.3	(30.61)	10.1	20.2	(20.4)
1998[a]	.11	27.4	30.1	(30.10)	11.1	19.2	(19.2)

Note: Expense ratio in column 1 is reported gross expense ratio as reported in TSP publications (before adjustment for forfeitures) plus 3 basis points imputed by authors for brokerage (trading) fees. Columns 5 and 6 are authors' estimates separating R&C from investment expenses. Investment expenses are assumed to be 3 basis points of trading costs plus 1 basis point for asset management, custodian, legal, and auditing fees related to investments. R&C costs are the remainder. TSP does not report its brokerage costs or breakdown of other expenses between investment and R&C.
a. Based on January–August, annualized
Sources: Thrift Saving Plan publications; authors' calculations.

The advantage of such a process is that workers have a clear-cut choice of investment portfolio—but choice is constrained in a way that is designed to keep fees low without sacrificing expected returns. This constraint may be a big advantage in an IA system where many small account holders are unaccustomed to evaluating multiple investment options and where it is important to avoid a high implicit contingent government liability. The disadvantages relate to limitations in the selection of portfolios, slow adaptation to change, and no competition. Workers who want a risk-return trade-off that is different from that permitted by the system's governing board or those who want active management cannot satisfy their preferences. Investment in enhanced index funds, high-yielding but risky venture capital, private equity, and new financial instruments are completely ruled out. Competitive pressures for good performance and innovation are limited once a portfolio is chosen since, for any given portfolio (and even across portfolios), there is no choice of manager. These disadvantages could be mitigated by increasing the number of benchmarks available and selecting two or three companies to run the funds for each benchmark. The larger the asset base, the more feasible this becomes.

In developing countries where the pension system is a major source of long-term capital, financial markets are not efficient, and few attractive financial instruments and benchmarks are available, a heavy concentration on passive investment may not be feasible or desirable. Thus, as was the case with the Bolivian model, this approach is promising but must be used with caution.

Open Entry and Price Ceilings: Sweden

Still greater product variety could be achieved, while retaining low fees, by allowing open entry subject to a price ceiling imposed by a central authority. Sweden recently established an IA system using this type of approach. Five million workers are expected to participate, contributing 2.5 percent of wages. This funded system is supplementary to a large unfunded "notional" defined contribution pillar, to which workers contribute 16 percent. For a full-time worker, annual contributions to the IA system will amount to US$600 per year, and about 16 billion kronor, or US$2 billion per year, are expected to flow into the system. Money began to accumulate in an unallocated pool in 1995, so when allocations to individuals and funds begin in 2000, total assets will be about US$10 billion.

All mutual funds that operate in the voluntary market (several hundred funds) are free to participate providing they agree to the net fee schedule set by the public agency that administers the system (the premiepension-smyndigheten, or PPM). Subject to this proviso, workers can select the fund of their choice. After studying the industry's production function to determine the size of fixed and variable costs, the public agency has just promulgated the fee schedule that it plans to impose. It is a complex schedule that attempts to mimic the cost function and the fee schedule that would be charged in the institutional market. It depends on the expense ratio charged by the fund to the general public in the voluntary market (as a proxy for asset class and quality) and the magnitude of contributions that it attracts in the mandatory system (table 7.14 and figure 7.3). A sliding scale was used so that price would track declining marginal and average costs. It also cushions the risk of participation for funds that are uncertain they will attract a large volume of assets, thereby encouraging diversity while restricting excess profits from those that are more successful (MPIR Investment Research AB 1998).

Mutual funds in the voluntary market in Sweden charge varying amounts ranging from 0.4 percent to more than 2 percent. As of 1997 the average fee plus trading commissions was 1.5 percent, similar the figure in the United States (Dahlquist, Engstrom, and Soderlind 1999). Funds will charge the same fees in the mandatory system but are required to pay a rebate to the PPM, which passes it back to workers. The rebate to the PPM is higher for high-cost funds and more popular funds. Funds that attract

Table 7.14. Fee Ceilings in Swedish IA System
(percentage of assets)

Marginal Fee Kept by Mutual Funds by Tranche of Assets They Attract in IA System[a]

Million KR	Marginal fees	VOLFEE = 200	VOLFEE = 150	VOLFEE = 40
0–70	0.40 + 0.75 (VOLFEE – 0.40)	1.60	1.23	0.40
70–300	0.35 + 0.35 (VOLFEE – 0.35)	0.93	0.75	0.37
300–500	0.30 + 0.15 (VOLFEE – 0.30)	0.56	0.48	0.32
500–3000	0.25 + 0.05 (VOLFEE – 0.25)	0.34	0.31	0.26
3000–7000	0.15 + 0.05 (VOLFEE – 0.15)	0.24	0.22	0.16
7000 +	0.12 + 0.04 (VOLFEE – 0.12)	0.20	0.18	0.13

Average Fee Kept by Mutual Funds by Total Fund Assets They Attract in IA System

Million KR	VOLFEE = 200	VOLFEE = 150	VOLFEE = 40
70	1.60	1.23	0.40
150	1.24	0.97	0.38
500	0.87	0.71	0.35
1000	0.61	0.51	0.30
3000	0.43	0.38	0.27
7000	0.32	0.29	0.21
15000	0.25	0.23	0.17

Note: This table shows the share of the mutual fund's fee in the voluntary market (VOLFEE) that it is permitted to charge in the mandatory IA system, depending on the assets that it attracts in the IA system. Fees are all expressed as a percentage of assets. One $US = 8.2 kronors. Panel A shows marginal fees, panel B shows average fees. Based on current rates, an additional 0.2 percent fee is estimated to be charged to cover trading costs (brokers' commissions). This is charged as a deduction from net assets. While this is the current fee, competitive forces may push it lower in the new system.
Source: PPM.

large sums from the mandatory system are left with a net marginal fee of less than 20 basis points and a net average fee of 20–30 basis points. Such fees will likely rule out intensive marketing since cost would exceed incremental net revenues. These net numbers are roughly similar to fees that large institutional investors in the United States pay for management of domestic assets.

This method could not be used, however, unless some other arrangements were made to cover R&C costs, for these costs will exceed the permissible fees in the early years of the new system. Many mutual funds would be unwilling to participate if they had to cover R&C expenses out of their allowable fee. The Swedish system avoids this problem by centralizing collections, record-keeping, and most communications—charging all workers an additional asset-based fee to cover these costs (thereby cross-subsidizing low earners) and amortizing expenses over a 15-year period (thereby spreading fixed costs over many cohorts). R&C costs are expected to be 0.3 percent at the beginning, eventually dropping to 0.1 percent. To avoid the cost of setting up a new collection system, the central tax authorities collect contributions together with other taxes and eventually pass them on to the PPM. The PPM records these contributions, aggregates the contributions of many individuals, and moves them in omnibus accounts to the mutual funds chosen by workers. Indeed, the funds will not even know the names of their individual members—a procedure know as

Figure 7.3. Average Fees Paid by Worker and Kept by Fund in Swedish System

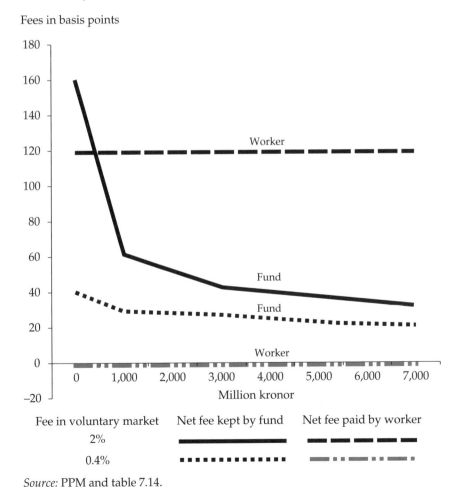

Fees in basis points

Source: PPM and table 7.14.

"blind allocations." The PPM will process all fund switches. These features reinforce the bulk buying power of the public agency and further discourage sales commissions.

The rebate collected from the funds is distributed back to the workers, according to a formula set by the PPM. One might expect (and high fee funds preferred) that the rebate would go back to workers in the originating fund, on grounds that net price paid by workers would then equal net fee received by fund, and both would approximate marginal cost. However, the PPM proposed (and low fee funds, that tend to be associated with unions, preferred) to give each worker back the same amount (as a percentage of assets invested) regardless of which fund he or she had chosen. This would drive a wedge between net price paid by workers and received by funds. Workers who chose low-fee funds would get back far more than the rebate paid by their fund, while workers in high-fee funds would continue to pay high fees that their funds would not keep. If the net fee received by each fund approximates its marginal cost (which is the intent), the net price paid by consumers would differ from marginal cost and, in making their allocation decisions, consumers would not be taking real marginal cost into account (figure 7.3).

The high fee funds and their potential consumers obviously opposed the PPM proposal. The net outcome, therefore, was a political compromise: part of the rebate will be returned on a group basis and part on an individual basis. Thus the system will redistribute across consumers in ways that are not obvious or obviously equitable. This controversy about how to distribute the rebate exemplifies the value judgements and/or political pressures to which price control systems are subject, sometimes at the expense of efficiency. It is not clear whether this redistributive fee-cum-rebate schedule will prove to be politically sustainable.

The Swedish system also illustrates some of the pitfalls of a price control system that stem from the difficulty in promulgating an efficient and equitable fee schedule for a differentiated industry. Experience in other industries warns that "incorrect" prices may be set and quality deterioration may occur under price controls. For example, it remains to be seen which funds will be willing to enter the system under these terms. If the price has been set too low, few if any funds would choose to participate. For example, in Kazakhstan a very low unstable fee ceiling of 1 percent of contributions plus 10 percent of investment returns has contributed to limited participation by private investment companies.[9] And those that do participate may provide inferior service. While many funds appear to be interested in Sweden, the nature of the participating companies will be skewed by the fee structure. Most likely bond, large cap, and index funds investing in Sweden and other industrialized countries will participate, while actively managed small cap and emerging market funds that have more expensive production functions may be reluctant to join. Thus price controls are implicitly pushing the system toward certain assets and passive investing, although these were not explicit goals at the outset.

How much is actually saved by this complex system? Under the current formula, the average fee that the consumers will pay and the funds will keep depends on the distribution of assets in the mandatory system, which is not yet known, since the system only began operation in the year 2000. Suppose that the demand and supply effects described above shape consumer choice so that 75 percent of all assets accrue to low-fee funds while 25 percent of assets are divided equally among the others. Then, the net average fee paid by consumers (including trading commissions and R&C costs) will be about 0.8 percent of assets annually, compared with 1.5 percent in the voluntary market. Total saving will equal 0.7 percent of assets. In the long run, as R&C costs fall, total savings rise to 1 percent (table 7.15).

As in the case of TSP, much of this potential saving is due to incentives that change the mix of funds and shift consumers toward low-cost funds. A smaller proportion is due to cost cuts for the given funds, stemming from fee ceilings that discourage marketing expenses. A final portion of the

Table 7.15. Average Annual Fees as Percentage of Assets for Alternative IA Systems

	Retail	*Institutional*
Latin America	Chile	Bolivia – Competitive bidding
Start up	9.39	3.00
Current	1.36	3.00
Lifetime simulation	0.76	0.54
Sweden	Mutual funds	IA systems – price ceilings
Current	1.50	0.80
Long run	—	0.50
United States	Mutual funds	Hypothetical IA systems
Active	1.50	0.64
Passive	0.32	0.16
		TSP (competitive bidding, passive)
		0.11

Note: See text and tables, especially tables 2, 6, 7, 12, and 13 for derivation of these numbers. Lifetime simulations are derived from tables 2 and 6. These numbers include imputed brokerage commissions (trading costs) and custodial costs. Numbers for Sweden are guestimates, based on assumption that average fee kept by participating mutual funds will be 0.3 percent of assets in short run, 0.2 percent in long run. PPM costs are 0.3 percent in short run, 0.1 percent in long run; trading and other costs = 0.2 percent of assets.

lower fee is attributable to greater bargaining power of the PPM, which keeps price in the mandatory sector close to marginal cost. The saving is not nearly as much as the TSP achieves, mainly because the Swedish fees are high enough to accommodate greater choice, including active management. Thus the Swedish model would be a possibility for other countries that want to provide considerable choice in their IA system while also achieving modest cost reductions—but the dangers of price ceilings discussed above are also real.

Constrained Choice: Is It a Good Choice?

An overarching characteristic of these approaches is constrained choice for the worker. The government organizes the market and constrains choice in every mandatory system, albeit with different objectives. In Chile and most other Latin American countries with decentralized schemes, pension funds must abide by detailed regulations controlling their investment portfolios, designed to reduce financial market risk and regulatory difficulty, rather than to minimize costs. As a result, marketing costs are high and returns have not been maximized, but potential disasters have been averted (Srinivas and Yermo 1999). Moral hazard problems have potentially been reduced, thereby making government guarantees of benefits less costly.

The IA models used in Bolivia, Sweden, and the TSP preserve private competitive fund management and worker choice, but they constrain choice with the object of reducing administrative costs and eventually increasing pensions. Preliminary evidence suggests that in the long run they will cut costs to less than 0.6 percent and in some cases to less than 0.2 percent of assets per year (table 7.15). If gross returns are not affected negatively, such fee reductions could raise pensions by 10–20 percent relative to the retail market.

To evaluate whether these cost and fee reductions are desirable, it is important to analyze their origin. We have identified three major sources: changes in investment portfolios and strategies, lower costs of managing a given portfolio, and redistributing by cost-shifting and cutting oligopoly profits. The first source has the largest impact on fees, especially in countries with efficient financial markets and passive investment opportunities. The second source, operating mainly by minimizing marketing and start-up expenditures, is available in developing countries as well. Cost-shifting involves distributional trade-offs between long-run and short-run fees and between fees in the voluntary and mandatory markets. The reduction in profits is probably the least important since, in many countries and in a global financial market, in the long run these will be small in any case.

Potential gains may also be achieved by centralizing the R&C function, although this is less clear.

Changes in Portfolios

All three cases severely limit the range of portfolios available to workers, ruling out "expensive" portfolios in assets such as small cap stocks and emerging markets, and instead directing workers toward index funds in liquid domestic instruments. Innovation and new product development is discouraged or ruled out. TSP does this most strongly and directly; about 90 percent of its fee saving is attributable to this constraint on asset allocation. Sweden does it indirectly by setting price ceilings that will restrict the supply of "expensive" funds and cross-subsidies that will push demand toward cheaper funds. Developing countries such as Bolivia that lack well-functioning index funds and liquid securities markets have much less access to this source of cost saving. Of course, they also lack access to a wide set of financial instruments necessary for diversified active investment, and availability is the main factor constraining their portfolios. This may, however, become an additional rationale for the development of new instruments, more accurate indexes, disclosure rules that will enhance market efficiency, and international diversification using index funds (see the Shah and Fernandes essay in chapter 9).

These constraints on asset classes are predicated on the assumption that the judgement of many workers about the relationship between fund performance and fees is imperfect, and that cost saving, which is certain, should take precedence over workers' expectations about returns, which are highly uncertain, in a mandatory scheme. The evidence cited above supports the idea that many small, and even large, investors are poorly informed. Constraining investment choice at the start of their new systems facilitates the concept of learning by doing, which is probably the most effective form of education, by limiting the mistakes people can make. It makes government guarantees of benefits potentially less costly by diminishing moral hazard problems.

But these restrictions decrease the adaptability for individual risk-return preferences to informed workers as well as the fund's incentive to innovate and are, therefore, not an unmitigated gain. The agents who set these restrictions may not always act in the workers' best interests. Additionally, individuals may have a smaller sense of "ownership" and a larger sense of being taxed if their choice of investment strategies is constrained. The risk to the government of being responsible for a bailout in case of investment failure may be greater when it has "endorsed" a small number of investment portfolios and managers. These dangers can be alleviated by allowing greater choice, but at a cost in terms of higher price (Sweden versus TSP).

Marketing Cost Reductions

All three cases achieve further economies by investing assets through the institutional market to a limited group of companies and centrally negotiating fees for large money blocks. Bolivia and the TSP set a small number of slots for investment companies a priori and auctioned off operating rights to the lowest qualified bidder. The competitive bidding process determined price. In Sweden the public agency predetermined a low price structure. The quantity of companies willing to accept these terms remains to be seen, but a small number is expected to dominate the market. The low fees and limited entry dampen marketing costs and excess capacity that might otherwise exist at start-up. Given the large fixed costs and declining average costs in the industry, it will always be tempting for funds to spend more on advertising and sales commissions to increase their market share as long as the attainable fee is higher than marginal cost.[10] When the fee is exogenously decreased, the incentive to spend on marketing will similarly decline, helping to sustain the low fee.

As discussed earlier, marketing provides both accurate and misleading information to consumers, incentives for good performance, and a large element of zero-sum game competition. Reductions in marketing expenditures are efficient if the zero-sum game component is cut while the useful information is not cut. It seems likely that the socially optimal amount of marketing is less in a mandatory IA system than in the voluntary market. Since the total investable amount is predetermined by law; marketing is not needed to induce people to save or to attract these savings to financial markets. While marketing imparts information, investment companies and brokers have a clear incentive to impart misleading information that is in their rather than the consumer's interest. This could be a big problem in a new mandatory system with many small inexperienced investors. In such a system it is important to provide other less biased, less expensive sources of information such as government publications and the popular media. The incentives for good performance and innovation imparted by marketing could continue to be provided in the voluntary marketplace. Reducing marketing expenses in the mandatory systems may be more problematic in countries with low tax collection capacities and fewer alternative sources of information, particularly those that wish to use marketing as a tool to increase coverage and reduce evasion.

Cost-Shifting

The third source of the fee savings is due to cost-shifting and is mainly a short-run and distributional effect: maintaining the burden of fixed costs in the voluntary rather than the mandatory systems and shifting part of the initial capital costs in a new system to later cohorts. For example, in Sweden entry is open only to firms that operate in the voluntary market, and the fee schedule aims at charging marginal cost. The public agency is using a 15-year amortization period for R&C, while a private company would probably expect a positive return in five years. Since the benefits of an IA system accrue disproportionately to younger generations, which have more opportunity to accumulate savings, it seems reasonable that much of the fixed costs should be shifted to them as well—but obviously this involves a value judgement. Obtaining lower fees through an all-or-nothing offer for large blocs in oligopolistic markets likewise reduces price in the mandatory system without a corresponding impact on real resource cost—it shifts fixed costs to the voluntary sector or cuts oligopoly profits.

Centralizing Collections and R&C: Does This Help?

The institutional approach is likely to imply centralized collections and record-keeping. Centralized collections enable money to be aggregated and moved in large blocs without the identity of the worker being disclosed, and centralized record-keeping allows the investment function to be more contestable in the rebidding process. Both TSP and Sweden separate collection and R&C responsibilities from investment responsibilities and turn the former over to a central agency. In Bolivia, where only two asset managers operate, virtual centralization through private companies has been achieved, but this has not been separated from the investment function. Is this desirable?

Besides its role in making the rebidding process more contestable, centralized record-keeping has other cost implications. It facilitates economies of scale and standardization and avoids the compatibility problems that could arise when a member switches funds and information systems. It enables provision of a basic level of service without competitive pressures to upgrade to a more costly level. Workers can more easily have multiple accounts without multiple costly records and with the entire lifetime record in one place upon retirement. Centralization also has a redistributive potential—it permits a cross-subsidy to small accounts of low earners, which may be deemed socially desirable in a mandatory scheme. But the downside is the possibility that the central R&C office may have little incentive for accuracy and efficiency if it has a monopoly.

Centralized collections enable the IA system to piggyback on existing tax collection systems, thereby avoiding the cost of setting up a new collection system and reducing incremental paperwork costs to employers. But piggybacking involves a large time cost and, hence, an opportunity cost. An average of 9 months will pass in Sweden each year before the contributions will be attributed to individuals and allocated to funds, during which time participants simply earn the risk-free government rate. If the government rate is 3 percentage points lower than the rate that investors would otherwise have earned, this opportunity cost is equivalent to a charge of 2.25

percent of contributions, or 0.11 percent annually of assets. We have not added this amount into our total cost calculations, but it should be considered—the advantages are not cost-free.

Centralized collections may also facilitate compliance, since a single collection agency has responsibility for tracking contributors and, therefore, for identifying evaders. Individual pension funds have little incentive to report evaders, since they will simply lose a potential future customer. But the centralized agency may also have little incentive, since it doesn't keep the money. The outcome here obviously depends on governance capacity and social norms, and we have little empirical evidence on actual outcomes.

Centralized collections and record-keeping may be handled through a public agency or may be contracted out to a private company or clearing-house in a competitive bidding process. Croatia is attempting the latter approach. Using a public agency may not be a good option for countries that have weak tax collection mechanisms and distrust of government. For example, this approach probably was not feasible in Chile at the start of its reform. Centralization via a contracting process has the advantage of introducing price and quality competition into the choice. The government or an association of pension funds could run the bidding process in order to make the winner more accountable. Even if centralization is not required from the start, the system is likely to move in that direction if subcontracting is permitted, which is not the case in Chile, due to scale economies. Most mutual funds in the United States (except the largest fund complexes) turn their R&C functions over to an external "transfer agent," and two transfer agents dominate the entire industry—evidence of natural market adaptation to scale economies. Many Australian funds contract out the account administration function to a few large R&C companies (Bateman 1999). We might expect such procedures to develop in other mandatory pension systems, if they are permitted. The pros and cons of alternative R&C arrangement obviously require further empirical study, as countries experiment with alternative systems.

Other Caveats and Pitfalls

The institutional approach to IA systems involves other caveats and pitfalls besides those already mentioned. First, in a centralized competitive bidding process, the "wrong" number of firms may be chosen, resulting in over- or underconcentration relative to the least-cost point. Or in a system of price ceilings, the wrong price may be chosen, resulting in under-or oversupply.[11] Second, there is the need to build performance incentives into the initial contract. It is likely that whatever performance and service characteristics are not explicitly mentioned will be given scant attention by the winning bidders who want to maximize their profits subject to the contractual constraints. Market competition provides continual implicit incentives for good performance in ways that matter to consumers. Innovation is encouraged. Competition bidding makes some of the incentives explicit ex ante and disregards the others—the essence of incomplete contracts. The greater the choice for workers and the contestability at the rebidding stage, the smaller is this problem. Moreover, the less confidence one has in the ability of workers to evaluate fund behavior, the smaller is this problem—and different analysts probably have different views on this subject. Empirical evidence on the performance of asset managers who are chosen under different procedures might throw some light on this issue.

Further along these lines, a competitive bidding process is inflexible in the face of unforeseen contingencies that have not been spelled out in incomplete contracts. One such unforeseen contingency occurred in Bolivia when the parent companies of the two winning investment managers merged in a global merger process.; the two winners became one, and the duopoly became, effectively, a monopoly.

Whether a monopoly or duopoly is involved, effective regulation is essential. But one or two large winners in a competitive bidding process may capture the regulators; the "regulated" may be in a stronger bargaining position than the regulators. Corruption in the bidding process and collusion afterwards is a related possibility (Valdes 1999a). A further problem is that a small number of large funds may exert a dominant control over small capital markets rather than helping to develop these markets further. These considerations may lead a country to choose a larger number of winners at the primary bidding stage than would be chosen on the basis of scale economies alone. Further concentration would then be achieved via the market at the secondary stage of competition for workers—but this would increase marketing costs as each "winner" tries to increase its market share.

A final problem occurs at the rebidding stage. Every competitive bidding process must specify a credible rebidding procedure. But the first winners may have a big competitive advantage over potential contestors in such markets. This is particularly the case if they have already invested in fixed costs and can, therefore, underbid new entrants who would have to cover such costs. A short-run bidding competition can thereby become a long-run monopoly, with little regulation or contestability. A large part of the fixed costs consists of the database of affiliates to the system. The rebidding contest can be enhanced by separating the R&C function from the asset management function and vesting ownership of the membership database in the system itself, rather than in the firms that carry out the investment or R&C functions.

The greater the choice, the smaller are these dangers, but the smaller also presents the opportunity for depressing administrative costs. We thus face a trade-off between reducing administrative costs, on the one hand, and increasing continuous incentives, adaptability, and political insulation, on the other. It seems plausible that the terms of this trade-off depend on the size of the system and the governance capacities of the country. The larger the contribution base, the greater the choice that can be allowed while still benefiting from low costs. Thus Sweden is likely to have the same long-run costs as Bolivia despite the fact that it offers greater choice, because of its larger average account size. The TSP has lower fees than Sweden, both because it has a larger asset base and because it constrains choice to a much greater extent.

A careful writing of the bidding contract—specifying performance targets and rewards, rebidding procedures, and a mechanism for handling exceptional contingencies—can minimize these pitfalls. The more responsible the governance of the country, the more likely that contracts will be carefully written and enforced, and thus the lower the political risks of operating through the institutional market. While competition and choice always have a role to play, countries with well-developed financial markets and good governance have available to them a wider range of options, including lower cost options.

Conclusion

We began this chapter by asking: What is the most efficient way to set up an IA component of a social security system? How can IA systems that consist of many small accounts garner the cost advantages obtained by the large investor in the institutional market? To answer these questions we compared costs in the retail market with those in the institutional market, including several IA experiments that aggregate these small accounts into large money blocs in setting price and market access.

Since these systems are new, the evidence is still fragmentary. Thus far it is promising. It appears that investing IAs through the institutional market with constrained choice can achieve substantial cost savings. This could raise final accumulations and pensions by 10–20 percent. Typically, these systems aggregate contributions, specify a small number of winning funds among which workers can choose, and use a competitive bidding process to set fees (although Sweden reverses this process and sets fees, allowing competition to determine quantity).

These fee reductions have been achieved by (i) changing the range of investment strategies faced by workers, (ii) cutting costs, and (iii) shifting costs or shaving profits. The largest observed fee reductions stem from a product mix change: constraining choice to investment portfolios and strategies that are inexpensive to implement, such as passive management (as in TSP). This requires access to well-developed financial markets and has an offsetting disadvantage for investors who would have preferred different portfolios. A process of price setting that cuts incentives for marketing (as in Bolivia and Sweden) and avoids excess capacity at the start of new systems (as in Bolivia) achieves the largest cost reductions for a given portfolio. This is likely to work best if the collection and record-keeping functions are separated from the investment function, which facilitates blind allocations and competition at the rebidding stage. The third effect is distributional: increased bargaining power in an all-or-nothing deal is used to maintain fixed costs in the old voluntary market, to partly transfer them to future cohorts through extended amortization, and to keep oligopoly profits low.

Any system of constrained choice imposes costs in terms of satisfying individual preferences, decreasing market incentives, and increasing the risk of political manipulation, corruption, collusion, and regulatory capture. Investment contracts are bound to be incomplete with respect to performance incentives and adaptability to unforeseen contingencies, and rebidding procedures pose a further problem. Trade-offs are therefore involved between administrative costs and other less certain and less tangible costs.

Probably the least-cost alternatives and trade-offs are available for industrialized rather than for developing countries. Industrialized countries have access to existing financial institutions, lower trading costs, passive investment opportunities, and more effective governance. For these reasons, they can save more than 1 percent per year by constraining choice and operating through the institutional market. In developing and transitional countries, particularly those with small contribution and assets bases, investment costs are likely to be higher and the opportunities for reducing fees lower. In particular, reducing fees through portfolio constraints may not be a realistic option in the short run for countries that have limited access to passive management or to large liquid asset classes. For these countries, the main cost-saving measure may be competitive bidding for a limited number of entry slots, which results in lower costs and fees for a given portfolio. Based on the experience of Bolivia, this offers the possibility of reducing costs substantially, especially at the start-up phase—providing government has the capacity and will to carefully construct and enforce the contract.

A total constraint on choice implied by a single centralized fund has led to poor net outcomes for workers and misallocated capital in many countries (see chapter 6), while the retail market option has led to substantial administrative costs. The institutional approach is an intermediate option that retains market incentive while offering the opportunity for significant cost saving. Hence, it represents an option that policymakers should seriously consider when establishing their mandatory IA systems—providing choice is not constrained "too much."

Notes

1. We wish to thank Gary Ferrier of the University of Arkansas, who collaborated on an earlier related paper, and Deepthi Fernando and Marianne Leenaerts of the World Bank for their excellent research assistance. We also thank Peter Agardh of MPIR, Stefan Ackerby of the Swedish Industry Ministry, Hans Jacobson of the PPM, and Pia Nilsson of the Swedish Association of Mutual Funds for the useful information they provided, and Augusto Iglesias for his helpful comments and criticisms of an earlier draft.

2. All these numbers are two to three time higher using PPP conversion rates.

3. We estimated average brokerage costs on the basis of a subset of funds that reported these data for 1997. The unweighted and weighted averages were 26 and 12 basis points, respectively. This measure probably understates full trading costs for two reasons: (1) for some assets trading costs are netted out of gross returns rather than reported separately, and (2) the impact of large buy and sell orders upon price are ignored. Brokerage costs reported here refer to the cost of trading securities and do not include brokers' commissions for selling fund shares, commonly known as front and back loads, which we annualize and treat as marketing costs. We estimated annualized front-loaded sales commissions as 0.2 times the front-loaded commission on new sales. We used an annualization factor of 0.2 to convert a onetime fee into its annual present-value equivalent, assuming that the average investment is kept in the fund for seven years and the discount rate is 10 percent, corresponding to the high rate of return over this period. The annualized fee is not very sensitive to the discount rate. Earlier data indicated that a seven-year average holding period is reasonable (Wyatt Company 1990).

4. The total investor expense ratio calculated here is very similar to the total shareholder cost ratio calculated by Rea and Reid (1998), although they use slightly different datasets and definitions. The most important differences are that they deal only with equity funds (which are more expensive than bond funds), and they do not include brokerage (trading) fees in their measure of investor costs. Their simple average cost ratio is 1.99 percent, and their asset-weighted average is 1.44 percent, which are very similar to our numbers of 1.85 and 1.43 percent, respectively. According to their calculations, marketing fees are 40 percent of total costs.

5. We did not use the "total investor cost ratio" as our dependent variable because reliable data were not available for holding periods by fund or on brokerage costs for many funds in the data set.

6. However, personal pension plans in the United Kingdom and master trusts in Australia, where workers have greater choice, have higher costs.

See Bateman (1999); Bateman and Piggott (1999); Blake (2000); Daykin (1998); Queisser and Vittas (2000); chapter 8 of this volume; and data from Financial Services Board of South Africa.

7. If the first stage is centralized, there is one group and one competitive bidding process for the entire labor force; here problems of potential corruption and collusion may raise costs and lower returns. If there are multiple groups in the first stage, the groups may be predetermined (closed) or open. Most employer-sponsored plans are predetermined group plans; here the principle-agent problem may reduce net returns. Alternatively, groups may be open and competitive; here advertising between groups for members may raise costs. The final section of the text further discusses the pitfalls of a centralized approach.

8. Another 20 basis points are paid to Citibank, which serves as international custodian for all the funds. In Chile the AFPs cover the custodial fees.

9. In Kazakhstan the pension fund is responsible for R&C. It contracts out the asset management function to investment companies, which are allowed to charge 0.15 percent of contributions plus 5 percent of nominal investment income. The pension fund keeps the remainder. The part of the fee that is based on investment returns will be high in good years and in inflationary periods, but very low in poor, noninflationary years. So far there are 11 pension funds, some tied to particular employers, plus one state pension fund with the majority of affiliates. There are three asset managers, including one multinational that is trying to develop other business in Kazakhstan.

10. Corroborating evidence about the cost savings when marketing is eliminated comes from Australia: the "industry funds," which are nonprofit and have a captive membership stemming from a collectively bargained retirement plan, charge fees that are less than one-third the level of for-profit "master trusts," which compete in the retail market with heavy sales expenses (0.53 percent of assets for the industry funds versus 1.9 percent for the master trusts; Bateman 1999; Bateman and Piggott 1999). This fee differential is due in part to marketing expenses in the master trusts but not the industry funds. The low-cost occupational plans in the United Kingdom, Switzerland, and South Africa, referred to earlier, also benefit from low marketing expense in the absence of worker choice.

11. If price is set too low, entry may be too limited or service and quality of entrants too constrained. If it is set on the wrong base, as in Kazakhstan, it may restrict entry and create incentives for nonoptimal investment behavior. If it does not adequately distinguish among asset classes, "expensive" assets may be excluded from the market; this may have occurred in Sweden.

References

Note: The word *processed* describes informally reproduced works that may not be commonly available through libraries.

Bateman, Hazel. 1999. "The Role of Specialized Financial Institutions in Pension Fund Administrations." Processed.

Bateman, Hazel, and John Piggott. 1999. "Mandatory Private Retirement Provision: Design and Implementation Challenges." Processed.

Blake, David. 2000. "Does It Matter What Kind of Pension Scheme You Have?" *The Economic Journal* 110(461): F46–81.

CONSAR (Comisión Nacional del Sistema de Ahorros para el Retiro). 1997. Tabulations.

Cost-Effective Management, Inc. (CEM). 1997. "Cost-Effectiveness Pension Fund Report, prepared for CALPERS.

Dahlquist, Magnus, Stefan Engstrom, and Paul Soderlind. 1999. "Performance and Characteristics of Swedish Mutual Funds 1993–97." Stockholm School of Economics.

Daykin, Christopher. 1998. "GAD Survey of Expenses of Occupational Pension Schemes." London: Government Actuary's Department.

Elton, E. J., M. J Gruber, S. Das, and M. Hlavka. 1993. "Efficiency with Costly Information: A Reinterpretation of Evidence from Managed Portfolios." *The Review of Financial Studies* 6(1): 1–22.

Gruber, Martin J. 1996. "Another Puzzle: The Growth of Actively Managed Mutual Funds." *Journal of Finance* 51(3): 783–810.

Guerard, Yves, and Martha Kelly. 1997. *The Republic of Bolivia Pension Reform: Decisions in Designing the Structure of the System.* Montreal: Sobeco, Ernst and Young LLP.

Ippolito, Richard A. 1992. "Consumer Reaction to Measures of Poor Quality: Evidence from the Mutual Fund Industry." *Journal of Law and Economics* 35: 45–70.

James, Estelle, and Robert Palacios. 1995. "Costs of Administering Public and Private Pension Plans." *Finance and Development* 32(2): 12–16.

James, Estelle, Gary Ferrier, James Smalhout, and Dimitri Vittas. 1999. "Mutual Funds and Institutional Investments: What Is the Most Efficient Way to Set Up Individual Accounts in a Social Security System?" Processed.

Lipper, Michael. 1994. "The Third White Paper: Are Mutual Fund Fees Reasonable?" New York: Lipper Analytical Services.

Malhotra, D. K., and Robert W. McLeod. 1997. "An Empirical Analysis of Mutual Fund Expenses." *Journal of Financial Research* 20(2): 175–90.

Malkiel, Burton G. 1995. "Returns from Investing in Equity Mutual Funds 1971 to 1991." *Journal of Finance* 50(2): 549–72.

Maturana, Gustavo, and Eduardo Walker. 1999. "Rentabilidades, Comisiones y Desempeno en la Industria Chilena de Fondos Mutuos." *Estudios Publicos* 73: 293–334.

Mitchell, Olivia. 1998. "Administrative Costs in Public and Private Retirement Systems." In M. Feldstein, ed., *Privatizing Social Security*. University of Chicago Press.

MPIR Investment Research AB. 1998. "Utformning av ersattningsmodell inom ramen for preipensionssystemet—analys och forslag." ("Design of Compensation Model within the Framework of the Premium Pension System—Analysis and Proposal"). Stockholm. Processed.

Muralidhar, Arun S., and Robert Weary. 1998. "The Greater Fool Theory of Asset Management or Resolving the Active-Passive Debate." WPS98-020. World Bank, Washington, D.C.

Patel, Jayendu, Richard J. Zeckhauser, and Darryll Hendricks. 1994. "Investment Flows and Performance: Evidence from Mutual Funds, Cross-Border Investments, and New Issues." In R. Sato, R. Levich, and R. Ramachandran, eds., *Japan, Europe, and International Financial Markets: Analytical and Empirical Perspectives*. New York: Cambridge University Press.

Pozen, Robert. 1998. *The Mutual Fund Business*. Cambridge, Mass.: MIT Press.

Queisser, Monika, and Dimitri Vittas. 2000. "The Swiss Multi-Pillar Pension System: Triumph of Common Sense?" World Bank, Washington, D.C. Processed.

Rea, John D., and Brian K. Reid. 1998. "Trends in the Ownership Cost of Equity Mutual Funds." *Perspective* 4: 1–15. Washington, D.C.: Investment Company Institute.

Sirri, Erik R., and Peter Tufano. 1997. "Costly Search and Mutual Fund Flows." Processed.

Srinivas, P. S., and Juan Yermo. 1999. *Do Investment Regulations Compromise Pension Fund Performance? Evidence From Latin America*. World Bank, Washington, D.C.

Valdés-Prieto, Salvador. 1999a. "Fiscal and Political Aspects of Transitions from Public to Private Pension Systems." Processed.

———. 1999b. "Las comisiones de las AFPs: Caras o Baratos?" *Estudios Publicos* 73: 255–91.

Von Gersdorff, Hermann. 1997. *The Bolivian Pension Reform*. Financial Sector Development Department. World Bank, Washington D.C.

Wyatt Company. 1990. "Investment Company Persistency Study Conducted for the National Association of Securities Dealers." Processed.

8

Administrative Costs under a Decentralized Approach to Individual Accounts: Lessons from the United Kingdom

Mamta Murthi, J. Michael Orszag, and Peter R. Orszag

INDIVIDUAL ACCOUNTS ARE PERHAPS THE MOST controversial component of the current debate over public pension reform across the globe. The administrative costs associated with such accounts are particularly contentious, with proponents claiming that costs will be relatively low and opponents claiming the contrary. The debate also involves the gross rate of return likely to be earned on individual accounts and other potential benefits of such accounts. This chapter focuses exclusively on the cost issue and does not discuss benefits. In particular, our purpose is to document the lifetime costs on an individual account for a typical worker in the United Kingdom and not to conduct a full cost-benefit analysis.

The administrative costs associated with any system of individual accounts can be broken down into three components:

- The *accumulation ratio* captures fund management and administrative costs for a worker contributing funds to a single financial provider throughout his or her career. As this study finds and as previous studies also have documented, this factor has reduced the value of an account in the United Kingdom by an average of 25 percent over an individual's working years.
- The *alteration ratio* measures the additional costs of failing to contribute consistently to a single financial provider over an entire career. Most previous analyses have ignored the costs of transferring funds from

one financial provider to another or stopping contributions. The evidence suggests that such costs are significant. In the United Kingdom, this factor has reduced an account's value by, on average at least 15 percent over a career.

- The *annuitization ratio* reflects the costs of converting an account into a lifetime annuity upon retirement. In the United Kingdom, this factor has reduced the value of an account at retirement by approximately 10 percent, on average, for the typical worker.

Taking into account interaction effects, these estimates indicate that, on average, various fees and costs have historically consumed between 40 and 45 percent of the value of individual accounts in the United Kingdom.

High costs in the United Kingdom appear to be related to a number of distinguishing features:

- The U.K. system involves privately managed, decentralized accounts and annuities. The U.K. system of individual accounts is privately managed and highly decentralized. Such systems tend to be substantially more expensive than centralized systems (see, for example, James and others 1998; National Academy of Social Insurance 1998).
- The U.K. system of individual accounts is voluntary. In the United Kingdom, individuals can choose whether to participate in the system of individual accounts and annuities. Such choice may lead to increased complexity and, therefore, potentially higher administrative costs.
- Until very recently, the United Kingdom did not regulate fees on individual accounts, although it did introduce new disclosure requirements on fees and a new training and compliance regime in 1995. The lack of fee regulation produced a wide variety of fees, many of which consumers do not fully understand, and has also facilitated front-loaded costs that impose additional costs on individuals' switching accounts. Regulating the fee structure may address some of these concerns, albeit at the potential cost of reduced supply (if the fee regulations are too restrictive, providers may be unwilling to offer accounts to some customers).
- Other institutional differences may affect costs. Any comparison between experiences in two countries inevitably ignores at least some institutional differences, so we must be careful in extrapolating from the U.K. experience to other countries. In particular, the sales process in the United Kingdom is highly regulated, with a principle of "polarization" so that independent advisers and salespeople must either sell the product of one company or sell products of all providers. While polarization may lead to more clarity for consumers, it also may restrict competition, thereby raising costs.[1]

It is thus not straightforward to extrapolate from the voluntary, privately managed individual accounts in the United Kingdom to a possible system of individual accounts elsewhere, especially if that system is mandatory and centralized. Nonetheless, the U.K. figures vividly warn that if individual accounts were adopted elsewhere, careful attention must be paid to the design of those accounts to ensure that administrative and other costs are not unduly high. Indeed, because of the historically high costs of pensions, the Labour government in the United Kingdom has recently implemented a pension reform in which a new form of individual account, the stakeholder pension, will be introduced in April 2001, in which charges will be restricted to 1 percent of funds under management per year.

This chapter examines in detail the costs associated with individual accounts in the United Kingdom. It comprises five sections: (i) background on the U.K. pension system, which outlines the structure of U.K. pension program and provides the context for the rest of the chapter; (ii) a taxonomy for evaluating fees, which presents a framework for evaluating charges both during a working career and during retirement; (iii) cost ratios in the U.K. individual account system, which result from the application of the framework to data from the United Kingdom and estimate how much of an individual account's value various costs consume; (iv) sources of provider costs; and, (v) summary and conclusions.[2]

Background on the U.K. Pension System

The pension system in the United Kingdom is complicated.[3] It consists of two tiers: a flat-rate basic state pension, and an earnings-related pension. The government provides the first tier, which is not related to earnings. The second tier, which can be managed by an individual, his or her employer, or the government, depends on an individual's earnings history. For a majority of workers in Britain, the government does *not* manage this second tier. Instead, for most workers, the second tier consists of either employer-based or individual-based private pensions. In this sense, the U.K. pension system is at least partially privatized, one of the few such examples in the industrialized world and the only example in the G-7 countries.

Basic State Pension

The first tier of the U.K. pension program is called the basic state retirement pension (BSP). The BSP is a pay-as-you-go system. Under the BSP, a portion of the National Insurance Contribution (NIC) payroll tax finances a flat-rate benefit for retirees. In other words, once a worker qualifies by working for a sufficient number of years, this basic benefit does not vary with the worker's earnings level.[4] The full benefit payments amount to about £65 per week per person. Currently, about 10.6 million pensioners (or virtually the entire population of retirees) receive a basic state pension. Such pensions provide about one-third of total income for retirees, a figure that is set to decrease over time because the BSP is indexed to prices instead of wages (the other components of the pension system are effectively indexed to wages).

The State Earnings-Related Pension Scheme

The second tier of the U.K. system offers three different alternatives to workers. Roughly one-quarter of British workers currently choose the most basic option, the State Earnings-Related Pension Scheme (SERPS). When it was first introduced in 1978, SERPS was relatively generous. Over time, however, reforms have made the program less attractive, especially to middle- and upper-income workers.[5] The maximum SERPS benefit is currently about £120 per week, and the average benefit is under £20 per week. The majority of Britons who remain enrolled in SERPS today earn less than £10,000 annually.

Workers who opt out of SERPS do not accrue SERPS benefits and, therefore, pay lower payroll taxes. Since their subsequent pensions are in effect not financed out of NIC taxes, the government provides a payroll tax rebate to reflect reduced future SERPS payments. They can then use the tax rebate to finance an employer-provided pension or an individual account. The two opt-out options are the following:

- *Individual Accounts.* Since 1988 one way to achieve contracted-out status has been through a personal pension. Since these "personal pensions," as they are called in the United Kingdom, are similar to the individual accounts being debated elsewhere in the world, in this chapter we refer to personal pensions as individual accounts. About 25 percent of workers in the United Kingdom are currently enrolled in individual accounts.
- *Employer-Based Pensions.* About half of all workers participate in an employer-sponsored pension plan (often referred to as an "occupational pension") and are thereby contracted out of SERPS. Occupational pensions can be either defined-benefit (DB) or defined-contributions (DC) plans.

To summarize, roughly one-quarter of workers belong to SERPS, one-quarter opt out of SERPS and into personal pensions, and one-half opt out of SERPS and into employer-based pensions.

Individual Accounts in the United Kingdom

The most relevant highlights of the system of individual accounts in the United Kingdom are the following:

- The government's payroll tax rebate finances contributions into individual accounts. Roughly half of account holders also contribute an additional amount on top of the government rebate. Indeed, the individual accounts examined in this chapter involve contributions of between £1,000 and £2,500 a year, and most tax rebates are under £1,000. To the extent that at least some of the costs associated with individual accounts are fixed, costs would consume an even larger percentage of smaller accounts than our estimates suggest.
- A variety of firms offer individual accounts in the United Kingdom, but insurance firms dominate the market.[6] Although the personal pension market is open to all providers, only insurers can offer certain types of related products.[7]
- The U.K. pensions market has a large number of providers. Competition among them is keen, as underscored by the withdrawal of several high-profile firms from the market. For example, Fidelity withdrew from the personal pension market in 1993 and transferred its plans to another provider. Citibank also pulled out of the market at about the same time. Despite these prominent withdrawals, the overall number of providers has not changed much until recently, when the imminent introduction of fee caps forced a number of more expensive providers to leave the market.
- Competition in the U.K. pensions market has sometimes been taken to the extreme, as evidenced by the "mis-selling" controversy arising from misleading advice that some financial firms provided about personal pensions. A desire to gain additional customers, at least in part, motivated this advice.
- The pressures induced by strong competition have not resulted in low costs. A number of features of the U.K. system make it expensive for providers; these features include the need to provide advice as well as complications involving tax compliance checks.

Annuity Markets in the United Kingdom

The SERPS program in the United Kingdom automatically provides an inflation-adjusted annuity to beneficiaries. Holders of individual accounts, however, must purchase an annuity if they want to avoid outliving their savings. Furthermore, the annuity must be defined in real (inflation-indexed) terms if they want to ensure that inflation does not erode those savings.

The regulations governing when an annuity must be purchased in the United Kingdom are complicated and depend on whether tax rebates alone or tax rebates and additional contributions funded the individual account:

- The portion of an individual account funded by tax rebates must be fully annuitized. The annuity must be purchased at some point between age 60 and age 75. The annuity payments must be the same for men and women for any given age of annuitization: providers *cannot* provide lower annual payments to women to reflect their longer life expectancies.
- The portion of an individual account funded by additional contributions does not have to be entirely annuitized. In particular, up to 25 percent of the accumulated balance from this component of the individual account can be withdrawn tax-free in a lump sum. If the account holder retires before the age of 75,[8] the rest of the account can be distributed in one of three ways: (i) an annuity purchased from a life insurance company, (ii) an annuity purchased from the provider of the individual account, or (iii) an income drawdown facility, under which the retiree withdraws specific amounts of money while most of the balance continues to earn market returns. At age 75, regardless of which option is initially chosen, the balance of the account must be converted into an annuity.[9]

Workers do not have to begin receiving the two components of the individual account—the part funded by tax rebates and the other part funded by additional contributions—at the same time. If workers die before annuitizing their account, the balance of the account enters their estate.

A Taxonomy for Evaluating Fees

This section presents a taxonomy for analyzing costs to the individual account holder within a system of individual accounts. We define and decompose the so-called charge ratio. We then use the decomposition to study costs in the U.K. system.

The Charge Ratio

We define the charge ratio as a measure of how much of an individual account's value is taken up by administrative charges and other costs. In particular,

$$\text{Charge ratio} = 1 - \frac{IA_c}{IA_{nc}}$$

where IA_c is the value of the individual account with charges and other costs, and IA_{nc} is the value of individual accounts without charges and other costs.

Since the value of the account with charges cannot be greater than the account without charges, the charge ratio varies between zero and one, with higher costs corresponding to higher values of the charge ratio. At one extreme—no fees of any form—the charge ratio takes the value zero. At the other extreme, where charges are so high that they consume the entire value of the pension, the charge ratio is equal to one. In practice, we would expect to observe values between the two extremes.

The costs associated with providing individual accounts, which are reflected in the charge ratio, arise from several sources:

- *Customer Acquisition.* Acquiring customers through sales, advertisement, and payment of commission to financial advisers can be very expensive. These are the most significant costs faced by providers.
- *Fund Management Charges.* Pension providers pay fund managers to oversee their investments. Usually, fund management charges do not represent a substantial fraction of total personal pension costs, especially in the United Kingdom, where fund managers typically earn lower salaries than their counterparts in the United States.
- *Regulatory and Compliance Costs.* Ensuring that accounts are sold properly can be expensive for both the private sector and regulators. Penalty fees for failing to observe regulatory requirements can also be significant. For example, it is estimated that about US$18 billion in compensation will need to be paid by U.K. insurers and independent advisers to cover mis-sold individual accounts.
- *Business Maintenance Costs.* Record-keeping and administration of accounts require resources. Information technology systems require expensive infrastructure and training investments.
- *Selection Effects.* In a voluntary account system, individuals who choose to have individual accounts will likely have different characteristics from the rest of the population. As has been noted elsewhere, both active and passive "adverse selection" play an important role in the annuity market: those purchasing annuities tend to have longer life expectancies than the population as a whole. Such adverse selection may result in significantly lower annuity rates, even if the insurance companies are not earning profits, given the characteristics of those choosing to annuitize. A lower annuity rate will show up in the charge ratio through the annuity ratio (see description below).

It is also important to note that we focus on the financial costs to consumers, not the resource costs to society. In many situations the two concepts may not be identical. For example, selection effects are of a somewhat different nature than many of the other costs listed above. Most of the accumulation costs, for example, likely represent direct resource costs to society, whereas selection effects represent indirect costs (by discouraging individuals from participating in the insurance market). We nevertheless include selection costs, as our focus is on financial costs to the consumer.

Decomposing the Charge Ratio

The charge ratio can be broken down into three components, corresponding to (i) the losses from administrative and other costs during a working life, assuming that contributions are made consistently to a single financial provider (accumulation ratio), (ii) losses from failure to contribute consistently to a single provider during one's working life (alteration ratio), and (iii) losses upon retirement from converting the account into an annuity (annuitization ratio).

- The *accumulation ratio* (ACR) captures fund management and administrative costs while the worker is contributing funds to an individual account throughout her career. It assumes that the contributions are made on a consistent basis to a single financial provider.
- The *alteration ratio* (ALR) measures the costs from altering contributions, that is, not contributing consistently to a single provider, during a working career. It captures the additional costs of switching an accumulated account balance to an alternative provider, of leaving the accumulated account balance with the original provider but diverting new contributions to an alternative provider, or of leaving the accumulated account balance with the original provider but stopping contributions altogether (for example, because of a withdrawal from the labor force or a switch to an occupational pension). It does not include the ongoing costs of holding an account with a single provider (which the accumulation ratio captures). Most previous analyses have ignored the costs of altering contributions and, thus, implicitly assumed an alteration ratio of 1.0.
- The *annuitization ratio* (ANR) reflects the losses from annuitizing an account upon retirement. It measures the ratio of private annuity yields to theoretical yields from population mortality tables and captures both adverse selection and administrative cost loadings on private annuities.

The charge ratio can be expressed as a function of these three ratios and the percentage of the account that is withdrawn as a lump sum (LS) upon retirement:

$$\text{Charge ratio} = 1 - \frac{\text{IA}_c}{\text{IA}_{nc}} = 1 - \text{ACR} \cdot \text{ALR} \cdot \left((1 - \text{LS})\text{ANR} + \text{LS} \right)$$

where ACR is the accumulation ratio, ALR is the alteration ratio, ANR is the annuitization ratio, and LS is the fraction of the accumulated account taken as a lump sum upon retirement. With this framework, we can see that almost half of an individual account's value could be lost through charges. As explained in more detail below, reasonable figures for the United Kingdom are an accumulation ratio of 0.75, an alteration ratio of 0.85, and an annuity ratio of 0.90. Assuming no lump-sum withdrawal, the charge ratio is:

$$\text{Charge ratio} = 1 - 0.75 \cdot 0.85 \cdot 0.90 = 0.43.$$

The total charge ratio is thus 0.43, so that over a worker's career and retirement, charges and other costs dissipate 43 percent of an individual account's value.

Cost Ratios in the U.K. Individual Account System

This section provides evidence on each of the three cost ratios outlined in the taxonomy presented in the previous section. For each of the three component ratios, we use actual data from 1988 (when individual accounts were introduced) to 1998, whenever available. The multiple ways in which costs are imposed on consumers complicated our task. As one commentator noted, "Pension plans have a bewildering array of charges, including bid/offer spreads, reduced allocations of premiums, capital units and levies, annual fund charges, policy fees and penalties on transfers, early retirement, and other events" (Chapman 1998). Our approach is designed to provide a comprehensive metric capturing all these various methods of passing along costs to the holders of individual accounts.

Accumulation Ratio

The accumulation ratio reflects what most commentators mean by "administrative costs." It measures the ratio of an individual account's value immediately prior to retirement to its value if no charges had been incurred throughout the worker's career. It assumes that the worker does not change providers.

The accumulation ratio measures the losses in the value of an individual account from charges such as annual management fees (as a percentage of the account's balance) and fixed charges (pounds per year). Perhaps the most familiar of these types of fees is the first: an annual fee equal to some percent of the account's balance, often expressed in terms of "basis points." A fee of 100 basis points is equivalent to 1 percent of the account's balance. Given assumptions about the account's balance and the time horizon, other types of fees can be expressed in terms of an annual management fee and vice versa (for further discussion of the relationship among various types of fees, see, for example, Diamond 1998).

Although expressing the fees in terms of annual basis points may be most familiar to investors, that form is not necessarily the most insightful. In particular, the accumulated effects of charges over many years may not be immediately obvious. We therefore express fees in terms of the accumulation ratio, which provides a useful summary of their effects over an entire career. An alternative, but fundamentally equivalent, approach is to compute an "annual charge equivalent" that captures all costs and expresses them on an annualized basis (see Rea and Reid 1998).

To compute the impact of fees on the accumulation ratio, it is necessary to make specific assumptions about the account's value over time (for example, what rate of return it earns, how quickly the contribution level increases, etc.). For this purpose, we employ the Minimum Funding Requirement assumptions published by the Faculty and Institute of Actuaries in the United Kingdom (Guidance Note 27). Under this set of assumptions, which are used to establish the minimum funding requirements for pensions, the inflation rate is assumed to be 4 percent per year; the nominal rate of return on equities, 9 percent per year; and nominal wage growth, 6 percent per year. Table 8.1 shows the effect on the accumulation ratio from various fees, applying the Minimum Funding Requirement (MFR) assumptions on wage growth and returns and assuming someone works 40 years, earns £14,000 at the start of his or her career, and contributes 10 percent of earnings to the pension. As seen in the table, annual management fees of 100 basis points reduce the value of an individual account by slightly more than 20 percent over a typical working life.

Drawing on data from a financial services publication in the United Kingdom, *Money Management*; Investment Intelligence (a data source for independent financial advisors); and other sources, we have constructed a detailed database of the fees charged by personal pensions in the United Kingdom. In particular, U.K. providers of individual accounts are required to publish figures showing the impact of administrative charges.[10] Specifically, providers apply a mandated set of assumptions and publish the projected account values after all their charges have been imposed. Using the same set of assumptions, the no-charge value of the account can be computed, and the charges, therefore, can be inferred by comparing the no-charge and postcharge values.

Using these data, we have computed the accumulation ratios for each year over the past decade.[11] In particular, comparing the no-charge value for an account held for 40 years with a single provider to the value of that same account after charges had been subtracted provides the accumulation cost for that provider, which is then expressed relative to the final account

Table 8.1. Simulated Impact of Fees on Accumulation Ratio over 40 Years

Annual management fees (basis points, as percentage of account balance)	Fixed annual charges (pounds per month)	Accumulation ratio
0	0	1.00
20	0	0.95
50	0	0.89
100	0	0.79
150	0	0.71
0	£2	0.99
20	£2	0.94
50	£2	0.88
100	£2	0.78
150	£2	0.70

Note: Simulations assume a 40-year contribution history for an individual whose starting annual wage is £14,000, and who contributes 10 percent of earnings to a personal pension. Wages are assumed to grow at 6 percent per year; inflation is 4 percent per year; and investment returns are 9 percent per year (Minimum Funding Requirement assumptions). The precise timing of fees within a year, as well as compounding effects over a year, mean that the management fee numbers are slightly different from annualized basis point reduction in yields.
Source: Authors' calculations.

balance. Averaging across providers produces the figures in table 8.2. The (unweighted) average of the 40-year accumulation ratio is 0.72 over the past decade.[12]

We have also examined our results for sensitivity to the underlying assumptions about the wage profile, wage growth, investment returns, and inflation. While using different assumptions changes the precise estimate, it does not change the broad orders of magnitude. Our conclusion is that a figure of 0.75 for the accumulation ratio, slightly above the average level over the past decade and consistent with the figure for 1998, is a conservative estimate from the U.K. experience.

Alteration Ratio

The accumulation ratio assumes that a worker holds an individual account with the same provider over her or his entire career. In reality, however, many individuals stop making contributions to a single financial provider at some point in their career. Such funding "alterations" can arise in the following situations:

- *Transferred account.* Workers switch both their accumulated balances and their new contributions to another financial provider.

Table 8.2. Management Fees and Accumulation Ratio, Unweighted Average over Providers, 1989–1998

Year	Average annual management fees (basis points)	Accumulation ratio (assuming 40-year career)
1989	149.2	0.71
1990	151.4	0.71
1991	152.6	0.71
1992	155.6	0.70
1993	148.7	0.71
1994	147.1	0.72
1995	137.8	0.73
1996	131.1	0.74
1997	127.9	0.75
1998	124.0	0.75
Average, 1989–98	*142.5*	*0.72*

Source: Money Management and authors' calculations. Additional assumptions and caveats as in table 8.1.

- *Paid-up account, new contributions to different provider.* Workers maintain their accumulated balances with the original provider (leaving that account "paid-up") but divert new contributions to a new financial provider. That is, *new* contributions are paid into the account held with a new provider, but the existing account remains with the original firm.
- *Paid-up account, no new contributions.* Workers maintain their accumulated balances with the original provider (again, the account is paid-up), but stop contributions altogether, perhaps because they leave the labor force, switch jobs and join an occupation pension, or their earnings fall below the lower earnings limit for contributions into the second tier of the U.K. system.

These events impose additional costs on consumers, and the accumulation ratio, therefore, does not capture all the costs associated with building up an individual account over a career. To incorporate the effects of changing contribution patterns during a working career, we define the concept of the alteration ratio, which measures the loss to an individual account's value purely from such changes. The product of the accumulation ratio and the alteration ratio provides a measure of how much of an individual account's value all charges absorb—including annual management fees, front loads, fixed annual fees, and transfer charges—before retirement and annuitization.[13] The annuitization ratio then measures additional costs to the individual from annuitizing the account. Analyses that rely solely on the accumulation ratio implicitly assume that alteration costs are zero.

Data on the duration of accounts held with the same financial provider illustrate the importance of the alteration ratio. As table 8.3 indicates, of the regular-premium individual accounts (those requiring ongoing contributions) sold by company representatives and held with financial companies in 1993, 14.5 percent had lapsed within one year, 25.4 percent had lapsed within two years, 33.8 percent has lapsed within three years, and 39.4 percent had lapsed within four years. Thus, roughly 40 percent of the individual accounts held in 1993 had lapsed within four years.[14]

Although it is difficult to extrapolate from the experience of a subset of the population over a very short time horizon, the dramatic number of lapses over a relatively short horizon highlights their potential importance. We have used the 1993-97 data to project the lapse rate over longer time span. The results are shown in figure 8.1, which plots the percentage of accounts remaining active with the original provider ("persistency") as a function of the number of years since the account was opened.[15] The projection suggests that roughly half of the accounts will have lapsed within five years, and almost all of the accounts (more than 99 percent) will lapse at some point over a 40-year career. In other words, individuals may be expected to change their provider (or stop contributing) at least once in their working life. This is not an unreasonable prediction given the existing evidence on lapse rates. Moreover, it is not inconsistent with other studies of alteration behavior. For example, Chapman (1998) estimates that "only about one in six keep their plans up to maturity." His data are for a 25-year horizon. Over 25 years, our projection would suggest that 5 percent—rather than 17 percent—of accounts would remain with their original provider.

Analysis of company data indicates that the majority of lapses occur from paid-up accounts, rather than from transferred accounts, and that the percentage has been increasing over time. Table 8.4 shows the share of lapses in each year due to paid-up accounts relative to the total (paid-up plus

Table 8.3. Percent of Lapsed Individual Accounts

Beginning year	Ending year			
	1994	1995	1996	1997
1993	14.5	25.4	33.8	39.4
1994	n.a.	14.9	25.3	33.2
1995	n.a.	n.a.	13.4	13.4
1996	n.a.	n.a.	n.a.	12.6

n.a. Not applicable.
Note: Data are for regular-premium pensions sold by company representatives.
Source: 4th Personal Investment Authority's Persistency Survey.

Figure 8.1. Persistency of Regular Premium Personal Pensions

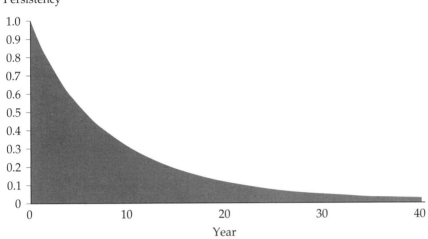

Source: Authors' calculations.

transferred). The proportion of accounts going paid-up has increased from two-thirds to four-fifths. Industry interviews also confirm this picture. While the proportion of paid-up accounts has been rising, we cannot

Table 8.4. Lapses by Cause of Lapse

Year	Percentage of new lapses due to paid-up accounts (relative to paid-up plus transferred)
1988	65.6
1989	61.8
1990	58.1
1991	62.2
1992	66.8
1993	70.0
1994	74.5
1995	76.7
1996	77.6
1997	79.3

Note: Paid-up numbers are constructed using line 26, column 4, of Form 46 from the Thesys DTI returns. Transfers are estimated as a sum of lines 24, 25, column 4, from the same form. In constructing the paid-up ratios, we summed over U.K. linked and U.K. nonlinked business and weighted by the average business in force for each class (an average of lines 11 and 39, column 4, from Form 46). We thank Chris O'Brien of Royal and Sun Alliance Life and Pensions for assistance with these calculations.
Source: Thesys database and authors' calculations.

confirm whether accounts go paid-up because new contributions are diverted to an alternative provider or whether contributions to individual accounts cease.[16]

The overall alteration ratio is thus complicated, both because a lapse can occur for different reasons (transferred to another provider, paid-up with new contributions to another provider, and paid-up with no new contributions) and because the cost associated with events within these broad categories depends significantly on the timing of a worker's lapse and on the structure of fees. In order to obtain insight into the alteration ratio, our approach is to examine each source of alteration costs in turn, initially assuming that all lapses obtain from that source. In the discussion below, we focus on one case only: in which lapses occur because workers transfer new contributions to alternative providers.[17] Studying costs in a situation where workers make new contributions to an alternative provider is useful because it typically yields the lowest cost to the consumer. It therefore provides a basis for arriving at a conservative estimate of the alteration ratio.

When an individual has a paid-up account and directs new contributions to an alternative provider, the original account normally still incurs charges. As Sumpter (1999) notes, "paid-up funds generally do not escape charges. The fund is still subject to management fees and, in some cases, administration charges, despite the fact that the client has stopped paying premiums. Some providers maintain the same level of charges, some reduce them, while others increase them."

In a case in which the individual diverts new contributions to alternative providers, the alteration ratio will be less than 1.0 if, for example, (i) the old or new provider imposes a fixed annual fee on the respective accounts, or (ii) the old or new provider front loads annual management or other fees on accounts. If however the only type of fees in both accounts is a constant annual management fee, the alteration ratio will be 1.0 regardless of how many times a worker switches between such accounts.

In order to estimate the alteration ratio when accounts go paid-up and new contributions are made to another financial provider, we assume that a worker opens an account with firm A and contributes to that account for some period. Then the worker leaves the accumulated balance with firm A (the account is paid-up) and makes all new contributions to firm B. If any of the above factors are present, the fees on the two accounts will be higher than the fees for a single account held with firm A throughout the worker's career. To compute the alteration ratio for this worker, we therefore compare the value upon retirement of the two accounts to the value of a single account had it been held with firm A for the worker's entire career. The difference, if any, is reflected in the alteration ratio.

More specifically, we construct a "typical" financial firm. For each year that an account is held with that typical financial firm, the firm imposes charges equal to the average (unweighted) charge across all providers for an account of that duration.[18] A worker going paid-up with his or her existing financial firm retains the funds in a regular-premium policy, and the charges associated with that regular-premium policy remain the same as they would with ongoing contributions. New contributions are paid to the typical financial firm, in another regular-premium policy. The final value of the two regular-premium policies are then compared to the value that a single regular-premium policy would have obtained and the additional charges are inferred.[19]

Using this methodology, we compute the alteration ratio for different ages at which an account is paid-up and contributions switched to a new provider. These are reported in table 8.5. As with the accumulation ratio, we assume a 40-year horizon.

The next step is to combine the various alteration costs with our projections for switching behavior to compute an average alteration ratio. In particular, we first simulate a large number of switching paths on the basis of our persistency model (based on the 1993–97 persistency data extrapolated over a longer period of time), assuming that all lapses occur because individuals divert contributions to alternative providers. For each such path, we then compute the alteration ratio as in table 8.5. Finally, we weight each alteration ratio by the probability of its associated switching path. The result is an overall average alteration ratio of 0.83.

Our discussion so far suggests that if lapses occur solely because of accounts being made paid-up, with new contributions deposited in a new account, the average alteration ratio is 0.83. Although we do not discuss the other two cases in this chapter, our findings suggest that (i) if lapses occur

Table 8.5. Illustrative 40-Year Paid-Up with New Contribution Ratio for Various Scenarios

Paid-Up Ages (age at making first account paid-up, age at second account paid-up, age at third account paid-up, etc.)	Paid-up with new contribution ratio
30, 39, 40	0.86
30, 31	0.91
30, 35, 40	0.85
30, 35, 40, 43	0.81
40, 41, 47	0.88
47, 48	0.93
40, 45, 50, 60	0.85

Note: These illustrations apply Minimum Funding Requirement assumptions (see table 1).
Source: Authors' calculations.

solely because of transfers, the average alteration ratio is 0.70, and (ii) if lapses occur solely because of accounts being made paid-up, with no new contributions, the average alteration ratio is generally even lower, depending
on when the contributions stop. In fact, for identical switching scenarios,
we find that transferring the accumulated balance to a new provider is generally more costly than going paid-up and diverting new contributions to
an alternative provider. This is consistent with the fact that more accounts
go paid-up than transfer. (The intuition for higher transfer costs is as follows. Where account balances are transferred to an alternative provider, we
assume the accumulated balance is transferred into a single-premium policy with the typical financial firm, and new contributions are paid into a
regular-premium policy with the same firm. This will result in higher costs
as, in general, a new single-premium policy will have somewhat higher
charges than an older regular-premium policy. For further discussion, see
Murthi, Orszag, and Orszag 1999a.)

Based on these findings, what would be a reasonable estimate of the alteration ratio? Given inherent uncertainties in the data and other factors (see
below), we prefer to err on the side of being conservative. We therefore adopt
a figure of 0.85 for the alteration ratio, which seems modest given U.K. experience. The alteration ratio may be significantly lower (that is, alteration costs
may be significantly higher) for many workers than the figure we adopt.

Our estimates quite clearly depend on the projected persistency data and
on other assumptions. Our data are for persistency of accounts sold through
the insurance companies. Persistency is somewhat higher for pensions
sold through different channels (for example, independent financial advisors rather than the insurance companies themselves). Greater persistency would raise the alteration ratio. Furthermore, although transfers lead to
higher costs than going paid-up and diverting new contributions to alternative providers, these costs have been falling over time. We are also aware
that most lapses occur because of accounts going paid-up, and that if contributions continue after the original account is paid-up, the average alteration ratio is 0.83. All this would seem to suggest that 0.85 is a reasonably
conservative estimate of the alteration ratio in the United Kingdom.

Combining our estimates of the accumulation ratio and the alteration
ratio suggests a total cost during a typical working life of 36 percent of an
account's no-charge value $(1 - 0.75 \cdot 0.85 = 1 - 0.64 = 0.36)$. Our estimates
are consistent with evidence from other studies. For example, Chapman
(1998) concludes that the annual charge equivalent to accumulation and
alteration costs would amount to 250 basis points per year, or about 42 percent over a typical 40-year career. Shuttleworth (1997) argues that "about
30 percent to 50 percent of the monies accumulated in a personal pension
are absorbed by charges if it is discontinued before middle age."
Shuttleworth's figure, which is based on accounts into which contributions

are no longer made, combines accumulation and alteration costs. Our comparable figure is less than the midpoint of his range.

Before leaving this section, it is worth pointing out that we are focusing solely on the cost to consumers; altering funding patterns imposes additional costs on consumers but may also have benefits, such as if individuals move toward high-yielding funds. An examination of any such benefits is, however, beyond the scope of this chapter.

Annuitization Ratio

A final source of charges and other costs is the purchase of an annuity upon retirement. Retirees who are concerned about outliving their savings have an incentive to purchase an annuity, which provides some sort of payment for every year that the annuitant (or the annuitant's dependent) is alive, in exchange for a lump-sum payment up front.

As noted above, the costs associated with annuities (the annuitization ratio) are distinct from those associated with accumulating the balance to be annuitized (the product of the accumulation and transfer ratios). For those who have accumulated retirement funds in an individual account, the purchase of an annuity provides insurance against depleting the account before death. Such insurance is costly, however, for two reasons:

- *Adverse Selection.* Those purchasing annuities are likely to have longer life expectancies than the general population—both because of socioeconomic reasons and because of individual behavior—that the annuity price will reflect in a competitive market. This adverse selection effect means that if someone with the typical life expectancy wishes to purchase an annuity, he or she must pay a premium relative to the actuarial fair price. That premium reduces the value of her annuity, relative to a no-charge and actuarially fair level.[20] This cost to the typical individual, however, does not measure the profit to the provider, the utility loss to the consumer, or the resource cost to society from the selection effect in the annuity market.[21] Rather, it merely represents a financial loss for the typical person, if he or she decided to purchase an annuity, relative to an actuarially fair annuity.
- *Cost Loadings.* In addition, annuity provision involves administrative costs, mortality risks, and other burdens for providers. The annuity value may therefore also be lower than its no-charge, actuarially fair level because of these costs. On the other hand, annuities also provide a form of insurance to life insurance companies, since they are negatively correlated with life insurance payouts. On net, we believe that the pure cost loading on annuities is relatively small in the United Kingdom. Poterba and Warshawsky (1999) reach similar conclusions for the annuities market in the United States.

The United Kingdom's long experience with compulsory annuitization of pension funds, along with the existence of inflation-indexed annuities that are less common or nonexistent in many other countries, provides a unique setting to investigate the operations of private annuities markets and policy lessons. The U.K. annuities market has been the subject of recent work by Brown, Mitchell, and Poterba (1999), Finkelstein and Poterba (1999), and the authors of this chapter (Murthi, Orszag, and Orszag 1999b). For example, as described in our paper on annuities, we have compiled data from Investment Intelligence into a database of annuity prices, with the data extending back in some cases to 1976. Using these data, we have computed annuity ratios for a wide variety of annuity types and in various years. The annuity ratio computations are very sensitive to mortality and interest rate assumptions. Here, we focus primarily on the most recent annuitant life figures and apply the Bank of England's term structure as well as corporate bond term structures for interest rate projections. This approach has the substantial advantage of relying on very recently published mortality tables; the insurers presumably do not have much additional information.

Our main findings are the following:

- The annuity ratios lie in the range of 0.85–0.90. Selection effects, that is, the higher than average longevity of the annuitant population, account for much of this cost. Our estimates suggest selection effects account for between one-half and two-thirds of the annuitization cost for the typical worker.[22] The remaining cost is due to other factors, including the administrative costs of life insurance companies. These findings are also consistent with those of Finkelstein and Poterba (1999).

- The costs of annuitization vary significantly by product type, particularly between nominal and real annuities. The average retiree can pay an additional 8–10 pence in the £ for purchasing inflation protection in addition to longevity insurance.[23] It is difficult to relate these additional costs to the additional risks borne by insurers, since insurers in the United Kingdom may cover their inflation risk by investing in inflation-indexed government bonds. The higher costs may have to do with selection effects. Since the real payout does not fall over time with inflation-indexed annuities, such annuities would tend to attract those with higher expectations of longevity. This possibility is not something we were able to investigate fully, as we did not have annuitant tables by product.

- There is no trend in value for money of annuities, at least not in the last five years.

- There is some evidence of price stickiness in the annuities market, with some providers adjusting their rates sluggishly in response to changes in interest rates.

We proceed by assuming that a reasonable estimate of the annuitization ratio for the United Kingdom is 0.90.

Sources of Provider Costs

Our focus thus far has been on the charges incurred by the typical worker. The examination of the sources of costs from the perspective of providers offers further insight into administrative costs. This perspective is the subject of ongoing research; this section provides some of our preliminary findings.

Provider costs for pensions can be divided into three main components:

- *Acquisition Costs.* These include the costs of new business, which include commission to advisers, compensation to salesforces, and any advertising costs.
- *Administration Costs.* These costs involve administering ongoing business, including information technology infrastructure costs and back- and front-office management.
- *Asset Management Costs.* These are the costs of managing assets.

Of these three sources of costs, asset management costs are the smallest component. Wholesale asset management costs are as low as 10 basis points, or 0.1 percent of the funds under management. Industry interviews confirmed that asset management costs for providers were typically below 15 percent of total costs. Passively managed funds are slightly less expensive than actively managed funds, but the overall share of asset management costs in total costs for large institutional investors is small enough that any cost differential between passive and active management does not significantly affect the costs of the retail product.[24]

To assess the other costs in more detail, we examine the statutory regulatory returns (the DTI, or insurance regulatory, returns), which contain information on insurance company expenses, called "Expenses Payable" (Form 40, line 22). This item covers all expenses incurred "in the administration of a company and its business," including commissions paid on the sale of its products and costs associated with the management of policies. Policy management includes policy administration and management of the firm's portfolio of assets. Reported expenses are divided into five categories: commissions related to the acquisition of business, other commissions, management expenses related to the acquisition of business, management expenses related to the maintenance of business, and other management expenses. The data are thus most useful for disaggregating costs into *acquisition costs* (commissions and other acquisition-related expenses) and *administrative costs* for ongoing business. As it turns out, acquisition costs are the most important component of provider costs.

Since larger companies are likely to have higher absolute expenses, we normalize expenses by examining expenses relative to assets under management (called an expense ratio). In table 8.6 we examine expense ratios for three years: 1997, 1994, and 1989. The data cannot be disaggregated by line of business (life, pensions, health, etc.), so the ratios represent costs of all types of business lumped together. However, regression analysis (not reported here) suggests that companies that do more pensions business have higher expense ratios, so it is possible that our estimates are a lower bound on the cost of personal pensions alone. We restrict the sample to companies with positive premium incomes from pensions business. This gives us 158 companies in 1997, 161 in 1994, and 178 in 1989.

Table 8.6. Life-Office Expenses (Selected Years)

All companies	1997	1994	1989
Average expense ratio (basis points)	139	194	238
Expense ratio - first quartile (basis points)	96	123	174
Expense ratio - third quartile (basis points)	166	227	270
Average share of business acquisition in total costs (percent)	65	69	73
Average share of commissions in total costs (percent)	31	32	33
Sample size	158	161	178
Companies with commission-free sale			
Average expense ratio (basis points)	47	72	100
Expense ratio - first quartile (basis points)	8	40	45
Expense ratio - third quartile (basis points)	59	82	148
Average share of business acquisition in total costs (percent)	50	52	56
Average share of commissions in total costs (percent)	0	0	0
Sample size	30	22	22

Note: 1. All averages are weighted. 2. Expense ratio is defined as Total Expenses (Form 40, line 22) over Admissible Assets (Form 9, line 21). Total Expenses covers only "ordinary branch" business, as "industrial branch" business is distinct (door-to-door sales, small premiums) and significantly more expensive. 3. The share of business acquisition costs is the sum of Commissions (Form 41, line 41), Other Commissions (Form 41, line 42), and Management Expenses related to Acquisition (Form 41, line 43), over Total Expenses (Form 41, line 49). The share of commissions is given by Commissions (Form 41, line 41), and Other Commissions (Form 41, line 42), over Total Expenses (Form 41, line 49). All expenses are net of reinsurance.
Source: Thesys database and authors' calculations.

In 1997 life-offices reported expenses of 139 basis points, on average, for every £ they managed. Two factors are worth noting about the overall expense ratios. First, reported expenses have been falling over time: they were higher in 1994 (194 basis points) and even higher in 1989 (238 basis points). Second, the expense ratio varies significantly across firms. For example, in 1997, a quarter of companies reported expense ratios below 96 basis points, and another quarter had expense ratios above 166 basis points. Examining the data more closely, we find that higher assets under management tend to be associated with lower expense ratios, suggesting economies of scale in the life and pensions business.

Sales expenses, particularly commissions, contribute significantly to costs. In 1997 nearly two-thirds of the reported expense ratio consisted of business acquisition costs. The share of business acquisition was even higher in earlier years. A large portion of business acquisition consists of commissions, which account for almost one-half of all business acquisition costs and 30 percent of total costs. The importance of commissions in overall costs vividly manifests itself when we confine our attention to companies with commission-free sales (see bottom half of table 8.6). In 1997 there were 30 such companies in our sample. The average expense ratio for this group, 47 basis points, is only one-third the ratio for the full sample. The share of business acquisition in total costs for these firms is smaller than for the full sample, but still high (50 percent). Clearly, even without commissions, life-offices spend a significant proportion of all expenses on acquiring new business.

Another possible metric for examining expenses is costs per policy or costs per new policy, rather than costs per £ under management. The average cost of writing a new policy was £329 in 1997, £333 in 1994, and £299 in 1989. These costs are very sensitive to the amount of new business, since a large portion of costs is fixed. For example, to sell policies, life-offices need to hire staff, advertise, prepare and distribute sales information, and invest in computer systems. The average cost of writing a new policy appears to be much lower for commission-free providers. It was £63 in 1997, £38 in 1994, and £20 in 1989.

Turning from the cost of new policies to the cost of all policies, we find the average cost of a policy in force was £38 per policy (£30 for commission-free providers) in 1997, £31 (£13 for commission-free providers) in 1994, and £36 in 1989 (£38 for commission-free providers).

It may also be useful to consider these absolute costs relative to premiums or the average value of the contract. However, the fact that individuals can either purchase regular-premium policies (which require periodic contributions until maturity) or single-premium policies (which require a one-off contribution) complicates such an analysis. Single-premium policies tend to be much larger in size, so treating single and regular policies as identical runs the risk of constructing an average that is representative of neither. We therefore construct an average using 10 percent of premiums from single-premium policies, which is a standard practice in the industry.

We find that the cost of putting a new policy on the books relative to the annual premium was 64 percent in 1997, 87 percent in 1994, and 81 percent in 1989. These magnitudes go some way towards explaining why providers are keen to front load charges. Once in force, the average cost of a policy as a proportion of annual premium was around 11 percent in 1997. It was 10 percent in 1994, and 9 percent in 1989.

Several providers (such as Equitable Life) do not front load charges. Because of the high front-end costs of policies, they therefore bear the financial risks of early lapses, as well as the capital costs of reserving against these risks. A move to prohibit front-loaded fees (such as that behind the U.K. government's recent Stakeholder reforms) without any change in the front-loaded nature of provider costs would imply increased capital requirements and risks for providers.

Summary and Conclusions

This chapter has provided an overview of costs in the U.K. personal pension and annuities markets. Those costs are significant, reducing the value of an individual account by more than 40 percent relative to its no-cost level. To summarize, we conclude that reasonable estimates of the three components of the charge ratio are (i) accumulation ratio: 0.75, (ii) alteration ratio: 0.85, and annuitization ratio: 0.90. Taking in account interaction effects, these estimates suggest an overall charge ratio of 0.41.

Potential Criticisms

The figures presented here are clearly subject to several criticisms. Perhaps most importantly, they are partly based on unweighted averages (giving an equal weight to each provider, regardless of market share) and are dependent on specific assumptions regarding stock returns and nominal wage growth. In the face of such potential criticisms, we note the following:

- Whenever possible, we have checked the unweighted averages against their properly weighted (weighted by market share) analogues. The differences are not empirically significant.
- We have adopted standard government assumptions regarding stock returns and wage growth.
- We have "rounded up" all our figures. In particular, our estimates of all three component ratios are conservative. The average accumulation

ratio over the past decade, for example, was 0.72, rather than the 0.75 figure we adopt. Our projected alteration ratio was particularly conservative, since we assumed a value of 0.85 despite an underlying alteration ratio of 0.70 if all lapses result from transfers; 0.83 if all lapses result from old accounts going paid-up and new contributions being made to alternative providers, and 0.68 if all lapses arise from contribution halts. Finally, the annuity ratio was 0.85–0.90, rather than the 0.90 figure we adopt. Using the actual estimated figures rather than the more conservative ones we have applied, the total charge ratio would range from 49 percent to 58 percent, relative to the 43 percent resulting from our conservative final figures.

- Broader historical analysis conducted by James (1999) supports our forward-looking estimates. James compares the net return on unit trusts and life insurance companies between 1988 and 1997 to the market return on their underlying assets and imputes the fees imposed on consumers. He concludes that the fees are equivalent to a charge of roughly 300 basis points per year.

- Finally, we have studied costs for relatively high contribution rates because we have based our estimates on contribution levels *above* the minimum government rebate level. Assuming some economies of scale, the charge ratio is likely to be higher than our figures suggest for individuals contributing only the government tax rebate to their individual accounts (see, for example, Budden 1997 on the share of rebate-only accounts consumed by charges).

Given these precautions, our results are unlikely to be grossly misleading. Thus, our conclusion is that the U.K. experience with individual accounts involves high administrative and other costs.

Lessons for Other Countries

As noted in the introduction, individual accounts can be organized in a variety of ways. The U.K. experience should help to refute the argument that competitive pressures will automatically reduce costs in the decentralized approach. At the same time, the U.K. experience may be relatively special because of the underlying complexity of the U.K. system.

Whatever the benefits of the services provided by financial firms to their customers, the costs embodied in the voluntary, privately managed U.K. system with unregulated charges are high. Indeed, as we have noted above, the approach has lost favor in Britain: The U.K. government has capped charges at 1 percent of funds under management in its new Stakeholder Pensions and ruled out front-loaded charges.

Notes

1. Polarization is currently under review by the U.K. government. London Economics (2000) provides an economic analysis of the effects of various alternatives to polarization.

2. A companion paper examines the annuities market in the United Kingdom in more detail (see Murthi, Orszag, and Orszag 1999b).

3. For more detailed discussion on the features of the U.K. pension system, see Budd and Campbell (1998); Liu (1998); Blake and Orszag (1997); and, especially, Blake (1995).

4. To be eligible for full payment, men must have paid NIC contributions for 44 years, and women for 39 years. Partial payments are available for those contributing for fewer years.

5. For a description of the reforms, many of which were designed to encourage movement to either employer- or individual-based pension systems, see Liu (1998).

6. The historical dominance of life insurance funds in this market may change as a result of the introduction by the U.K. Treasury of new pooled investment fund management vehicles called Individual Pension Accounts.

7. For example, only insurance firms can offer annuities, waiver premia for disability insurance, and tax-advantaged life insurance policies. Partly in response to the mis-selling episode, however, the historical dominance of insurance companies may be slowly changing. Non-traditional providers, such as Virgin Direct; supermarkets; or the retail chain, Marks and Spencer, have recently entered the market. Also note that foreign providers from Europe, Australia, and Canada and their subsidiaries have a significant presence in the market.

8. Individuals designate a retirement age, normally required to be between 50 and 75, for their individual accounts.

9. There are a wide variety of annuity types, including level annuities, which pay the same amount in pounds for the term of the annuity; unit-linked annuities, which pay an amount linked to stock prices for the term of the annuity; index-linked annuities, which pay an amount linked to the retail price index for the term of the annuity; and with-profits annuities, which pay an amount linked to the profits of the provider. Other choices include whether the annuity is single life or joint; minimum guarantee or not; and the frequency of payment (monthly, quarterly, annual, etc.). The annuities market thus presents a wide variety, perhaps a bewildering variety, of choices for retirees.

10. For a description of the current requirements, see Financial Services Authority (2000).

11. The *Money Management* data assume that the pension is held for up to 25 years, whereas the Investment Intelligence data assume up to a 35-

year horizon. We have converted the 25-year and 35-year figures to 40-year equivalents, so that the horizon is consistent with a full working life. The fact that the fee structure tends not to change significantly toward the end of the published 25- or 35-year horizon facilitates the conversion process.

12. For various data-related reasons, it is easier to take unweighted rather than weighted averages. This procedure may lead to biased results if fees are systematically related to market share. However, indirect evidence from other sources, along with preliminary additional analysis of our data, suggests that any such bias is minimal. If anything, taking unweighted averages may be responsible for some portion of the rise in the accumulation ratio in recent years as the market has seen the entry of a large number of commission-free providers, who do not (yet) have substantial market share.

13. Murthi, Orszag, and Orszag (2000) document the extent of front loading of charges historically in the U.K.

14. A lapse means that contributions are no longer being made to the account and that it has either been transferred to some other provider or become paid-up.

15. We use a Weibull hazard to estimate persistency. For the selected parameter values, the hazard rate shows negative duration dependence: the longer the account has been held, the less likely it is to lapse.

16. Overall in 1997 there were 21.9 million pension policies in force in the life insurance industry. This far exceeds the number of active accounts, so that some people will have several accounts.

17. Murthi, Orszag and Orszag (1999a) discuss the other two cases in greater detail.

18. To compute fees in each year, we compute the forward after-charge yield for each provider and compare that after-charge yield to the precharge yield assumed in the regulatory filings. The difference is then attributed to fees. We then average across all firms, giving an equal weight to each provider. Weighting by assets does not substantially affect the results.

19. Alteration costs arise solely from any costs that depend on the duration of an account held with the typical financial firm. Diverted accounts have shorter durations (upon retirement) than nondiverted accounts.

20. There are two sources of the adverse selection effect worth noting: adverse selection in the distribution of those who choose to purchase an annuity relative to the population as a whole, and adverse selection within the pool of annuitants in the distribution of annuities purchased. In other words, those with longer than average life expectancies may be both more likely to purchase an annuity (one source of adverse selection) than the overall population and also more likely to purchase a higher-valued annuity (another source of adverse selection) than other annuitants with shorter life expectancies.

21. For a discussion of utility gains from the purchase of annuities, see, for example, Mitchell and others (1997).

22. Annuity ratios using annuitant life tables are in the range of 0.95–0.97.

23. Annuity ratios are typically 0.08–0.10 lower for retail price indexed annuities than for level annuities.

24. It is important to note that the results for passive management versus active management may be fundamentally different at the retail level.

References

Note: The word *processed* describes informally reproduced works that may not be commonly available through libraries.

Blake, David. 1995. *Pension Schemes and Pension Funds in the United Kingdom.* Oxford: Clarendon Press.

Blake, David, and J. Michael Orszag. 1997. *Towards a Universal Funded Second Pension.* Available at ftp://www.econ.bbk.ac.uk/pub/review.ps.

Brown, J. R., O. S. Mitchell, and J. M. Poterba. 1999. "The Role of Indexed Bonds and Real Annuities in an Individual Accounts Retirement Program." NBER Working Paper No. 7005. National Bureau of Economic Research, Cambridge, Mass.

Budd, Alan, and Nigel Campbell. 1998. "The Roles of the Public and Private Sectors in the U.K. Pension System." In M. Feldstein, ed., *Privatizing Social Security.* Cambridge: National Bureau of Economic Research.

Budden, Robert. 1997. "Money Down the Drain?" *Money Management* (January): 46–53.

Chapman, John. 1998. "Pension Plans Made Easy." *Money Management,* November.

Diamond, Peter. 1998. "Administrative Costs and Equilibrium Charges with Individual Accounts." Processed.

Financial Services Authority. 2000. The Conduct of Business Sourcebook.

Finkelstein, Amy, and James Poterba. 1999. "Selection Effects in the Market for Individual Annuities: Evidence from the United Kingdom." NBER Working Paper No. 7168. National Bureau of Economic Research, Cambridge, Mass.

James, Estelle, Gary Ferrier, James Smalhout, and Dimitri Vittas. 1998. "Mutual Funds and Institutional Investments: What Is the Most Efficient Way to Set Up Individual Accounts in a Social Security System?" Paper presented at NBER Conference on Social Security, December 4, 1998.

James, Kevin. 1998. "The Price of Retail Investing in the U.K.." Financial Services Authority. Processed.

Liu, Lillian. 1998. "Retirement Income Security in the United Kingdom." ORES Working Paper No. 79. Washington DC: Social Security Administration.

London Economics. 2000. "Polarisation and Financial Services Intermediary Regulation." Report prepared for Financial Services Authority. Available at http://www.fsa.gov.uk/pubs/other/polar.pdf.

Mitchell, O., James Poterba, Mark Warshawsky, and Jeff Brown. 1997. "New Evidence on the Money's Worth of Individual Annuities." NBER Working Paper. Forthcoming.

Murthi, Mamta, J. Michael Orszag, and Peter R. Orszag. 1999a. "The Charge Ratio on Individual Accounts: Lessons from the U.K. Experience." Birkbeck College Working Paper No. 99-2. Available at http://www.econ.bbk.ac.uk/ukcosts.

_____. 1999b. "The Value for Money of Annuities in the U.K.: Theory, Experience and Policy." Available from www.econ.bbk.ac.uk/annuities.

_____. 2000. "The Maturity Structure of Administrative Costs: Theory and U.K. Experience." Available from www.econ.bbk.ac.uk/ukcosts.

National Academy of Social Insurance. 1998. "Evaluating Issues in Privatizing Social Security, Report of the Panel on Privatization of Social Security." Available at http://www.nasi.org.

Poterba, James, and Mark Warshawsky, 1999. "The Costs of Annuitizing Retirement Payments from Individual Accounts." NBER Working Paper No. 6918. National Bureau of Economic Research, Cambridge, Mass.

Rea, John, and Brian Reid. 1998. "Trends in the Ownership Cost of Equity Mutual Funds." Investment Company Institute, *Perspective* 4(3).

Shuttleworth, John L. 1997. "Operating Costs of Different Forms of Pension Provision in the U.K.." Coopers and Lybrand LLP.

Sumpter, Jane. 1999. "Lifestyles of the Young and Mobile." *Money Management*, February.

9

The Relevance of Index Funds for Pension Investment in Equities

Ajay Shah and Kshama Fernandes

The Idea of Index Funds

IN THE DECADES OF THE 1960S AND THE 1970S, many studies indicated that actively managed funds, which seek to obtain excess returns by actively forecasting returns on individual stocks, do not actually obtain statistically significant excess returns. This was consistent with the hypothesis of "market efficiency," which suggested that obtaining excess returns should be difficult in a competitive market.[1]

This research suggested a superior investment strategy: the index fund, a portfolio that passively replicated the returns of the index. The most useful kind of market index is one in which the weight attached to a stock is proportional to its market capitalization. Index funds are easy to construct for this kind of index, since the index fund does not need to trade in response to price fluctuations. Trading is only required in response to issuance of shares, mergers, and so on.

The first index fund dates back to 1972. In the following years, the indexation industry grew at a dramatic pace. However, exact data about the size of the industry is hard to obtain. Table 9.1 summarizes some evidence about the size of the index fund industry. Index funds are arguably one of the most successful ideas to have flowed into the real world from academic economics.

In an ideal world, where trading is frictionless and dividends are obtained by shareholders on the exact ex-dividend date, the index fund would exactly replicate the returns on the index (inclusive of dividends). A variety of events necessitate trading by the index fund: issuance of shares by a company (which raises the weight of the company in the index), addition or deletion of companies from the index, reinvestment of dividends,

Table 9.1. The Size of the Indexation Industry

		Assets under indexation (US$ billion)			
Manager	Total	U.S. equity	U.S. bonds	Intnl. equity	Intnl. bonds
Barclays Global Investors	407	288	73	45	0.3
State Street Global	207	122	27	58	0.3
Bankers Trust	156	131	4	22	0.0
TIAA-CREF	96	84	0	12	0.0
Sum of above four	866	625	104	137	0.6
Total of 55 managers	1323	952	210	156	1.0
Four-firm concentration (percent)	65	66	50	88	60

Note: It is safe to suggest that this survey missed many smaller index fund managers and many index funds outside the United States. Hence the total size seen here is an underestimate, and the four-firm concentration ratio seen here is an overestimate.
Source: A survey of index fund managers run by the magazine *Pensions & Investments*, February 22, 1999.

etc. In the real world, trading imposes transaction costs upon the index fund, and dividends are not obtained exactly on the ex-date.

When a security trades at an "ideal" price of $\bar{p}$, purchasers ultimately pay a slightly higher price p_b. The percentage degradation faced here, $100((p_b/\bar{p}) - 1)$ is referred to as the "market impact cost." Index maintainers make their calculations assuming that all trading is done at zero market impact cost; index funds always suffer impact cost and thus generate inferior returns. Suppose we have a time-series of returns on an index (inclusive of dividends) of r_t, and the index fund experiences a time-series of returns of $r_t{'}$. Then the annualized standard deviation of $r_t - r_t{'}$ is termed "tracking error."

Tracking error summarizes the extent to which the index fund is able to accurately track the index. Index fund managers seek to minimize tracking error. From the viewpoint of an investor, an index fund that experiences a large tracking error is a source of risk because it might not replicate the returns on the index in the future.

The Rationale for Index Funds

Traditional fund management has been based on the premise that the fund manager adds value through continuous efforts at improving risk-adjusted returns by forecasting returns. Index funds are counterintuitive in that they make no such effort. The index fund manager makes no attempt at returns forecasting; his or her only goal is to replicate index returns. The arguments for why might index funds may be more attractive can be sum-marized in relation to two basic issues:

- *Market efficiency.* If markets are fairly efficient, it would prove diffi-cult for active managers to obtain excess returns, after considering the higher fees and costs that they have to run up.
- *Agency problems.* The principal-agent problem between investors and money managers presents special difficulties owing to the unob-servability of the fund managers' ability and effort.

The relative ease with which the principal can monitor the fund man-agement activities of the agent, in the context of index funds, is one factor that underlies the growth of index funds.

Does Active Management Yield Excess Returns?

Active management represents an attempt to obtain excess returns. In doing so, active managers must expend resources on the enterprise of fund management and incur transaction costs in trading.

Table 9.2. Costs and Expenses of Equity Funds
(percentage)

	Large cap U.S. equity	Large cap non-U.S. equity	Small cap U.S. equity	Emerging market equity
Commissions, taxes	0.07	0.28	0.25	0.51
Bid/offer, market impact	0.23	0.50	0.75	1.08
Total trade cost	0.30	0.78	1.00	1.59
Turnover				
Active	150	150	150	150
Passive	8	10	50	20
Trade cost				
Active	0.45	1.17	1.50	2.39
Passive	0.02	0.08	0.50	0.32
Difference	0.43	1.09	1.00	2.07
Management/custody fees				
Active	0.45	0.55	0.75	1.20
Passive	0.05	0.20	0.08	0.55
Ongoing costs				
Active	0.90	1.72	2.25	3.59
Passive	0.07	0.28	0.58	0.87
Difference	0.83	1.44	1.67	2.72

Note: This table shows a comparison between the expenses and transactions costs incurred by actively managed funds, as compared with index funds
Source: Cheung (1999).

Table 9.3. The Coefficient of the "Index Fund" Dummy in Regressions that Explain the Expense Ratio

Year	Coefficient	t–statistic
1992	−18.93	−1.69
1993	−32.45	−3.12
1994	−41.66	−5.3
1995	−34.16	−4.8
1996	−38.31	−5.8
1997	−39.47	−8.9

Note: James and others (2000) have a series of cross-sectional regressions exploring the determinants of the expense ratio in the Morningstar database. These regressions control for the following variables: assets, squared assets, average number of shareholders, assets per shareholder, assets in fund complex, three-year net return, three-year gross return, three-year standard deviation, dummies for five asset classes, a dummy variable if the fund targets institutional investors, the initial investment, variables expressing loads and the 12b1 fees (in the United States), turnover, a dummy variable for advice from a bank, and fund age. This table shows the results for the coefficient of the "index fund" dummy (measured in basis points) in these regressions.
Source: James, Smalhout, and Vittas (2000).

Index funds feature lower expenses by avoiding the expenditures in information collection and processing required in returns forecasting. Table 9.2 shows evidence about the expenses and fees of index funds as compared with actively managed funds, where index funds hold an advantage of 0.83 to 2.72 percent per year through lower expenses. Table 9.3 summarizes some empirical evidence from the essay by James, Smalhout, and Vittas in chapter 7, using linear regressions that seek to explain the expense ratio of funds in the Morningstar database. After controlling for a variety of factors that influence expenses, we see that index funds incur lower expenses by around 30 to 40 basis points per year.

As a broad regularity, index funds tend to engage in smaller trading volumes as compared with actively managed funds, which also helps enhance returns through lower costs of transacting. Table 9.2 shows some U.S. evidence about the transactions costs incurred by index funds as compared with actively managed funds, where index funds hold an advantage of between 0.43 to 2.07 percentage points per year through lower transactions costs.

We may note here that the large-cap stocks on the U.S. stock market are among the largest companies in the world. The situation in many developing countries may be closer to the evidence shown for the medium-cap and small-cap universes of the U.S. stocks market.

In the fund industry, index funds are a highly contestable area owing to product standardization. If an active manager (for example, Warren

Buffet) is highly successful, and supports high fees, it is not clear how a com
petitor can offer a comparable competing product. In contrast, if one index
fund on a given index commands high fees, it is easy for entrants to offer
sharply comparable products and, hence, lead to a reduction in fees.

Low fees and expenses are not an end in themselves. The higher fees and
expenses of actively managed funds might be justified if markets were inefficient enough so that excess returns were obtained, in excess of these fees
and expenses. For instance, the perception that prospective returns are higher often justifies paying higher management fees and transactions costs in
small-cap, illiquid asset classes. Hence the most important issue in evaluating index funds is the ultimate returns delivered to the investor, net of
fees and expenses.

Tables 9.4 through 9.6 summarize the historical experience with index
funds as opposed to active managers. Table 9.4 shows that the index fund
in the United States lagged behind index returns by 40 basis points; however, actively managed funds lagged behind index returns by the larger
margin of 110 basis points. In table 9.5 we see that in four major asset classes

**Table 9.4. A Performance Comparison: Evidence from the United
States over 1976–97**

Product	Average returns, 1976–97 (percent)
Returns on S&P 500	15.2
Returns on S&P 500 index fund	14.8
Return on general equity funds	14.1

Note: This table summarizes the U.S. experience with index funds as compared to actively
managed funds. Over this 21-year period, the S&P 500 index outperformed the S&P 500
index fund by 0.4 percent per year, and it outperformed the average actively managed
fund by 1.1 percent per year.
Source: Figure 5 in Bogle (1998).

**Table 9.5. Mutual Funds that were Outperformed by their Respective
Indexes**

Category	Benchmark index	Period	Percent of funds that underperformed
General equity funds	Wilshire 5000 Index	1986–95	65
International equity funds	MSCI-EAFE Index	1986–95	73
Emerging markets funds	MSCI-Emerging Markets	1993–95	88
Bond funds	Lehman Brothers Bond Index	1986–95	77

Note: In four major asset classes, we see that the predominant outcome was for the active
fund to underperform its benchmark index. This regularity holds for equities invested outside the United States and also in developing countries.
Source: Lipper Analytical Services.

Table 9.6. Performance of the Median Active Manager When Compared with Indexes

Category	Median manager	Index	Difference
U.S. equity (S&P 500)	21.97	24.15	–2.18
U.S. small cap (Russell 2000)	15.20	11.86	3.34
Non-U.S. equity (MSCI EAFE)	10.46	9.50	0.96
Emerging markets (IFC composite)	–8.23	–8.70	0.47

Note: Performance over the five-year period, ending on December 31, 1998, of the median active manager as compared with the market index. For example, in the universe of emerging market equity, the median manager lost 8.23 percent, while the index lost 8.7 percent, so the median manager was 47 basis points ahead.
Source: Russell, cited in Cheung (1999).

the majority of actively managed funds lagged behind their benchmark indexes, including two categories outside the United States: the classes of "international equity" and "emerging markets" investments.[2]

Agency Problems

We can obtain important insights into the appeal of index funds by focusing on the principal-agent relationship between the investor and the fund manager. How is the investor to choose among competing fund managers? How is the agent to monitor the fund manager and ensure that the actions of the fund manager are in his or her best interest?

Fund management is a complex process in which agency problems could surface at many levels. There are many decisions in which the fund manager could choose to act in ways counter to the best interest of the investor (Shah 1999), such as the following examples:

- The fund manager could choose to buy stocks in which he or she has a personal interest. Sometimes fund managers allow manipulative cartels to use the assets of the fund, for which they may receive private benefits.
- The fund manager could "front-run" against the fund, buying stocks on his or her personal account immediately before doing so on behalf of the fund.
- The fund manager could choose trading mechanisms that yield superior private rents instead of choosing the trading mechanism that yields the lowest transactions costs.
- The fund manager has choices about custodial and administrative services that might not be made in a cost-minimizing fashion.

It is difficult for an investor, or a trustee, to ensure that the fund manager is making these decisions in his or her best interest. Monitoring performance, therefore, is the prominent device to exercise control. The investor would select fund managers who have exhibited the highest returns in the past and fire fund managers who fail to perform.

A naive comparison of returns across alternative funds is an inefficient way to measure fund manager ability when there are differences in the levels of risk adopted by different funds. The inherent randomness of market returns suggests that a casual comparison of returns should give way to a formal statistical test in comparing fund managers. This leads us to the enterprise of scientific performance evaluation efforts.

Mutual fund performance evaluation as yet suffers from many conceptual difficulties (Roll 1977). In addition, the statistical efficiency of existing performance evaluation procedures is limited, owing to the poor signal-to-noise ratio whereby genuine ability in fund management tends to get drowned in the noise of market fluctuations Bodie, Kane, and Marcus (1989, p. 735), provide an example of a fund manager who has substantial skill—he adds returns of 0.2 percentage points per month (that is, in excess of 2.4 percentage points per year). It turns out that if the standard procedure of measuring the "alpha" of the fund manager were employed using monthly returns, we would need to observe the results of his fund management for 32 years before we can reject the null hypothesis of no ability ($\alpha = 0$) at a 95 percent level of significance.[3] This makes it difficult for investors to identify and adequately monitor fund managers. This signal-to-noise ratio would be at its worst in developing countries, where stock market returns tend to be more volatile.

This poor signal-to-noise ratio becomes a particularly contentious issue when anyone other than an individual makes decisions about the choice of a fund manager for the individual. Consider a situation in which a pension fund committee selects an active fund manager. This poor signal-to-noise ratio reduces the ability of the committee to identify the manager with the best ability. When ability is relatively hard to measure, there is a greater role for political lobbying in determining the choice of the manager. Alternatively, signals such as pedigree, size, or years of experience are often used as proxies for ability, reducing the contestability of the market for money management services.[4]

Once a manager is chosen, suppose the returns prove to be below the index at a future date. The pension fund committee would then be relatively vulnerable to accusations of having chosen the wrong fund manager. This factor also generates a bias towards hiring fund managers who fare well on signals such as pedigree, size, or years of experience, which helps the committee to produce a plausible defense for their actions in the future, if the need arises.

The literature on performance evaluation has posed a significant challenge to the proposition, held by all active managers, that the active manager is capable of adding value. In similar fashion, there are legitimate concerns about the proposition, held by most sponsors, that the plan sponsor is capable of selecting the active manager(s) who will add value in the future.

These problems are an important motivation for the growth of index funds, particularly in situations like pension investment. Comparing alternative index fund managers is relatively straightforward—it essentially involves comparing the tracking error that they have produced. It also makes it easier for individuals to obtain accountability from an institution such as a pension committee: poor asset returns should be directly linked to poor returns on the index.

The Mechanics of Index Funds

The stereotypical view of index funds is that their management is a trivial task. Yet, in practice, there are significant challenges in the creation and operations of an index fund.

Unlike active managers, who make no promises about future returns, index funds promise to replicate the returns of a publicly observable index. If the index rises by 20 percent, and if the index fund reports 19 percent returns, then the investor is entitled to be suspicious about how 100 basis points of returns were lost. This level of scrutiny and accountability makes index fund management a challenge.

Choice and Construction of Index

In many countries "widely prevalent" stock market indexes exist. In this case the modern development of the financial sector, in the direction of index funds or index derivatives, almost automatically proceeds using these widely prevalent indexes. These market indexes often present a host of awkward difficulties in modern applications.

In most cases, these market indexes were created years ago in an environment with limited information access, poor computation, and limited knowledge of financial economics. All three factors are much altered today. Modern electronic stock exchanges, which use anonymous trading with computerized order matching, offer a wealth of information about market liquidity. The revolution in computational power at ever lower prices has made it possible to embed complex computational procedures into day-to-day index management. Finally, research into index funds and index derivatives through the decade of the 1980s and '90s sheds new light upon the issues in index construction.

The difficulties with many traditional stock market indexes may be summarized as follows:

- When some stocks in the index are inadequately liquid, this contaminates the information represented by the index and makes it harder to use the index for financial products such as index funds or index futures.

- An illiquid stock contaminates the information content of the index via "stale prices," where the computation of the index at time t_2 is forced to use information about a trade on an illiquid stock at t_1, $t_1 < t_2$.
- Illiquid stocks make it difficult to trade the entire index as a portfolio and significantly hamper the viability of index funds and index derivatives. For example, it is fairly inconvenient to undertake program trades for all 500 components of the Standard & Poor (S&P) 500 index, and approximation of the index using 150–300 stocks is a common procedure. Similarly, stock market indexes for developing countries created by agencies such as the International Finance Corporation (IFC) are often highly impractical when it comes to using them for index funds or index futures.

The procedures for "managing" the stock market index often leave much to be desired. The composition of an index should evolve over the years, reflecting changes in the economy, and the procedures through which this takes place should be immune to special interests. Many traditional index maintainers have shown a weakness in this area. In many countries, index maintainers do not even produce a variant of the market index inclusive of dividends.

Every stock market index is a trade-off between diversification and liquidity. Small market indexes tend to be illiquid and underdiversified; large market indexes tend to be well diversified and illiquid. Yet there are sharply diminishing returns to diversification. Most randomly chosen portfolios in a country prove to be extremely highly correlated with each other, as long as they are highly diversified. Hence, as long as adequate diversification is obtained, the identity of specific stocks in the index is not too important as far as the risk/return character of the index is concerned.

Shah and Thomas (1998) suggest that choosing highly liquid stocks to form a well-diversified index could be a useful strategy. There are two aspects to market liquidity: *market impact cost* (the degradation in price faced when placing a market order) and *market resiliency* (the time taken for the market to revert to its original state after an order is placed). Measuring and characterizing market resiliency is still an unsolved research problem. However, on electronic exchanges market impact cost can be accurately measured. Shah and Thomas (1998) use this in their method for index construction. Table 9.7, which is reproduced from their paper, summarizes the market impact cost in doing program trades on alternative indexes in India. The National Stock Exchange (NSE)-50 index, in which low market impact cost in doing index program trades is explicitly a goal, has substantially lower market impact cost as compared with alternative indexes.[5]

Table 9.7. Impact Cost in Portfolio Trades for Alternative Stock Market Indexes in India

Index	Market cap. (Rs. trillion)	Impact cost (%) at trans. size (Rs. million)		
		5	10	20
BSE-30	1.96	0.35	0.46	0.67
Barings India Index	1.59	0.29	0.36	0.50
IFC India Index	2.62	0.53	0.65	0.89
MSCI India Index	2.67	0.53	0.64	0.87
NSE-50	2.21	0.29	0.36	0.49

Note: Average impact cost (in percent), in 1997, on India's National Stock Exchange (NSE), for doing program trades for alternative stock market indexes. The NSE-50 index, which explicitly factors market impact cost into the index construction, proves to have significantly lower market impact cost.
Source: Authors' calculations.

Stock market indexes that use methods such as these would be well suited for the implementation of index funds and index derivatives. The reduced market impact cost when doing program trades on the index leads to reduced tracking error for index funds.

Table 9.8 gives an international perspective on the transactions costs faced in doing program trades on a given index. In each case it is assumed that a series of trades are done through one trading day, in order to buy the desired "basket size." In the United States the spot market supports transactions of around US$5 million with a total cost of 0.21 percent. When the index futures market is used, the size of the basket rises to

Table 9.8. Trading Costs on Spot Market for Some Market Indexes

Index	Basket size ($ million)	Commission (percent)	Market impact cost (percent)	Total (percent)
US: S&P 500	5	0.057	0.150	0.207
US: S&P 500 futures	100	0.005	0.012	0.017
US: S&P Midcap	5	0.100	0.300	0.400
US: Russell 2000	5	0.150	0.655	0.805
India: NSE-50	5	0.200	0.250	0.450
India: Nifty Junior	2	0.200	0.800	1.000

Note: This table shows the transactions costs faced in buying index baskets for some alternative market indexes. These numbers assume that the basket is traded over a maximum of one day.
Sources: U.S. data from exhibit 3 of Chiang (1998); Mason and others (1995); Data on India from author's experiences (1999).

US$100 million, and the cost drops to one-twelfth of this. The costs faced in obtaining baskets of less liquid stock market indexes, such as the S&P Midcap or the Russell 2000, are much higher. In a developing country, India, the main stock market index (NSE-50) supports much smaller basket sizes: around US$5 million can be obtained in a day at a market impact cost of 0.25 percent. The next tier of less liquid stocks in India, the Nifty Junior index, faces a higher market impact cost of 0.8 percent for obtaining US$2 million in a day.

Some related evidence on the importance of index construction is presented in table 9.9, which summarizes the tracking error obtained by the "synthetic index fund" strategy using alternative indexes. In all countries the local index yields a lower tracking error than the *Financial Times*/Standard & Poor indexes or the Morgan Stanley Country Indices (MSCI). The reasons for this are not immediately apparent; it may be because local indexes are more sensitive to local market liquidity. Regardless of the sources of this difference in tracking error, this evidence underlines the importance of local indexes as a vehicle for index funds and index futures.

Table 9.9. Tracking Error for Synthetic Index Funds

	Annualised tracking error		
Index	*Local*	*FT/S&P*	*MSCI*
TSE 35	2.92	5.26	5.58
Nikkei 225	3.06	7.14	8.20
Nikkei 300	2.61	2.97	2.92
TOPIX	2.94	3.14	4.24
Hang Seng	5.20	7.06	6.88
All ords	3.11	3.52	4.25
STOXX 50	2.76	3.66	3.75
Euro STOXX 50	2.82	4.50	4.25
FTSE 100	2.25	2.54	2.50
CAC 40	1.59	3.47	2.80
DAX	1.17	3.54	4.39
SMI	1.10	2.06	2.51
AEX	1.30	4.70	6.34
IBEX 35	2.37	2.58	2.91
MIB 30	2.00	3.55	3.74
OMX	2.18	3.67	3.11

Note: This table compares the annualized tracking error obtained with a synthetic index fund, using three alternative indexes for each country.
Source: Table 4 (p. 5) from Goldman Sachs Equity Derivatives Research (1999).

Methods of Implementing Index Funds

At first glance, implementing an index fund appears straightforward: the index fund is supposed to buy stocks with the correct weights and trade in response to changes in the index set or when any of the index stocks issue new capital (see Liesching and Manchanda 1990 for a survey of relevant techniques). In practice, implementing index funds proves to be a significant challenge, especially when the underlying stock market index has been poorly designed.

The simplest method through which index funds are implemented is "full replication," where the portfolio held by the index fund is the same as the index. Such an index fund will replicate the returns of the index, subject to the caveat of transaction costs in trading.

Many countries have market indexes with design flaws, and one of the most common problems is that of a market index containing highly illiquid stocks. Sometimes, a market index for a sector innately suffers from high transaction costs in trading when the entire sector is only made up of illiquid stocks. When some or all index components are inadequately liquid, index funds that use full replication can suffer from a large tracking error owing to the large transactions costs faced in trading the entire index. One path for the implementation of an index fund, in this situation, consists of holding a portfolio p´ that is different from the index portfolio p in which (i) the transactions costs associated with implementing p´ are much lower than those faced with the true index p, and (ii) the correlation between p and p´ is high. In general, the portfolio p´ should be chosen by explicitly solving a mathematical programming problem to minimize the tracking error.[6] If the liquidity of index components is sufficiently "unbalanced" so that some components are disproportionately more liquid than others, such an index fund might obtain a lower tracking error compared to a fund that uses full replication.[7]

The third strategy for implementing an index fund is to utilize stock index futures. Suppose an index futures product requires placing \$x of collateral to support a position of \$100. Then it is possible to replicate the returns on an index portfolio worth \$100 by adopting a long position on the index futures market for \$100, and investing the residual cash 100-x in riskless government securities (Mason and others 1995). This is called the "synthetic index fund." In the United States, which has the most liquid index futures market in the world, the synthetic index fund has an annualized tracking error of around 0.46 percent (Goldman Sachs Equity Derivatives Research 1999).

In most markets this yields slightly higher returns than the index for two reasons: (i) the rate of return embedded in the index futures basis is slightly higher than the riskless rate of return because of the credit risk of the futures clearing corporation, and (ii) the residual cash 100-x is often invested in slightly risky securities, such as short-rated AAA corporate bonds, which yield slightly higher returns.

Evaluating the Alternative Implementation Strategies

Full replication is feasible when the liquidity of the stocks that make up the index supports low-cost program trades on the complete index. The methods for index construction in Shah and Thomas (1998) orient toward index funds implemented through full replication. Full replication requires the least sophistication in terms of analytical and computational abilities in the fund industry.

When stock market indexes suffer from illiquid index components, optimization-strategies can be useful; however, they require considerable sophistication in terms of quantitative finance.

When liquid index futures markets are available, synthetic index funds are often an excellent option. In mature markets the transaction costs faced when trading the index using the index futures market can be as low as one-tenth to one-twentieth of the transaction costs faced when trading shares on the spot market. Holding a position on index futures involves lower custodial and administrative costs, especially in markets with primitive settlement systems where physical share certificates are still in use. On the contrary, the index futures implementation will forgo revenues from stock-lending that the full replication fund enjoys.

Implementation through index futures is particularly attractive when the market index suffers from disproportionately illiquid index components: the index futures market offers a single, liquid, tradable product. The user of the futures market would be relatively shielded from the illiquid index components.

The weaknesses of this implementation strategy are twofold:

- The first problem is that index futures contracts expire, and the index fund would need to reestablish this position on the next available contract, a process called "rollover." If an index fund has assets of US$100 billion, it would need to execute trades worth either US$100 billion or US$200 billion on the index futures market every few months. This is in sharp contrast to an index fund that is implemented using full replication: a fund with assets of US$100 billion would typically undertake a trading volume of US$1 billion to $5 billion in a year. Large index funds would suffer considerable transaction costs when doing this rollover, for even the highly liquid index futures markets are not adequately liquid to support such large transactions. Hence, the largest of index funds have often been limited to full replication strategies. There is an element of active management in the rollover process. If a rollover can be timed carefully for an instant in time when the near contract is expensive and a far contract is cheap, then the rollover can actually yield excess returns. However, this gives us an element of active management inconsistent with the goals of index funds.

- Furthermore, at the level of the economy, the index futures implementation has a basic weakness, since index futures are in "net zero supply": for each buyer of a futures, there has to be an equal and opposite seller. If we think of 50 percent of the gross domestic product of a country being invested in index funds using index futures, it will prove to be hard to find sellers who would be at the opposite end of the trades (Rubinstein 1989). If index futures markets are used by index funds on this scale, we could observe breakdowns in the market efficiency of the index futures market and enhanced tracking error for these index funds.

In the real world all three implementation strategies have a useful role to play, depending upon the situation. Ideally, if index construction is done soundly in a country, then full replication should be the mainstream implementation strategy used by the bulk of indexed assets. Index futures often seem attractive for individual index fund products, but considerations of the economy as a whole (as in the context of the pension sector) relegate implementation strategies using index futures to the margin in efficiently coping with incremental assets moving in or out of index funds. Optimization-based strategies could be useful for extending the universe of indexation beyond the most liquid assets, or when faced with badly designed market indexes.

The Enabling Market Infrastructure for Index Funds

The conventional analysis of index funds is generally based on treating the stock market index and the equity market as a given, and analyzing the usefulness and implementation of index funds. For example, in the United States, the S&P 500 as an index, and trading based on the "specialist" on the NYSE as a market design have existed for many decades; research on index funds in this context has treated the S&P 500 and the NYSE as givens.

From the viewpoint of policy, it is useful to examine the question from a different perspective: what is a market infrastructure that can best enable index funds? What aspects of the design of the financial system can be modified so as to help the implementation and usefulness of index funds?

Index

The most basic foundation of indexation is the stock market index. The treatment of index construction (see previous section) suggests that there are significant gains to redesigning market indexes using modern knowledge of financial economics, especially in countries with modern market infrastructure in the form of electronic order-matching.

Unfortunately, market indexes that have existed for decades are hard to displace from the public imagination. Even in a country with nearly 100 percent literacy, the poorly designed Dow Jones index plays an important role. Yet in many developing countries, where existing market indexes are not well respected, opportunities presently exist for successfully introducing a new index. Policymakers can play a role in this migration out of legacy indexes.

Electronic Trading

Implementing index funds obviously relies on an exchange in which orders are executed. Prior to modern technology, a variety of market mechanisms developed to address this problem: the specialist of the NYSE, the dealers of NASDAQ, the floor with "open outcry" at the futures exchanges in Chicago, and so forth.

From the early 1970s onwards (Black 1971), an important new idea of market design has arisen—using a computer to match orders in a market where economic agents *anonymously* post prices and quantities they desire. This has also been termed the "open electronic limit order book" (OELOB) market. It has significant theoretical appeal (Glosten 1994) and is the dominant form of market organization that exchanges have employed worldwide in the 1990s. In recent years, the research community has been able to obtain fresh insights into market liquidity on the OELOB market (Handa, Schwartz, and Tiwari 1998).

After a decade of debate and resistance, many traditional exchanges have moved from a labor-intensive market design to the electronic exchange— for example, the London Stock Exchange (LSE) in 1997 and the London International Financial Futures Exchange (LIFFE) in 1998.

In labor-intensive markets a "program trade" is difficult to execute, since human reaction time has low mean and high variance. If an index containing 100 stocks has to be purchased, it would require interacting with 100 (or more) humans. This is a complex and expensive affair. Even today, on the NYSE, executing program trades for the S&P 500 takes around two minutes; the index trader is exposed to the risk of market fluctuations within this time interval. In contrast, electronic exchanges make it convenient and efficient to place program trades. It is possible for an electronic exchange to execute 100 orders in a very short time, thus reducing the tracking error that results from purchases spread over different index levels.

The open electronic limit order book market is particularly valuable for index funds since it is transparent about prices *and liquidity*. An entire program trade can be priced before it is placed.[8] This is in sharp contrast with a traditional market such as the NYSE, where every program trade results in an unpredictable execution.

While the implementation of worldwide equity index funds has been greatly enabled by the spread of electronic exchanges in the 1990s, most bond markets continue to use primitive market institutions, presenting a significant hurdle to the growth of bond index funds.

Call Auctions

The "call auction" is a uniform price double auction where buyers and sellers compete in offering buy and sell prices for a stated interval of time (Economides and Schwartz 1995; Handa and Schwartz 1996). It is a trading procedure that aggregates the order flow over a period of time to produce greater liquidity and allows all buyers and sellers to obtain a single price (there is no "market impact cost" in the electronic call auction).

We can cite three examples of the use of the call auction:

- The NYSE "opening price" is obtained using (manual) call auctions on each of the underlying stocks. This makes it convenient for program trading to take place at the NYSE open. Market orders that are placed in the call auctions are guaranteed to obtain the exact opening index level. For this reason the S&P 500 futures settlement price is derived from the NYSE opening price of the *next day* after trading on the futures market has stopped.
- The Arizona Stock Exchange (http://www.azx.com) relies exclusively on electronic call auctions.
- In India, the National Stock Exchange begins and ends the day using an electronic call auction. This ensures that index traders can attain the opening and closing levels of the index at zero impact cost.

To the extent that index funds are able to execute program trades at zero impact cost using call auctions, it reduces the tracking error that they face.

Index Futures

Index futures reduce the transaction costs of doing large index trades. As seen in table 9.8, execution of basket trades for 20 times the basket size in the United States takes place at one-twelfth the cost. This clearly suggests that index futures have a major role to play in implementing index funds. To the extent that a country has a functioning index futures market, it would assist index funds in obtaining lower tracking error.

Negative Externalities of Indexation

The worldwide growth of index funds in recent decades has raised concerns about the externalities that this rise of indexation could impose upon the economy. These concerns reside in four areas: (i) distorted cost of capital for index stocks, (ii) inferior corporate governance, (iii) diminished market efficiency, and (iv) enhanced concentration in the fund industry.

Distorted Prices of Index Stocks

Many observers have expressed concerns about index funds "blindly" buying index stocks. If US$100 billion are in index funds on a given index, and if a stock enters the index with a weightage of 0.5 percent, then index funds would be forced to buy US$500 million of this stock. Conversely, index funds would be forced to sell shares of companies that are dropped from the index.

Could these activities significantly distort share prices? Do they result in elevated valuations and, hence, an unusually low cost of capital for index stocks? Does the growth of index funds thus contaminate the resource allocation produced by the stock market?

While these concerns may appear intuitively sound, they should be interpreted in the context of the actions of the rest of the market. If index funds purchased US$500 million of a given stock, and if the price of the stock rose above a "fair valuation," then many informed speculators would choose to sell that stock. If markets were efficient, we would see a reshuffling in the ownership pattern of the company, with many shares going from informed speculators into index funds; however, in the ideal efficient market, the impact on prices should be zero.

The event of addition or deletion of stocks from the S&P 500 index, with large index funds in the background, has given researchers many opportunities to study these effects, starting from the early work of Shleifer (1986) and Harris and Gurel (1986). Table 9.10 summarizes the evidence from Lynch and Mendenhall (1997). When Standard & Poor announces that

Table 9.10. Abnormal Price Fluctuations Owing to Inclusion/Exclusion in the S&P 500 Index

| | (% change in stock price) | |
	Addition	Deletion
From announcement date to effective date	+3.8	−12.7
From effective date to 10 days after	−2.3	+6.2

Note: This table presents evidence about abnormal stock price movements associated with addition or deletion from the S&P 500 index in the United States. The trading by index funds seeking to do full replication would have to be fully completed by the "effective date."
Source: Lynch and Mendenhall (1997).

a stock is added in the index, a future date when this announcement takes effect, called the "effective date" is announced in advance. Index funds that seek to do full replication would be forced to buy the stock by this date. From the announcement to this effective date, an abnormal price movement of +3.8 percent is observed; however, 2.3 percent of this is lost in the following 10 days. Hence the long-term price of inclusion in the S&P 500 is +1.5 percent. While this is a clear violation of market efficiency, it appears fairly benign in terms of not constituting a large distortion of stock prices or the cost of capital.

The evidence is less benign in the case of stocks that are dropped from the index: the selling by index funds generates a temporary drop of 12.7 percent, of which 6.2 percent is regained in the following 10 days. The permanent drop in price amounts to 6.5 percent.

Therefore, evidence exists that in a world with large indexed assets the prices and, hence, cost of capital of stocks is distorted depending on inclusion or exclusion from the index. However, these effects do not appear to be very large.

Inferior Corporate Governance

Some observers have criticized index funds on the grounds that index fund managers do not take interest in resolving the agency conflicts between shareholders and managers. Index funds are viewed as free riders on the corporate governance problem that other agents in the economy are expending resources upon.

This free-rider problem is present with any investor who chooses to ignore corporate governance issues. The implicit logic of the limited liability company is that it gives shareholders the right, not the obligation, to vote.

We can view failures of corporate governance as a violation of market efficiency. If a firm is producing inferior cash flows owing to improper incentives for managers, then there is an opportunity for an active portfolio manager to seize control of the company, modify its activities so as to attain higher cash flows, and benefit from these activities to the extent that the share price of the company goes up. The existence of these situations, and the importance of speculators who engage in such activities, is undeniable.

Diminished Market Efficiency

Index funds are criticized for not engaging in stock speculation, making forecasts about future returns, buying "undervalued" stocks and vice versa. If, in principle, the entire economy shifted to index funds, then market efficiency would undoubtedly deteriorate drastically. This is somewhat related to the previous issue; if the entire economy shifted to index funds, agency problems would be exacerbated.

It is useful to view index funds as the product of an equilibrium. In a world where numerous economic agents compete for speculative profits, a state approaching market efficiency is obtained. Index funds are useful in this state. The appeal of index funds is closely related to the extent to which competition among speculators makes it difficult to obtain excess returns from active management.

If, in a country, there were too few speculators and too many index investors, then the rates of return in active management would significantly exceed those obtained through indexation. As yet we probably have not encountered this situation in any country.

Concentration in the Fund Industry

Earlier we commented on the role of signals such as pedigree, size, and years of experience as proxies for fund management ability, in a world where it is difficult to identify genuine ability. This serves to reduce the contestability of the money management industry.

While this problem is an important motivation for index funds, insofar as index funds lend themselves to easier monitoring of the actions of fund managers, the pressures towards concentration of the fund industry are even more acute with index funds. The basic problem is that index fund management itself is a fixed cost activity. Once computer systems are set up for managing a small index fund, the same systems scale up to much larger assets. The costs of sales and distribution also prove to be lower, per unit of assets, for larger funds.

This phenomenon has led to remarkably low fees for large investors: in the U.S. market, fees of 0.01 percent per year are known to be prevalent for assets of US$1 billion. However, this phenomenon serves to throw up entry barriers against a new firm that seeks to manage index funds. Hence we see a pronounced concentration in the index fund industry, with four-firm concentration ratios in excess of 60 percent (see table 9.1). Each basis point of fees on a US$1 billion of assets is a revenue of US$10 million. The major indexers seen in this table probably earn significant monopoly rents.

This is one negative consequence of the rise of index funds. Active management, in contrast, does not suffer from increasing returns to scale to this extent. On the contrary, many active managers view the management of large assets as an important handicap that makes it difficult for them to obtain excess returns. There is empirical evidence suggesting that the "optimal" size for a growth fund in the United States is around US$1.5 billion, for a value fund, around US$500 million, and for a blend fund approximately US$2 billion (Indro and others 1999). These modest sizes are in sharp contrast with the index fund industry, where extremely large funds dominate.

Index Funds in Developing Countries

In the context of a developing country, the four central questions concerning index funds are the following:

- Given the prevalence of inferior market efficiency, are index funds relevant in developing countries?
- Are the benefits of index funds inaccessible in developing countries owing to the greater tracking error that is faced because of illiquid stock markets?
- What implementation strategies should be adopted for index funds in developing countries?
- What can developing countries do in order to better benefit from the supply of risk capital through index funds?

Are Index Funds Relevant?

Most studies on the returns from active management use data for Organization for Economic Cooperation and Development (OECD) countries. While accurate measures of the size of the indexation industry do not exist, the available evidence suggests that 88 percent of existing indexed assets are located in the United States alone. To what extent do the arguments and evidence about index funds, which are well established in OECD countries, relate to developing countries?

Research in recent years supports the idea that significant differences exist in the character of price processes in emerging countries as compared with those seen in OECD countries. Emerging markets are considered to have higher volatility, higher long-term returns, higher transaction costs, and greater predictability (Bekaert and others 1998). If market efficiency in developing countries is systematically inferior, there may be greater opportunities for active managers to add value in the fund management process. Hence the case for indexation may not readily scale from OECD countries to emerging markets.

THEORETICAL ARGUMENTS

At a basic level there are three aspects that could lead to inferior market efficiency because developing countries differ from OECD countries:

- *Information Access.* Inferior disclosure laws, and an ill-developed information business, imply that information access in developing countries is inferior.
- *Human Capital.* Inferior human capital may imply that there are fewer economic agents that can arbitrate away mistakes in observed prices.

- *Transactions Costs.* Market mechanisms in developing countries often impose high transactions costs, so that what appears to be a breakdown of market efficiency at a statistical level is not actually a profit opportunity. To the extent that inefficiencies are not exploitable, net of transaction costs, market efficiency *holds* in an economic sense. The efficient market's hypothesis is only a statement about the absence of arbitrage opportunities in an economy populated by rational, profit-maximizing agents. To quote Jensen (1978), "an efficient market is defined with respect to an information set Ft if it is impossible to earn economic profits by trading on the basis of Ft."

If these three factors are at work in producing inferior market efficiency in developing countries, it does not necessarily imply that active management is a superior alternative. If information access is poor, then active managers would similarly suffer from the lack of information. The inadequacy of skills in the financial sector in a country would equally apply to firms that seek to do active management, as they apply to individuals engaging in stock speculation. It is not clear that active managers would somehow be able to tap into superior human capital. Finally, if market inefficiencies exist owing to high transaction costs, these inefficiencies are not profit opportunities for active managers.

The second section of the chapter showed an important motivation for indexation: the agency problems between investors and fund managers. These problems are present to a greater extent in developing countries, where institutional development is inferior and law enforcement in the financial sector is highly limited. This is a particularly important motivation for indexation in developing countries where the institution of the corporation, and the mechanisms for overcoming principal-agent problems between investors and fund managers, are poorly developed.

When a pension committee has to make decisions on behalf of workers in developing countries, the risk of a poor decision by the pension committee owing to ethics lapses is acute, and indexation is correspondingly attractive even if the index is not ex-ante mean variance efficient.

EMPIRICAL EVIDENCE

If the above arguments are sound, then the empirical evidence should also favor index funds in developing countries. Empirical testing in this area suffers from several constraints, notably the lack of a well-defined "emerging markets benchmark" and the short time-series.

The evidence in table 9.5 suggests that 73 percent of equity funds that invest outside the United States underperform a benchmark index, and 88 percent of funds that invest in "emerging markets" underperform the index. These fractions are not particularly different from those seen with index funds in OECD countries.

These results from table 9.5 should be interpreted with caution, for the data series only runs from 1993 to 1995. In a recent working paper, Muralidhar and Weary (1998) summarize the evidence on active management in various asset classes. Table 9.11 summarizes their results. For example, for the U.S. large-cap sector they find that the average manager underperforms by 42 basis points, net of fees, and imposes a tracking error of 4.8 percent on the investor.

For non-U.S. equity we see significant value added by active managers when the MSCI Europe, Asia, and Far East (EAFE) index is used. However, if the "EAFE–Lite" index is used (which attaches a lower weight to Japan), the excess returns vanish.

For emerging markets equity, Muralidhar and Weary (1998) present evidence over a somewhat longer period, from 1992 to 1997. Using the MSCI Emerging Markets Global (EMG) Free index, they find that active managers add value to the extent of 190 basis points per year, at the price of a tracking error of 8.4 percent. However, , for the following reasons this evidence does not necessarily imply that active management is a superior strategy in emerging markets:

- As Muralidhar and Weary (1998) point out, all their evidence is somewhat biased in favor of active management owing to the selection bias in which the funds that survive for the full span are likely

Table 9.11. The Value Added by Active Management

Asset class	Performance of active managers			Benchmark index
	Returns (%)	Tracking error (%)	Information ratio	
US large cap	+0.42	4.8	0.0	S&P 500
US mid cap	+0.91	6.9	0.3	S&P Midcap
US small cap[a]	+2.94	8.9	0.4	Russell 2000
Non-US eq.[a]	+4.00	10.5	0.4	MSCI EAFE
Non-US eq.[a]	−0.15	6.5	0.0	EAFE - Lite
Emerging mkts. eq.[a]	+1.90	8.4	0.3	MSCI EMG Free

Note: This table summarizes the evidence of Muralidhar and Weary (1998) on the performance of active managers in various asset classes. For each asset class, it reports the average extent to which fund managers outperformed the benchmark (net of fees), the tracking error with respect to the benchmark, and the average information ratio (annualized excess return divided by tracking error).
a. The evidence pertains to five years (12/92 to 12/97); for other categories it pertains to a 10-year period (12/87 to 12/97).
Source: Muralidhar and Weary (1998).

to be the funds with better returns. They describe empirical evidence that suggests that correcting for this selection bias reduces the apparent returns of fund managers in the EAFE universe by 170 basis points per year.

- The MSCI EMG Free index is not well established as a sound benchmark covering the emerging markets universe (see, for example, Masters 1998).
- From a sponsor's point of view, the tracking error is also an important concern. When a sponsor hires an active manager in this universe, the one-year returns (relative to the benchmark) could lie between –14.6 and +18.4 percent. This poses significant risks for the sponsor.
- The average excess return seen here is a mean of a small sample of 33 fund managers. In an environment with high background noise (the weaknesses of the MSCI EMG Free index and the high tracking error), the statistical precision of this average could be limited.
- This environment, with a high tracking error, makes it difficult to select an active fund manager, and exposes the sponsor to the agency conflicts discussed in the second section. In this sense the ex post average excess returns of fund managers in this asset class are not easily identifiable in an ex-ante sense.

In chapter 7, James, Smalhout, and Vittas have a set of regression equations in which a variety of variables explain the net return of funds investing in various asset classes. The explanatory variables used here are assets, squared assets, number of shareholders, assets in fund complex, three-year standard deviation of returns, a dummy variable if targeted at institutional investors, the size of the initial investment, variables about loads and 12b1 fees (in the US), turnover, a dummy variable for "bank advised," the age of the fund, and a dummy variable if it is an index fund. The dataset used here is drawn from the Morningstar database.

Table 9.12 summarizes the evidence that these regressions offer on the "index fund" dummy variable, after controlling for all the other variables described above. This shows negative coefficients in three sectors: U.S. small caps, international, and emerging markets. However, none of these coefficients are statistically significant.

These results are somewhat biased against index funds insofar as the dataset suffers from selection bias. However, the numerical results do suggest that the null hypothesis—that the average returns from index funds are similar to the average returns from active management—cannot be rejected. This is in contrast with the U.S. large-cap asset class, where this hypothesis can be conclusively rejected in favor of the idea that index funds yield higher returns.

Table 9.12. The Coefficient of the "Index Fund" Dummy in Cross-Sectional Regressions Explaining Fund Returns

	U.S.			Emerging
	Large cap	*Small cap*	*International*	*markets*
Coefficient of "index"	+2.61	−1.27	−3.57	−3.72
t-statistic	4.26	−0.45	−1.29	−0.39
Number of funds	580	218	480	96
Adjusted R^2	16.94	11.04	8.79	30.34

Note: James and others (2000) have a set of cross-sectional regression equations explaining the returns of funds by asset class. This table shows the coefficient of the dummy variable "index fund" in these models.
Source: James and others (2000).

Are Index Funds Feasible?

Some observers have expressed concerns that the inferior stock market liquidity and the weaknesses of stock market indexes in developing countries will lead to significant tracking error in index funds.

The evidence in table 9.8 suggests that program trading on some stock market indexes in developing countries is feasible, although the basket size that can be obtained in a day is obviously much smaller than that seen in the United States. Index funds in developing countries are likely to be formed of much smaller assets than those seen in the United States; hence, this is not a key constraint. The Industrial Development Bank of India (IDBI) Mutual has an index fund on the NSE-50 index, which has an annualized tracking error of 0.35 percent.[9]

How Should Index Funds Be Implemented?

Developing countries are characterized by significant concerns about stock market liquidity, low skills in modern financial economics, and ill-developed derivatives markets.

The concerns about stock market liquidity would emphasize caution in terms of being able to execute program trades on the index basket. In developing countries, it is not safe to make assumptions about reliably trading even the stocks in the largest quartile. For example, the IFC India index, which is not conscious about market impact cost in program trades, suffers from a market impact cost that is 82 percent worse than that of the NSE-50 index, when doing program trades of Rs.20 million.

The weakness in skills in modern financial economics suggests that optimization-based procedures may be hard to implement. Even if skills and software were to be transplanted from external sources, the factor models that are required for these optimization-based procedures are typically based on the research literature going over decades. Such knowledge is typically not available in the literature in a developing country.

The weakness in index derivatives suggests that index derivatives would not play an important role in implementing index funds.

Hence, the simplest situation is one where an index fund is implemented using full replication, and the index is free of stocks that are disproportionately illiquid. The methods of Shah and Thomas (1998), described in the third section, are designed to produce an index that suits these needs.

For countries that already have index derivatives, index funds that use full replication can greatly benefit, on the margin, from using a liquid index futures market. Index options can be used to construct a variety of guaranteed return products (Mariathasan 1997).

In each country a research program on models of asset pricing would create the knowledge and understanding of factor models that would lead to optimization-based procedures in the future.

What Can Policymakers Do to Enable Index Funds?

The primary role that policymakers can play in enabling index funds is in terms of building the institutional infrastructure that helps index funds. This runs over the issues of index construction, electronic trading, program trading, call auctions, and index futures discussed in the fourth section. From the viewpoint of pension reforms, to the extent that equity investment by pension funds is channeled through index funds, it would generate greater development of human capital in this area and a constituency for the reforms that would lead to this market infrastructure.

Pension Investment in Equities

In this section we link the ideas presented above more directly with the questions and concerns of pension investments.

Harnessing the Equity Premium

The basic motivation for equity investment by pension funds is based on the "equity premium," the excess expected return offered by the equity market (Siegel 1998). On 70-year horizons for which stock market indexes are observed in OECD countries, the real rate of return on the equity index is around 5–6 percentage points in excess of the real rate of return on fixed income investments. The existence of the equity premium is consistent with economic theory in which investors who bear the risk of nondiversifiable fluctuations should be compensated with a premium in the form of higher expected returns; however, the size of the premium seems to be difficult to explain (Mehra and Prescott 1985; Seigel and Thaler 1997).

The equity premium provides a powerful justification for pension invest-ment using equities, particularly when considering the long time horizons faced in pension investment. Over a 30-year horizon, investing at 1 percent in real terms (a typical fixed-income asset) yields a return of 35 percent, while investing at 6 percent in real terms (a typical stock market index) yields a return of 474 percent.

The empirical evidence about the equity premium is entirely based on the growth of stock market indexes observed over past decades. Hence, investment in the equity index is a direct method of translating this evidence into an investment strategy. The viability of index funds, and their ability to operate at fairly low levels of tracking error, suggests that this is indeed a feasible investment strategy.

The "Active Management Premium"

More generally, we could ask the question: can an actively managed fund result in the core equity premium (the returns to the index) and an addi-tional "active management premium"? The empirical evidence (tables 9.4 and 9.5) seems to suggest that we cannot reject the null hypothesis that the active management premium is zero.

The issues discussed in the second section are particularly important in the context of pension investment and serve as a motivation for favoring index funds even if the active management premium were positive.

Sophistication of Workers

In individual-centric programs most workers are not sophisticated in understanding performance evaluation of money managers. They are ill equipped to consume the results of performance evaluation, and hire the fund manager with the best ability.

Three-Layered Agency Problems

If a layer of intermediaries—in the form of a pension committee—is intro-duced, we would have a two-tiered agency conflict in which workers would need to devise institutional mechanisms to encourage committee members *and* fund managers to work in the best interests of workers. Devising incentive-compatible arrangements in this situation is not easy. In either scenario index funds offer a way to sidestep these problems by offering clear accountability while staying in tune with the basic goal of pen-sion investment in equities, which is to harness the equity premium.

Political Risk of Investments in Equities

Many observers have commented on the quasi-nationalization that might be implicit in large-scale pension investments in equities. It is easy to imag-ine that 50 percent of the gross domestic product of many countries could be invested in equities. In this case there is a risk that government could use this control for political ends. This is particularly important in countries that do not use individual accounts or give workers a choice of the fund manager.

By limiting the discretion with fund managers, index funds are a way to reduce this political risk. If pension investments exclusively took place through index funds, then fund managers would have very little discretion about how they would pick stocks.

Conclusion

In conclusion, index funds are an important investment strategy for investors who seek to harness the equity premium. The case for index funds has often been phrased in terms of market efficiency and the observed inability of active managers to outperform the index over long periods of time. In addition, the agency conflicts between investors and fund managers are also an important motivation for index funds, which benefit from simple and unambiguous accountability.

The equity premium gives us a powerful motivation for equity investment by pension funds. In this context, index funds make it possible to sidestep the complexities of forming contracts and monitoring institutions to govern fund managers.

In developing countries that seek to use index funds in pension investment, there are avenues through which policymakers can improve the viability of index funds. The issues faced here are primarily those of market mechanisms used on the equity market and the construction of the market index. In many countries there are significant avenues for improvement in these areas, which will benefit market efficiency generally and the viability of index funds particularly.

Notes

1. We acknowledge the financial support of the World Bank for this work. We are grateful to Estelle James and Dimitri Vittas of the World Bank, Susan Thomas of the Indira Gandhi Institute for Development Research, the participants of the conference entitled New Ideas about Old Age Security (World Bank, Washington, D.C., September 1999), the participants of the conference entitled *Asian Masters of Indexing* (Singapore, September 1999), and the participants of the *IIIrd Capital Markets Conference* (Unit Trust of India Institute of Capital Markets, Bombay, December 1999) for many ideas and improvements.

2. The concept of an "emerging market index" still appears to have many difficulties (Masters 1998). Table 9.6 shows related evidence for a

comparable five-year period. There are fewer conceptual difficulties faced with a stock market index pertaining to one country. Many countries have yet to embark upon large-scale international diversification as a part of their pension reforms. The local stock market index is obviously best suited to purely domestic performance appraisal. However, much of the empirical evidence about the performance of active managers (for example, table 9.11) is derived from internationally diversified money managers. However imperfect, we should use this empirical evidence while applying care in interpretation.

3. A similar argument is found in Ambarish and Siegel (1996).

4. There is empirical evidence that suggests that active managers produce inferior returns when assets under management cross a certain threshold (Indro and others 1999). Hence, if size is used as a signal of ability, and a sponsor is biased towards selecting the largest of funds, then this could introduce a bias towards inferior performance.

5. The ongoing management of the NSE-50 index set may be summarized as the following rules:

- Every stock outside the index is screened for liquidity as follows. In a scenario in which it was indeed the 51st stock in the index, program trades are simulated for buying Rs.5 million of this hypothetical index. The market impact cost faced on this stock is measured. If impact cost is below 1.5 percent with a 90 percent probability, over the last six months, the stock is considered eligible.
- A stock inside the index set is deleted from the index when it fails this same test: when the impact cost on this stock (in doing index program trades worth Rs.5 million over the last six months) exceeds 1.5 percent with a probability of 10 percent or more. The largest available eligible stock is used as a substitute.
- An eligible stock from outside the index displaces the smallest stock inside the index, even if the smallest incumbent stock is adequately liquid, if the incoming stock is more than thrice the size of the smallest incumbent stock.
- These rules are applied every three months to govern index set changes.

6. Liu, Sheikh, and Stefek (1998) offer an exposition of this procedure. Blin (1997) provides an example of applying factor models to solving this problem, of finding a 10-stock portfolio that is maximally correlated with India's NSE-50 index. Harrison (1991) offers an example of applying this to obtaining an index fund in New Zealand.

7. There is relatively little research on tracking error. Part of the problem here is that accurate measurement of transaction costs, with the market mechanisms prevalent in the United States, is difficult. For example, Larsen and Resnick (1998) discuss tracking error obtained through optimization but assume that there are no transaction costs.

8. For example, at http://www.utisel.com/livefeed, the market impact cost for doing index trades in India is displayed in real-time. It is calculated off the limit order book, which is publicly visible on India's National Stock Exchange, an electronic exchange.

9. Nayak (1997) documents the experience of the first index fund running out of India, on the NSE-50 index.

References and Bibliography

Note: The word *processed* describes informally reproduced works that may not be commonly available through libraries.

Ambarish, R., and L. Siegel. 1996. "Time Is the Essence." *Risk* 9 (August).

Bekaert, G., C. B. Erb, C. R. Harvey, and T. E. Viskanta. 1998. "Distributional Characteristics of Emerging Market Returns and Asset Allocation." *Journal of Portfolio Management*, 24 (Winter): 102–16.

Black, F. 1971. "Towards a Fully Automated Exchange, Part I and II." *Financial Analysts Journal*, vol. 27.

Blin, J. 1997. "Risk Structure in Indian Stocks," in T. Waghmare, ed., *The Future of Fund Management in India—1997*. New Delhi: Invest India–Tata McGraw-Hill.

Bodie, Z., A. Kane, and A. Marcus. 1989. *Investments*, 1st ed. Boston: Richard D. Irwin, Inc.

Bogle, J. C. 1998. "The First Index Mutual Fund," in A. S. Neubert, ed., *Indexing for Maximum Investment Results*. Glenlake Publishing Company, Ltd.

Cheung, H. 1999. "Investment Styles and Approaches: Active and Passive." Presentation at the conference on Recent Trends in Institutional and Pension Fund Investment Management in Asia, organized by the World Bank and the Hong Kong Monetary Authority, Hong Kong.

Chiang, W. C. 1998. "Optimizing Performance," in A. S. Neubert, ed., *Indexing for Maximum Investment Results*. Glenlake Publishing Company, Ltd.

Economides, N., and R. A. Schwartz. 1995. "Electronic Call Market Trading." *Journal of Portfolio Management* 21(3): 10–18.

Glosten, L. R. 1994. "Is the Electronic Open Limit Order Book Inevitable?" *Journal of Finance* 49: 1127–61.

Goldman Sachs Equity Derivatives Research. 1999. "The Dynamics of Tracking Error in Synthetic Index Strategies." *Global Index and Derivatives Quarterly*, 1–11.

Handa, P., and R. A. Schwartz. 1996. "How Best to Supply Liquidity to a Securities Market." *Journal of Portfolio Management* 22: 44–51.

Handa, P., R. A. Schwartz, and A. Tiwari. 1998. "The Ecology of an Order-Driven Market." *Journal of Portfolio Management* 25: 47–55.

Harris, L., and E. Gurel. 1986. "Price and Volume Effects Associated with Changes in the S&P 500 List: New Evidence for the Existence of Price Pressures." *Journal of Finance* 41: 815–29.

Harrison, A. 1991. "New Zealand's Index Funds." *BARRA Newsletter*.

Indro, D. C., C. X. Jiang, M. Y. Hu, and W. Y. Lee. 1999. "Mutual Fund Performance: Does Fund Size Matter?" *Financial Analysts Journal* 55: 74–87.

Jensen, M. 1978. "Some Anomalous Evidence Regarding Market Efficiency." *Journal of Financial Economics* 6: 95–101.

Larsen, G. A., and B. G. Resnick. 1998. "Empirical Insights on Indexing." *Journal of Portfolio Management* 24: 51–60.

Liesching, R., and V. Manchanda. 1990. "Establishing the Fund," in E. Bishop, ed., *Indexation*. Euromoney Publications PLC.

Liu, S., A. Sheikh, and D. Stefek. 1998. "Optimal Indexing," in A. S. Neubert, ed., *Indexing for Maximum Investment Results*. Glenlake Publishing Company, Ltd.

Lynch, A. W., and R. R. Mendenhall. 1997. "New Evidence on Stock Price Effects Associated with Changes in the S&P 500 Index." *Journal of Business* 70(3): 351–83.

Mariathasan, J. 1997. "Guaranteed Return Funds," in T. Waghmare, ed., *The Future of Fund Management in India—1997*. New Delhi: Invest India–Tata McGraw-Hill.

Mason, S., R. Merton, A. Perold, and P. Tufano. 1995. "BEA Associates: Enhanced Equity Index Funds," in S. Mason, ed., *Cases in Financial Engineering*. Prentice Hall.

Masters, S. J. 1998. "The Problem with Emerging Market Indexes." *Journal of Portfolio Management* 24: 93–100.

Mehra, R., and E. Prescott. 1985. "The Equity Premium: A Puzzle." *Journal of Monetary Economics* 15: 145–61.

Muralidhar, A., and R. Weary. 1998. "The Greater Fool Theory of Asset Management, or Resolving the Active-Passive Debate." Technical Report No. 98-020. World Bank, Washington, D.C.

Nayak, P. J. 1997. "An India Managed Index Fund," in T. Waghmare, ed., *The Future of Fund Management in India—1997*. New Delhi: Invest India–Tata McGraw-Hill.

Neubert, A. S., ed. 1998. *Indexing for Maximum Investment Results*. Glenlake Publishing Company, Ltd.

Roll, R. R. 1977. "A Critique of the Asset Pricing Theory's Tests: Part I." *Journal of Financial Economics* 4: 120–76.

Rubinstein, M. 1989. "Market Basket Alternatives." *Financial Analysts Journal* 45(5): 20–29.

Shah, H. 1999. "Pension Fund Investments: Individual Choice versus Control." Technical Report. World Bank, Washington, D.C.

Shah, A., and S. Thomas. 1998. "Market Microstructure Considerations in Index Con-struction," in *CBOT Research Symposium Proceedings*. Chicago Board of Trade.

Shleifer, A. 1986. "Do Demand-Curves for Stocks Slope Down?" *Journal of Finance* 41: 579–90.

Siegel, J. 1998. *Stocks for the Long Run*. McGraw-Hill.

Siegel, J. J., and R. H. Thaler. 1997. "Anomalies: The Equity Premium Puzzle." *Journal of Economic Perspectives* 11(1): 191–200.

Waghmare, T., ed. 1997. *The Future of Fund Management in India—1997*. New Delhi: Invest India–Tata McGraw-Hill.

10

Regulation of Withdrawals in Individual Account Systems

Jan Walliser

MANDATORY PENSION SYSTEMS BASED ON individual accounts are spreading around the world.[1] Following the Chilean example of the early 1980s, many Latin American countries including Argentina, Colombia, Mexico, and Peru introduced individual account systems in the 1990s. Eastern Europe and the former Soviet Republics in Asia constitute a second region with major reform activity, although reforms have been less far-reaching than in Latin America. The major driving force behind most reform programs was the imminent financial problem of the countries' traditional pay-as-you-go systems.

Under the new systems, workers set aside earnings in individual accounts, which later replace some or all of the previously pay-as-you-go financed pensions. During the accumulation phase, workers invest a percentage of their income in approved investment products. Following retirement workers withdraw the accumulated assets to finance consumption in old age. In addition to the retirement income financed with individual accounts (second pillar), the government generally offers a general-revenue financed benefit (first pillar) in form of a basic pension or a welfare program for workers without sufficient resources.

Much of the initial interest in designing the new pension systems has naturally focused on the accumulation phase. Details concerning how much money to set aside, where to invest it, how to regulate investment companies and investment portfolios, and what type of survivor and disability insurance to establish have drawn much attention. The Chilean system, for example, features a 10 percent contribution rate for individual accounts and imposes fairly tight regulation on investment portfolios, investment returns, and charges.

With the maturity of individual account systems, policy questions surrounding the design of the withdrawal phase will require more attention.

Standard pay-as-you-go systems generally offer an inflation-indexed pension for the duration of a worker's life. Can private insurance markets offer such a pension—called a life annuity—at reasonable cost? What flexibility should retirees have in choosing insurance products that convert their retirement account balance into retirement income? What form of government oversight and regulation would strike a reasonable balance between the interests of retirees and taxpayers who finance income protection programs? These represent some of the core questions confronting policymakers in reform countries.

The major conclusions of the discussion are the following. Optimal income allocation in old age depends on a large number of factors, including the income received from other pensions, bequest motives and family arrangements, health and long-term care issues, housing, investment portfolio choices, and inflation protection. Therefore, weak observable life annuity demand in many industrialized countries does not necessarily indicate insurance market failure. Nonetheless, government regulation of the withdrawal of account balances should ensure an inflation-protected stream of income for the retiree and potential survivors that exceeds income available from government welfare programs. More flexibility for the choice of insurance product could be permitted for the remaining account balance, helping to tailor income streams to individual needs and arrangements.

This chapter proceeds in two sections. first it discusses issues of consumption in old age. Starting with a simple model, it outlines different model extensions and their impact on the optimal consumption choice. The first part also reviews the importance of insurance market failure vis-à-vis other explanations for observable weak life annuity demand. Drawing on the conclusions of the first section, the second part lays out options for policymakers and weighs their respective advantages and disadvantages.

Income and Consumption in Old Age

Pension programs seek to provide a stream of income in old age that is sufficient to meet consumption needs. To evaluate which insurance products and withdrawal regulations could help to meet retirees' needs, it is important to gain an understanding of optimal choices and how they vary in different settings. A variety of circumstances, including uncertainty about the life span, the functioning of insurance markets, family arrangements, health risks, and fluctuations in the rate of return can affect old age consumption.

A Simple Model of Consumption Allocation

Suppose workers reach retirement age with wealth W_t, which includes the savings in individual accounts. Workers would like to allocate this wealth over the remaining years of life to ensure that consumption needs can be met. In deciding how much to consume in each year, workers take into account that they might die at the end of year t with probability $(1 - p_{t+1})$ and might survive to year $t + 1$ with probability p_{t+1}. People are assumed to retire at age 65, and the maximum life span is 120 years. Also suppose that the only assets available in the economy are government securities with a fixed rate of return of r. For simplification, assume furthermore that a utility function with constant relative risk aversion governs consumption choices C_t. Under these assumptions, a worker solves the following optimization problem:

(1) $$\max_{c} \frac{1}{1-\gamma} \sum_{t=65}^{120} (1+\delta)^{65-t} C_t^{1-\gamma} \prod_{s=65}^{t} \pi_s$$

(2) $$s.t. \ C_t = (1+r)W_t - W_{t+1}$$

(3) $$W_{120} \geq 0$$

where γ represents the utility function parameter that determines the degree of risk aversion and δ stands for the pure rate of time preference, the discount factor for future utility.

The model can be solved using the following standard first-order conditions (Euler equations):

(4) $$C_{t+1}^{\gamma} = C_t^{\gamma} \pi_{t+1} \frac{(1+r)}{1+\delta}$$

As shown by equation (4), optimal consumption growth depends on (i) the risk aversion of the retiree, (ii) the rate of return that can be earned in the market, and (iii) the impatience of the retiree, which in this case is represented by both the pure rate of time preference δ and survival probabilities π. Generally speaking, more consumption is allocated to those periods in which a retiree is more likely to be alive.

Because a retiree is uncertain about the actual length of life, he or she must self-insure against longevity risk by always saving some wealth for the possible continuation of life. As a result those workers who die before the maximum length of life leave some unintended bequests—wealth they were unable to consume owing to early death. The size of those unintended bequests depends on the actual age at death and the risk aversion of the retiree. The more risk-averse a retiree (the larger γ), the flatter is the desired consumption path and the more wealth is allocated to years with low survival probabilities.

Suppose an insurance company offers retirees a contract that charges them a premium Z_t in period t, pays an annuity a_{t+1} in period $t + 1$ if the retiree survives, and nothing if the retiree dies. Accordingly, the retiree's budget constraint (2) changes as follows:

$$(5) \qquad C_t = (1+r)W_t - W_{t+1} - Z_t a_{t+1} + a_t$$

A retiree facing budget constraint (5) would decide to either purchase annuities with all of his or her wealth or hold his or her wealth entirely in bonds. The retiree has the choice between two assets, bonds and annuities, and which of the two instruments is held depends on the relative rates of return, that is, the relationship between the safe rate of return r and the price of annuities Z. If $1/Z$ exceeds $(1 + r)$, a retiree would only purchase annuities because he or she could receive a higher rate of return $1/Z$ through full annuitization.

Actuarially fair and frictionless annuity markets would charge retirees a price $Z = \pi/(1 + r)$. The insurance company, taking into account the death of an annuity buyer, collects the annuity with probability $\pi < 1$. The insurer thus charges a price that is smaller than the inverse of the rate of return, or equivalently $1/Z > (1 + r)$. Accordingly, in a world with perfect insurance markets all retirees should hold their entire wealth in annuities. The latter permits retirees to avoid unintended bequests and reap a higher rate of return. Yaari (1965) first formalized the observation that full annuitization remains optimal under these circumstances.

The insurance against life span uncertainty offered by annuities can substantially increase a retiree's utility. The consumption path with annuities can be solved using the following Euler equations:

$$(6) \qquad C_{t+1}^{\gamma} = C_t^{\gamma} \frac{\pi_{t+1}}{Z_t(1+\delta)}$$

If annuities markets are actuarially fair and $Z_t = \pi_{t+1}/(1 + r)$, the Euler equations collapse to an expression that is independent of survival probabilities and simply reflect the rate of return and the pure rate of time preference. In other words, in allocating consumption the retiree does not have to consider the risk that in some periods he or she would have very little wealth to consume because of an unexpectedly long life span. Figure 10.1 shows the consumption path for a 65-year-old male assuming (i) survival probabilities from the 1996 life tables compiled by the U.S. Social Security Administration, Office of the Actuary (1999),[2] (ii) normalized retirement wealth of 100 units, (iii) a pure rate of time preference of 1 percent, and (iv) an interest rate of 3 percent.[3]

Figure 10.1. Consumption Paths with and without Annuities Markets

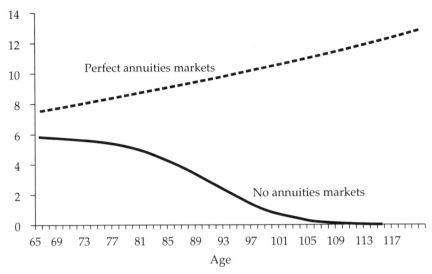

Note: $r = 0.03$, $\delta = 0.01$, $\gamma = 2$, 1996 life tables for the United States, retirement wealth normalized to 100.
Source: Author's calculations.

Table 10.1 illustrates the welfare gains arising from the existence of annuities markets for the same parameter values used for figure 10.1. Under those assumptions, men could gain between 65 and 110 percent of their original retirement wealth by having access to fair annuities, depending on the degree of risk aversion, and women could gain between 50 and 80 percent.

The large potential welfare gains from pooling longevity risk give rise to the question of why observable annuities markets are so small. In most

Table 10.1. Welfare Gains from Perfect Annuities Markets
(percent of wealth at age 65)

Gamma	Male	Female
2	65.8	51.6
4	78.8	60.8
10	96.9	73.5
20	108.5	81.5

Note: $r = 0.03$, $\delta = 0.01$, 1996 life tables for the United States.
Source: Author's calculations.

developed countries, many retirees hold substantial wealth in nonannuitized resources, and the market for private life annuities is very small. If there is so much to be gained from full annuitization, why are private annuities so unpopular? Three possible explanations emerge: (i) annuitization through government programs and employers, (ii) market imperfections, and (iii) additional factors determining consumption allocation in old age that are missing from the simple model outlined above. The latter two could also affect the regulation of the withdrawal phase in individual account systems.

Annuitization through Government Programs

Most industrialized nations already provide their retirees with annuitized resources through mandatory government programs or employer pension coverage. In the United States, for example, retirees generally receive income from old age and survivor Insurance and are covered by Medicare, the health insurance program for the elderly. Both programs reduce wealth bequests because they are financed by payroll taxes, which diminish income available for retirement saving. The resources that those programs offer depend on survival and can, therefore, cannot be turned over to potential heirs; in other words, by paying into the government retirement and health care system, potentially wealth bequests are transformed into annuitized wealth. Moreover, many employers offer private pensions, which constitute another form of annuitized wealth. An extensive study by Auerbach and others (1995) shows that the overall annuitization of American retirees ranged between 40 and 50 percent between 1987 and 1990. Similarly, a study by Gustman and others (1997) find that for the average U.S. household expected future government pension payments and expected future private pension payments account for 27 percent and 23 percent of net worth, respectively.

As suggested by the simple model presented above, government and private pensions do not alone explain why people refrain from annuitizing their remaining resources. In the model, annuitized resources diminish the amount of the potential wealth W bequest and increase the annuity stream a. Hence, the existence of government and private pension programs would lead to smaller disposable resources for retirees. In order to explain observed behavior, namely, the fact that very few people purchase private annuities in addition to pensions received from the government and employers, other aspects must be added to the model.

Studying the interaction between existing pension programs and annuity demand in industrialized countries is nonetheless important. First, those programs interact with annuities markets and may exacerbate market imperfections. Second, to the extent that observed behavior points at demand for annuities, it could give some indication about the demand for annuities in a system that replaces a government program with individual accounts.

Available empirical evidence for the United States does not support the notion that people wish to hold less annuitized wealth than offered to them by government and employers. In an actuarially fair insurance market, annuitization could be reversed through purchasing life insurance (Yaari 1965). Life insurance is a payment to one's heirs contingent on death, and purchase of life insurance, therefore, permits the conversion of a current stream of income into a lump-sum wealth payment. However, Brown (1999) finds that the pattern of life insurance holding does not support the conclusion that people attempt to offset mandatory annuitization by purchasing life insurance. Hence, the limited empirical evidence is consistent with the view that retirees value the annuities in their portfolios.

Market Imperfections

Insurance markets with imperfect information can give rise to adverse selection. An insurance is by definition a payment contingent on an uncertain event. Life annuities are income payments contingent on the annuitant's survival. Prices for annuities, as for other types of insurance, therefore, depend on an insurance company's assessment of the probability that an uncertain event occurs. However, the particular risk properties of an insurance customer may be unknown to the insurance company, although they are known to the customer. Because insurance is more attractive for the adverse risks (in the case of annuities, those with longer than average life expectancy), an insurance company cannot base its prices on probabilities for the average person but must raise its prices to account for the fact that bad risks purchase more insurance. That outcome, in turn, may reduce the attractiveness of insurance further for low-risk customers, who might decide to reduce their demand, necessitating further price increases by insurance companies, further reducing the attractiveness of insurance.

Rothschild and Stiglitz's (1976) seminal paper evaluated the equilibrium in insurance markets with adverse selection. They find that under certain assumptions insurance companies would segment the market into different risk classes, which would both receive insurance coverage at actuarially fair prices. However, insurers would restrict the insurance coverage of the good risks to avoid giving an incentive to bad risks to purchase the same contract. Eckstein, Eichenbaum, and Peled (1985) applied the Rothschild-Stiglitz insurance equilibrium to annuity markets. They show that mandatory annuitization might be Pareto-improving, and they argue that their finding supports Diamond's (1977) case for social old age insurance.

The Rothschild-Stiglitz equilibrium may, however, not describe annuity insurance markets well. As Rothschild and Stiglitz (1976) discuss in detail, their separating equilibrium relies on the assumption that insurers can restrict the quantity of insurance. While it is reasonable to assume that insurers can restrict basic insurance against automobile accidents or health problems because it makes little sense to purchase that insurance twice, quantity constraints may not be applicable to annuity insurance. Annuities offer a stream of income, and nothing prevents people from purchasing an income stream from different insurers to circumvent any quantity restriction. If insurers can control only prices and not the overall quantity, the price will be less favorable for low risks and more favorable for high risks than in a separating equilibrium. Moreover, the price will appear unfavorable for the average person in the population.

The economics literature shows that those who decide to purchase annuities live longer than average. Friedman and Warshawsky (1988, 1990) and, more recently, Mitchell and others (1999) demonstrate that life annuities in the United States tend to be more expensive than could be expected from average life expectancy. In particular, Mitchell and others calculate that for the average 65-year-old male, the value of an annuity stream is between 15 and 25 percent less than could be expected from average life tables. They also find that annuitants' living longer than the average American causes about half of that reduction, with overhead costs accounting for the remainder. Finkelstein and Poterba (1999) report that the value of voluntary annuities for 65-year-old males in the United Kingdom is between 10 and 15 percent lower than average life tables would predict. The annuitants' longer lives cause more than 60 percent of that reduction in value.

The observation that the value of annuity streams falls short of what would be considered actuarially fair for an average retiree could be attributed to two factors. The first, mentioned above, is adverse selection, which is the possibility that annuitants know more about their longevity than insurers and are thus more likely to purchase annuities. However, in both the United States and United Kingdom, longevity is tied to lifetime income, and richer people tend to live longer. Economic theory would predict that people with more income purchase more annuities. Thus, the fact that annuitants live longer than average could also reflect a second fact, namely, the income-mortality correlation. In other words, higher-income people buy more annuities because they have more wealth, and the observation that annuitants live longer than the average arises because higher-income people also tend to live longer.

Whatever the exact explanation for the observed longer lives of annuitants, the lack of actuarial fairness for the average retiree on its own cannot explain the small private annuity demand. Friedman and Warshawsky (1988) impose the observable gap between actual and actuarial fair annuities on a model similar to the one outlined above by increasing the price of annuities Z. They conclude that even in the presence of an annuity provided by a public pension program, prices would have to be much higher to prevent annuity purchases in the private annuities market. Walliser (2000) derives annuity prices endogenously in a simulation model of private annuity demand with heterogeneous agents and a public pension program. Such a model can reproduce observable differences between equilibrium annuity prices and actuarially fair prices (the so-called load factor) but does not drive people out of the annuities markets. Figure 10.2 shows the load factors for life annuities resulting from the interaction of optimizing agents differing in income and survival probabilities.[4] For example, the model produces equilibrium annuity prices for 65-year-old males that are about 8 percent higher than those derived from average survival probabilities. The magnitude of load factors corresponds to the load factors attributable to adverse selection found by Mitchell and others (1999). However, despite the lack of actuarial fairness for the average retiree, the model does not predict that people drop entirely out of the annuities market unless they wish to consume less than their public pension.

Figure 10.2. Percentage Increase in Annuity Prices for Males and Females over Actuarially Fair Prices (Load Factor) Generated by a Life-Cycle Model

Load factor in percent

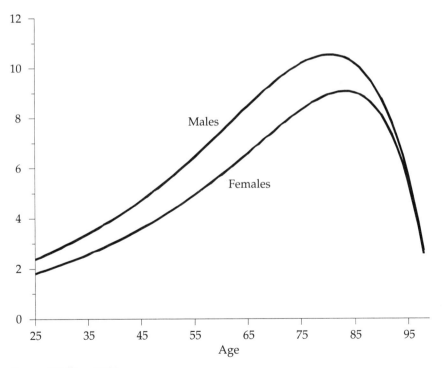

Age

Source: Walliser 2000.

Hence, market imperfections that raise annuity prices by the same per centage observed in the United States and the United Kingdom cannot on their own explain why people prefer to hold nonannuitized wealth.

A second possible imperfection of annuities markets stems from transaction costs. If renegotiating a contract every period involves sufficiently high transaction costs for the insurance company and the annuitant, long-term contracts may be an attractive option. Indeed, most annuity and life insurance companies face large costs from selling contracts through their sales force,[5] and most observable contracts are long-term arrangements. As Yagi and Nishigaki (1993) show, those contracts have the consequence that the annuitant may not be able to match the annuity payments to his or her consumption. Therefore, retirees must optimize their consumption path through additional saving at the interest rate r if they desire to increase consumption over time. Moreover, if annuity contracts are closed at one point in time, the rate of return an annuitant reaps from the contract will be constant over time rather than variable with conditional survival probabilities as in the model outlined above. As a result the annuitant would change his or her consumption path and allocate more consumption to the earlier years of retirement. Formally, a constant life annuity in an actuarially fair market would cost the following amount Z in each period t:

(7)
$$Z = \left(\sum_{t=65}^{120} (1+r)^{65-t} \prod_{s=65}^{t} \pi_s \right) / 56$$

The price Z for a constant annuity purchased at age 65 initially falls short of the time-varying price Z_t and later exceeds Z_t of an actuarially fair, time-varying annuity. As can be seen from plugging the constant price in equation (6), it would lead retirees to reduce their consumption growth and increase consumption earlier in life.

Bequest Motives and Intrafamily Insurance

Pensioners may want to leave bequests to their children or relatives for a variety of reasons. They might include, for example, their children's utility directly in their considerations, receive joy from giving money (without caring directly about the utility of their children), or use bequests as a disciplining device to receive attention and care in old age (Bernheim, Shleifer, and Summers 1985). Whatever the reason, the desire to bequeath reduces the incentive to annuitize wealth at retirement.

Consider the allocation of wealth between bequeathable and annuitized wealth with a joy-of-giving bequest motive as in Fischer (1973). Assuming, for simplification, that bequests enter utility in the same fashion as other consumption, the utility function (1) changes as follows:

$$(8) \qquad \max_{C,W} \frac{1}{1-\gamma} \sum_{t=65}^{120} (1+\delta)^{65-t} \left(C_t^{1-\gamma} + \frac{\eta_{t+1}}{1+\delta} W_{t+1}^{1-\gamma} (1-\pi_{t+1}) \right) \prod_{s=65}^{t} \pi_s$$

η_t stands for the relative utility weight of bequests made at the beginning of age t and W_t for the respective bequest, which equals nonannuitized wealth. The problem can be solved recursively from the last period of life when death is certain and the purchase of annuities would be irrational (see Fischer 1973, and Friedman and Warshawsky 1988). Figure 10.3 shows the paths of consumption and bequeathable wealth for different ages. With utility weights for bequests generating bequests of about four times annual consumption, actuarially fair annuity markets, and a risk preference parameter of two, about 60 percent of wealth would be annuitized at age 65. This share would fall with age. Moreover, overhead costs for annuities would reduce the attractiveness of annuities as would the existence of a social security program that provides annuity income (see Friedman and Warshawsky 1990).

Figure 10.3. Annuitized and Bequeathable Wealth in a Life-Cycle Model with Bequest Motives

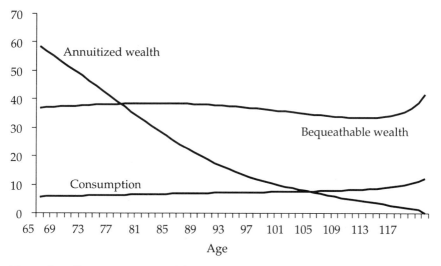

Note: = 0.03, δ = 0.01, γ = 2, 1996 life tables for the United States, retirement wealth normalized to 100.
Source: Author's calculations.

Family annuity contracts may be another reason why people refrain from purchasing private annuities. If family members jointly optimize their joint consumption path while taking into account individual survival probabilities, they could achieve substantial welfare gains over a situation without annuities markets. Kotlikoff and Spivak (1981) calculate that a two-person household with identical survival probabilities could achieve almost 50 percent of the utility level achievable with fair annuities markets.[6] The utility gain rises the more household members participate in the intrafamily insurance scheme, and those schemes could be more attractive if private annuities are costly owing to adverse selection or transaction costs.

Empirical evidence in the United States does not support risk sharing within extended families. Altonji, Hayashi, and Kotlikoff (1992, 1997) find that the pattern of consumption and income transfers between households belonging to the same extended family is not consistent with perfect risk sharing. However, the studies cannot rule out limited risk-sharing arrangements, for example, between couples, which would still crowd out life annuity demand, particularly in the presence of government and employer-provided pensions. Moreover, to the extent that families in less developed countries are larger and encompass several generations living together, implicit intrafamily insurance could be very important, with the concomitant decline in observable annuity demand.

Health and Long-Term Care Insurance

The discussion has thus far assumed that retirees face uncertainty about the length of their life. However, other risks loom in old age. In particular, health care spending and long-term care needs increase with old age. To the extent that insurance markets for health and long-term care insurance are imperfect, retirees might wish to keep a stock of nonannuitized wealth in order to meet sudden expensive medical care needs.

Significant extensions to the standard model are necessary to explain a rational nonpurchase of annuities. Simply adding health risks in a similar fashion as longevity risk to the above model without bequest motive would not reduce annuity insurance. If annuity contracts can be renewed annually, the retiree could still reap a higher rate of return by annuitizing all wealth notwithstanding the lack of health or long-term care insurance markets. However, as discussed earlier, transaction costs may lead to nonreversible long-term contracts. In that case, the retiree might not be able to meet the health care spending out of current income and might keep a buffer stock of nonannuitized wealth.

Lack of control over long-term care spending could also explain why retirees refrain from fully annuitizing their wealth. Richter and Ritzberger (1995) analyze a principal-agent model of long-term care insurance. If long-term care insurance is unavailable and retirees cannot control the quantity of care once they become frail, they must offer incentives to their caregivers to provide adequate care. If health risks and longevity risks are positively correlated, it can be shown that it is optimal not to annuitize all wealth. The result follows because holding nonannuitized wealth allows hedging against long-term care risks.

Portfolio Choice

Generally speaking, extending the model to include risky assets could not explain why people do not purchase annuities. The model outlined above assumes that only safe assets exist in the economy. Replacing a safe asset with a risky asset would not alter the analysis. The safe return r would simply have to be replaced with an expected rate of return, implying that the return to annuities would also be uncertain. If both risky and nonrisky assets coexist in the economy, annuities could be backed by a set of both assets reflecting the optimal portfolio allocation of the retiree, and full annuitization of wealth would remain optimal.

The portfolio of annuities may differ from the desired portfolio choices for two reasons. First, many governments offer some guarantees for annuity payments. In return for that guarantee, they impose certain portfolio restrictions on annuity companies to limit the risk of failure. As a result of those restrictions, fairly conservative investment portfolios could be required for annuities, and retirees might choose to purchase risky assets in addition to the annuity.

Second, the annuities backed by risky portfolios, so-called variable annuities that are offered in the United States, are investment-insurance hybrids. Because both the investment firm and the insurance firm charge fees, variable annuities tend to cost substantially more than investments in the underlying portfolio without an annuity component. As a result of the high costs, variable annuities have become more of a tax shelter for high-income savers than a product that insures against longevity risks.

Another portfolio risk stems from inflation. Few governments offer indexed bonds that could be employed to back an inflation-protected annuity. Moreover, in countries where they exist, the markets for inflation-indexed bonds are thin. As a result, very few annuity products protect against inflation risk. However, even if such products are widely available, as in the United Kingdom, they are reportedly not very popular among retirees. Brown and others (1999) calculate that the money's worth (expected discounted present value of the annuity divided by the price of the annuity) of inflation-indexed annuities in the United Kingdom is about 5 percentage points lower than the money's worth of standard annuities. That difference could be interpreted as the cost of inflation protection and is apparently more than many retirees will pay.

Policy Implications

The previous discussion demonstrates that the decision about consumption allocation in old age is complex and that many choices remain poorly understood. It is therefore difficult to draw a single conclusion or guiding principle from economic theory for the design of the withdrawal phase in individual account systems. Instead, policy recommendations for the design of the withdrawal phase in individual account systems should take into account a whole set of issues. How strictly withdrawals are regulated and which forms they take would depend on country-specific circumstances, including the way in which a society cares for its elderly and how large a role the government plays in providing a safety net and medical insurance.

The lack of annuity demand in industrialized countries is likely caused by a number of factors, and adverse selection is probably not the main reason why people refrain from converting their wealth into annuities. The evidence for the United States shows that annuitants have a longer life expectancy than those who do not purchase annuities. However, a similar outcome could result from the correlation between income and longevity and the link between the size of public pension benefits and longevity. Moreover, theoretical results reveal that unfavorably priced annuities alone could not explain the lack of demand. Bequest motives, self-insurance against health risks, the inability to adapt annuities exactly to the desired consumption stream, lack of inflation protection, and, most importantly, the existence of a public pension system all contribute to the weak demand for additional annuity coverage. Hence, regulating withdrawals should aim at more than simply avoiding adverse selection in annuities markets.

Regulation of the Withdrawal Phase

Most economists believe that the provision for old age consumption should be at least partly mandatory. The rationale for enforcing retirement savings is that workers may be myopic or would otherwise rely on publicly provided income support because the government cannot credibly commit to let retirees starve. That argument can be extended to the withdrawal phase of individual account systems. Insurance market imperfections would lend further support to government regulation of withdrawals.

A variety of insurance products could be considered to tailor withdrawals to a retiree's needs. In what way those products should be regulated depends on the size of other government programs, government guarantees for annuity firms, and equity considerations in annuity pricing.

Reasons for Government Intervention

Workers and retirees may be uninformed or myopic. Providing for old age and allocating savings requires forward-looking and rational choices.

Because of the complexity of choices, workers and retirees may fail to provide adequately for their retirement years. Bayer, Bernheim, and Scholz (1996) offer empirical evidence that educational support can markedly improve retirement saving choices. Similar arguments apply to the withdrawal of retirement savings. Moreover, retirees may simply be impatient and consume more of their retirement savings than would be considered prudent from a paternalistic perspective. Imposing rules on withdrawals would force retirees to act within boundaries set by the government.

The lack of forward-looking behavior may also result from explicit or implicit government income guarantees. If the government cannot credibly commit to ignore retirees without sufficient means, those with sufficient retirement savings may feel compelled to spend down their wealth and subsequently rely on government income support programs, a moral hazard created by government guarantees. Withdrawal rules would avoid the potential costs of a large retiree population drawing welfare benefits and ensure that retirement savings are used for consumption in old age.

Aspects of the insurance market may also warrant government intervention. First, government withdrawal rules may change the pricing of annuities by expanding the pool of annuitants and possibly limiting people from dropping out of the market based on private information. Accordingly, government intervention could limit adverse selection. Moreover, in many countries the government guarantees at least a portion of the annuity payments in case an annuity company fails. Because government guarantees could otherwise encourage overly risky investment strategies of insurance firms, some government regulation of insurance portfolios would be warranted.

Types of Withdrawals

The theoretical discussion in the second section focused on simple life annuities as a type of withdrawal. However, financial markets in industrialized countries have developed a whole set of annuity products. In general, those products can be distinguished by the following five characteristics (also see Poterba 1997):

- *The method of payment.* Some annuities must be purchased with a single premium (single premium annuities); others must be purchased with a series of annual payments (fixed-annual-premium annuities, flexible-premium annuities). Retirees in an individual account system would typically purchase their annuity with a single premium.
- *The number of people covered.* Annuities can be purchased for an individual (individual annuity) or several people (joint life annuities, joint and survivor annuities).
- *The waiting period for benefits.* Annuity payments can begin immediately after the purchase of the annuity (immediate annuity), or the

annuity can be deferred until a certain age is reached (deferred annuity). Both options could be attractive in an individual account system. Currently, individual accounts are typically converted into immediate annuities.

- *The nature of payouts.* Life annuities provide income until the death of the annuitant. A fixed-payments-certain life annuity provides payments until the death of the annuitant and also guarantees a certain number of payments even if the annuitant dies early. Refund annuities return a portion of the premium should the annuitant die before a certain date. Some annuities provide payments only for an agreed-upon fixed period of time so that payments may end before the death of the annuitant. Those annuities do not insure against life span uncertainty. They resemble so-called phased withdrawals, which divide the account balance according to the expected remaining life span.

- *The variability of payouts.* Annuity payouts can be fixed or variable. A fixed annuity guarantees a minimum payment. The "nonparticipating" fixed annuity pays a constant stream of annuity payments whereas a "participating" fixed annuity provides a guaranteed minimum payment and additional dividend payments that depend on the performance of the insurance company's investment portfolio. Variable annuities also rise and fall with the performance of the annuity insurer's investment portfolio, but they do not guarantee a minimum payment.

Issues in Regulating Withdrawals

For the reasons outlined above, economic analysts seemingly concur that some regulation of withdrawals is reasonable. However, such consensus does not cover the details of the regulation. The remaining part of this section addresses some specific questions that need to be answered.

Which portion of the account balance should be subject to withdrawal rules and which portion could be withdrawn in a lump sum? The portion of the account balance that should be preserved for withdrawal over time should depend on the generosity of other government old age income support programs. Imposing withdrawal rules on retirees has the ultimate goal of limiting the potential cost arising from government income support for the elderly. Hence, the withdrawal rules would have to cover only that portion of account balances sufficient to finance a level of retirement income above government welfare levels. For example, the Chilean government allows the lump-sum withdrawal of those funds that exceed the level necessary to purchase an annuity of 120 percent of the guaranteed pension level. Thus, retirees may reduce their income level compared to pre-retirement years by spending savings too quickly, but their income will remain high enough so that they do not qualify for government assistance.

How much higher the income from the individual accounts should be than a guaranteed minimum pension depends largely on the rules governing the income support system. Rules should be set so that the retirement income derived from individual accounts remains above guaranteed pension levels throughout retirement. For example, if guaranteed pension levels rise with productivity, they may catch up with income withdrawals from individual accounts if the latter are fixed in nominal terms. Moreover, pension guarantees may be smaller than what might be considered a comfortable level of consumption. Both reasons would support regulation that sets mandatory income withdrawal from individual accounts above the pension level guaranteed by the government.

Regulation could ensure participation in the insurance market and avoid any adverse selection. If only a portion of the account balance must be converted into an annuity or some other form of withdrawal, such regulation would effectively split the insurance market into one market for regulated withdrawals and one market for voluntary purchases. Clearly, both markets would interact. The market for regulated purchases would not be subject to adverse selection, but the market for voluntary purchases would likely be subject to even stronger adverse selection (Walliser 1997). Imposing a mandate on the entire account balance that would largely eliminate the voluntary market could avoid adverse selection but would restrict the flexibility of retirees to adapt income streams to their needs.

The extensiveness of the mandate depends, therefore, largely on the weight of the argument to ensure the functioning of insurance markets against the argument for flexible provision of retirement income. First, if the accounts provide a relatively small portion of overall retirement income, mandatory purchase of annuities or another form of withdrawal over time with the entire account balance would not restrict the ability to adapt income streams to consumption needs. (It would, however, affect the selection in the market for voluntary purchases.) If individual accounts accumulate a large proportion of worker's retirement wealth, more flexibility is warranted given the evidence that some generous pay-as-you-go pension systems may force retirees to hold too much wealth in annuities.[7] Second, the portion of the balance covered by the mandate hinges on the importance of the insurance market argument. Although people who participate in annuity insurance markets in the United States clearly live longer than other retirees, the extent to which private information about life expectancy causes this phenomenon is unclear. Further study of the experiences with newly emerging annuities markets is necessary to clarify that question. However, initial figures from Chile seem to indicate that annuities are a very popular withdrawal option (Valdés-Prieto 1998), especially among those with sufficient wealth to retire early.

Which Types of Withdrawal Should Be Permitted for the Regulated Withdrawal of the Account Balance?

One the major issue concerns whether to allow only life annuities or to permit other forms of withdrawal over time. Life annuities protect the retiree (and potentially his or her survivors) against the uncertainty about the length of life. Other products, which distribute the regulated portion of the account balance over a certain time span, do not offer such protection. For example, so-called phased withdrawals in Chile divide the remaining account balance (after a possible lump-sum withdrawal) over the expected length of life, taking into account the interest accrued over time.

Protecting government finances and ensuring participation in the insurance market would both suggest prohibiting phased withdrawals as alternatives to annuities. Because phased withdrawals do not protect against life span uncertainty, those with unexpectedly long lives could qualify for government assistance at the end of their life span. Moreover, phased withdrawals would allow those who expect to live only short lives to opt out of the annuities market and thus encourage adverse selection.

A second question concerns the types of annuities people should be allowed to purchase with the regulated portion of their account. As outlined above, annuities come in a variety of forms. Some annuities allow the refund of wealth to heirs, while others vary with the performance of capital markets. Refund- and period-certain annuities could raise the concern that they may lead to adverse selection in annuities markets because people who choose them presumably believe that they will not live long. They would therefore prefer to return some of the annuity premium to their heirs in exchange for a lower annual income payment. However, because those annuities protect the retiree against life span uncertainty, they do not raise any issue of moral hazard concerning government welfare programs. Thus, government could allow retirees to choose those options under the condition that the remaining income payments exceed the guaranteed pension by sufficient amounts. The resulting separation of the annuities market into subgroups would also support some self-selection of annuitants into risk classes.

Some restriction on the risk properties of so-called variable annuities is necessary. Most individual account systems impose some portfolio restrictions to limit the risk of losses, implicitly protecting the government's financial position. For the same reason, restricting the portfolio choices of retirees is in some ways warranted. One possibility would be to restrict the income variation to the portion of retirement income above the guaranteed minimum pension, similar to the fixed and participating annuities currently offered by the Teachers Insurance and Annuities Association in the United States. A fixed and participating annuity guarantees a minimum income payment for the remainder of life. The income is raised when the return of the underlying portfolio exceeds certain thresholds.

Inflation protection should be mandatory for at least the portion of accounts for which withdrawal over time is regulated. Otherwise, the real value of the pension could decline substantially and surprisingly, necessitating government support. To the extent that inflation protection is unavailable in the marketplace, the government might have to issue inflation-indexed securities to facilitate the market-provision of inflation-protected annuities. In some countries with limited financial market capacity for government securities, ensuring inflation protection may be a difficult task.

Withdrawals should ensure some form of survivor protection. Without sufficient regulation, some retirees could choose to tie the annuity only to their own survival. If their surviving spouses were without other means, the government would have to step in with income support. In essence, those retirees would free-ride on the government's income support program by choosing a higher annuity payment for themselves without protecting their survivors.

AT WHAT AGE SHOULD THE WITHDRAWAL BEGIN?

The withdrawal age poses the problems of portfolio risk and adverse selection. Unless the portfolio during the accumulation phase coincides exactly with the portfolio backing the life annuity, annuitization implies a portfolio change. Because of large fluctuations in equity markets, enforcing portfolio switches at one point in time may be perceived as unfavorable. However, it must be noted that unless equity markets have a mean-reverting property, predicting the market movement is impossible, and allowing retirees to choose the point of conversion themselves does not resolve the underlying portfolio risk. Thus, while allowing retirees to choose the age of conversion may give additional flexibility, it does not solve the portfolio risk problem. Instead, it encourages adverse selection because those with illnesses and shorter life expectancy will never annuitize their wealth or wait until the greatest possible age. The best solution to portfolio risk would be to limit the portfolio changes necessary at retirement by allowing annuity providers to offer variable annuities based on a variety of investment portfolios.

WHAT RESTRICTIONS IN PRICING ANNUITIES SHOULD BE IMPOSED ON ANNUITY PROVIDERS?

Annuity companies could attempt to separate annuitants into risk classes based on sex, marital status, forebears' longevity, income, and health habits. However, such pricing would cause conflicts between the protection of individual privacy and the informational demands of annuity insurers. For example, would insurance companies be able to use the results of genetic tests, or would that information remain private? The extent to which privacy remained protected would generally determine the ability of certain groups to reduce their annuity coverage based on private information about longevity prospects.

Equally difficult is the distinction between market separation and the perception of discrimination. For example, would insurers be allowed to sell differently priced annuities to men and women, or would unisex policies be required? Many may perceive it as discriminatory if women receive a smaller pension than men for an identical insurance premium. However, from a pure insurance perspective, a lower pension for women is actuarially fair because women tend to live longer than men, necessitating the provision of their retirement savings over a longer time span to provide income.

If annuitization is not mandatory, enforcing the same premium for different risk classes would make mandatory annuities unattractive to people with shorter life expectancy and exacerbate adverse selection. Specifically, if there are alternatives to full annuitization (phased withdrawals, for instance), those with shorter life expectancies might simply stay out of the annuities market, raising the price of annuities for other market participants.

If annuitization is mandatory, prohibiting the segmentation of annuitants into risk classes implies redistribution among different risk classes. If low-income retirees with shorter life expectancy pay the same price for an annuity as high-income people with above-average life expectancy, wealth is redistributed from the low-income retiree to the high-income one. If unisex annuities are required, resources will be implicitly redistributed from men to women, since women generally outlive men. Both types of redistribution could have substantial effects on the welfare of certain groups (Walliser 1997).

HOW SHOULD ANNUITY INSURERS' PORTFOLIOS BE REGULATED?

If policymakers implicitly or explicitly guarantee the annuity contracts offered by private insurers, regulation of annuity insurers' funds would be necessary to reduce the risk to the government. Annuity insurers are exposed to the risk that their investment portfolios underperform or their investments fail. As a result, a company may be unable to meet its obligations, and policymakers may feel obliged to assist retirees whose annuities' payments cannot be sustained. One possibility is to create some formal insurance for annuity companies. However, such insurance could lead to overly risky investment strategies of annuity insurers, unless it is properly priced or policymakers develop regulations to limit taking risks. Hence, if implicit or explicit guarantees are extended to annuity payments, policymakers might decide to restrict portfolio choices of annuity firms. Effectively, regulating the insurer's or the annuitant's investment choices (for variable annuities), as discussed above, constitute just two manifestations of the same issue: the entity that bears the risk may take on too much risk if the government offers guarantees.

Conclusions

Theoretical models of consumption in old age depend on a variety of factors, including uncertainty about longevity, health and long-term care, portfolio choices and risk, and bequests and intrafamily arrangements. Although there is considerable evidence that annuitants live longer than average retirees, the extent to which private information about life span uncertainty causes this phenomenon is unclear. As a result, the regulation of the withdrawals from individual accounts has to strike a balance between flexible arrangements that can accommodate individual circumstances and the reduction of adverse selection that may affect the pricing of insurance products.

Regulation should ensure a sufficient inflation-protected stream of retirement income with coverage of survivors. Annuitization of a portion of accumulated funds with some survivor coverage should be mandatory to reduce the government's exposure to welfare payments for retirees with insufficient means. However, some flexibility over the choice of annuities could be permitted, enabling retirees who expect shorter lives to purchase refund annuities. Funds exceeding the amounts necessary to finance a sufficient retirement income could be made available for lump-sum withdrawals. Such an option would allow the retiree to choose among a variety of withdrawal options and ensure that individual circumstances and needs could be met.

Notes

1. The views expressed in the chapter represent those of the author and not necessarily those of the International Monetary Fund. The author thanks Matthew Berger, Luis Cubeddu, Edouard Maciejewski, and Joachim Winter for helpful comments.

2. The life tables do not reflect future mortality changes. The results, therefore, should be interpreted as illustrative because they rely on a cross-section of survival probabilities.

3. For illustrative purposes, an increasing path of consumption is assumed for perfect annuities markets, resulting from an interest rate that

exceeds the pure rate of time preference. Alternatively, a flat or declining consumption path could be constructed by increasing the pure rate of time preference.

4. Another implication of his model is that the correlation between income and mortality, rather than classic adverse selection, causes a large proportion of the increase in annuity prices.

5. Warshawsky (1998) reports that in the state of New York sales commissions can be as large as the legally imposed limit of 7 percent of the annuity premium.

6. For a discussion of the demand for joint life annuities and the consumption allocation of couples, see Brown and Poterba (1999). Hurd (1999) discusses a life-cycle model for couples and the interaction between observable bequests and intrafamily insurance.

7. For example, Börsch-Supan (1994) shows that many German retirees save a substantial portion of their public pension income.

References

The word *processed* describes informally reproduced works that may not be commonly available through libraries.

Altonji, Joseph, Fumio Hayashi, and Laurence J. Kotlikoff. 1992. "Is the Extended Family Altruistically Linked? Direct Tests Using Micro Data." *American Economic Review* 82(6): 1177–98.
———. 1997. "Parental Altruism and Inter Vivos Transfers: Theory and Evidence." *Journal of Political Economy* 105(6): 1121–46.
Auerbach, Alan J., Jagadeesh Gokhale, Laurence J. Kotlikoff, John Sabelhaus, and David N. Weil. 1995. "The Annuitization of American's Resources: A Cohort Analysis." NBER Working Paper No. 5089. National Bureau of Economic Research, Cambridge, Mass.
Bayer, Patrick, B. Douglas Bernheim, and John Karl Scholz. 1996. "The Effects of Financial Education in the Workplace: Evidence from a Survey of Employers." NBER Working Paper No. 5655. National Bureau of Economic Research, Cambridge, Mass.
Bernheim, B. Douglas, Andrei Shleifer, and Lawrence H. Summers. 1985. "The Strategic Bequest Motive." *Journal of Political Economy* 93(6): 1045–76.
Börsch-Supan, Axel H. 1994. "Savings in Germany." In James M. Poterba, ed., *International Comparisons in Household Savings*. University of Chicago Press.
Brown, Jeffrey R. 1999. "Are the Elderly Really Over-Annuitized? New Evidence on Life Insurance and Bequests." Massachusetts Institute of Technology. Processed.

Brown, Jeffrey R., Olivia S. Mitchell, James M. Poterba, and Mark J. Warshawsky. 1999. "The Role of Real Annuities and Index Bonds in an Individual Account Retirement Program." NBER Working Paper No. 7005. National Bureau of Economic Research, Cambridge, Mass.

Brown, Jeffrey R., and James M. Poterba. 1999. "Joint Life Annuities and Annuity Demand by Married Couples." NBER Working Paper No. 7199. National Bureau of Economic Research, Cambridge, Mass.

Diamond, Peter A. 1977. "A Framework for Social Security Analysis." *Journal of Public Economics* 8(3): 275–98.

Eckstein, Zvi, Martin Eichenbaum, and Dan Peled. 1985. "Uncertain Lifetimes and the Welfare Enhancing Properties of Annuity Markets and Social Security." *Journal of Public Economics* 26(3): 303–26.

Finkelstein, Amy, and James M. Poterba. 1999. "Selection Effects in the Market for Individual Annuities: New Evidence from the United Kingdom." NBER Working Paper No. 7168. National Bureau of Economic Research, Cambridge, Mass.

Fischer, Stanley. 1973. "A Life Cycle Model of Insurance Purchases." *International Economic Review* 14(1): 132–52.

Friedman, Benjamin M., and Mark J. Warshawsky. 1988. "Annuity Prices and Saving Behavior in the United States." In Zvi Bodie, John B. Shoven, and David A. Wise, eds., *Pensions in the U.S. Economy*. University of Chicago Press.

———. 1990. "The Cost of Annuities: Implications for Saving Behavior and Bequests." *Quarterly Journal of Economics* 104(1): 135–54.

Gustman, Alan L., Olivia S. Mitchell, Andrew A. Samwick, and Thomas L. Steinmeier. 1997. "Pension and Social Security Wealth in the Health and Retirement Study." NBER Working Paper No. 5912. National Bureau of Economic Research, Cambridge, Mass.

Hurd, Michael. 1999. "Mortality Risk and Consumption by Couples." NBER Working Paper No. 7048. National Bureau of Economic Research, Cambridge, Mass.

Kotlikoff, Laurence J., and Avia Spivak. 1981. "The Family as an Incomplete Annuities Market." *Journal of Political Economy* 89(2): 372–91.

Mitchell, Olivia S., James M. Poterba, Mark J. Warshawsky, and Jeffrey R. Brown. 1999. "New Evidence on the Money's Worth of Individual Annuities." *American Economic Review* 89(5): 1299–1318.

Poterba, James M. 1997. "The History of Annuities in the United States." NBER Working Paper No. 6001. National Bureau of Economic Research, Cambridge, Mass.

Richter, Wolfram F., and Klaus Ritzberger. 1995. "Optimal Provision Against the Risk of Old Age." *Finanzarchiv* 52(3): 339–56.

Rothschild, Michael, and Joseph Stiglitz. 1976. "Equilibrium in Competitive Insurance Markets: An Essay on the Economics of Imperfect Information." *Quarterly Journal of Economics* 90(3): 629–49.

U.S. Social Security Administration, Office of the Actuary. 1999. *Annual Statistical Supplement to the Social Security Bulletin*. Washington, D.C.: Government Printing Office.

Valdés-Prieto, Salvador. 1998. "Risks in Pension and Annuities: Efficient Design." Social Protection Discussion Paper No. 9804. World Bank, Washington, D.C.

Walliser, Jan. 1997. "Privatizing Social Security While Limiting Adverse Selection in Annuities Markets." Technical Paper No. 1997-5. Congressional Budget Office, Washington, D.C.

————. 2000. "Adverse Selection in the Annuities Market and the Impact of Privatizing Social Security." *Scandinavian Journal of Economics*, 102(3): 373–79.

Warshawsky, Mark J. 1998 "The Market for Individual Annuities and the Reform of Social Security." *Benefits Quarterly* (3rd Quarter): 66–76.

Yaari, Menahem E. 1965. "Uncertain Lifetime, Life Insurance, and the Theory of the Consumer." *Review of Economic Studies* 32(1): 137–50.

Yagi, Tadashi, and Yasuyuki Nishigaki. 1993. "The Inefficiency of Private Constant Annuities." *Journal of Risk and Insurance* 60(3): 385–412.

11

Personal Pension Plans and Stock Market Volatility

Max Alier and Dimitri Vittas

SINCE THE EARLY 1980S THERE HAS BEEN a veritable explosion in personal pension plans. Such plans involve the accumulation of balances in individual accounts and their use in generating retirement income.[1]

Following the example of Chile, which pioneered systemic pension reform in developing countries in 1981, several other Latin American countries implemented similar reforms in the 1990s. These include Argentina (1994), Bolivia (1995), Colombia (1994), El Salvador (1998), Mexico (1997), Peru (1993), and Uruguay (1996). All of the reformed pension systems, despite considerable variation in scope and design details, entail as one of their main components the use of fully funded personal pension plans. More recently, several countries in economic transition, including Croatia, Hungary, Latvia, and Poland in Eastern Europe and Kazakhstan in Central Asia, passed legislation mandating personal pension plans as part of their national pension systems.

At the same time, there has been a growing use of defined contribution personal pension plans in various Organization for Economic Cooperation and Development (OECD) countries. In the United States, the authorization of individual retirement accounts (IRAs) by the Employee Retirement Income Security Act of 1974 stimulated the spread of personal pension plans. The authorization of employer-sponsored 401(k) plans in 1978 and the clarification of the tax treatment of these plans in the early 1980s provided a major boost. A further important development occurred in 1986 with the introduction of the Thrift Savings Plan for federal government employees. Although employer-sponsored defined contribution plans existed before the mid-1970s, 401(k) plans are now dominant. In the United States an early and highly successful example of personal pension plans is the system run by the Teachers Insurance and Annuities Association-College Retirement Equity Fund for college professors and teaching staff.

391

In the United Kingdom, as in other Anglo-American countries, specific industries once offered workers defined contribution plans, traditionally known as money-purchase schemes. Their use declined drastically after the high inflation of the 1960s. Defined contribution plans continued to be used on a small scale, especially in the form of additional voluntary contribution plans and pension plans for self-employed people. They became more widespread after 1988, when employees gained the right to opt out of both the earnings-related component of the state pension system and employer-sponsored pension plans. At the same time, companies in the United Kingdom as well as Australia, New Zealand, and South Africa started to convert their defined benefit plans into defined contribution ones, especially for new employees.

Among OECD countries, Australia and Switzerland stand out as the only ones that mandate employers to offer pension plans to all of their employees. Although employers are free to offer defined benefit plans, the minimum legal requirements are set out in terms of defined contribution plans, which has given a boost to the offer of defined contribution plans in these countries.

Finally, countries such as Malaysia and Singapore have long operated national provident funds based on individual accounts and defined contribution plans. Several other developing countries, especially in Africa and Asia, have also established provident funds.

The growth of personal pension plans has taken place despite the persistence of two major policy concerns regarding their ability to offer stable and adequate retirement benefits to covered workers. The first concern is that the plans transfer the investment risk of pension funds to participating workers and expose them to the volatility of financial returns. The second relates to the underdevelopment and apparent inefficiency of private annuity markets, even in the most advanced industrial countries, let alone in the developing world.

Traditional critics of pension reform have argued that because of the volatility of both equity and bond markets, personal pension plans would be unable to provide a satisfactory pension to all retiring workers. In fact, in countries such as Greece and Hungary that have suffered from repeated episodes of hyperinflation, widespread concern exists that a catastrophic collapse of capital markets might completely wipe out the real value of accumulated balances and leave retiring workers without any income. High inflation would also exact a heavy price from the annuity market. Hyperinflation would either erode the value of nominal annuities or lead to the insolvency of insurance companies. In either case, pensioners would be deprived of their regular income.

Finally, emphasis should be placed on the importance of maintaining low inflation and a stable macroeconomic environment for the successful operation of pension systems that rely on personal pension plans. But even with reasonable price stability, fluctuations in equity and bond returns could cause large differences in replacement rates for different cohorts of workers. Historical data from the United States show that replacement rates would have been highly volatile if extreme investment strategies involving undiversified portfolios (all equities or all bonds) had been followed.

This chapter, using the longest available data set (from the United States markets),[2] focuses on the impact of market volatility on investment returns and replacement ratios under various stylized scenarios.[3] It does not discuss the problems facing annuity markets.[4]

There are three aspects of the volatility of investment returns as it affects the replacement rates offered by personal pension plans: (i) fluctuations in annual returns and their impact on the replacement rates of different cohorts of workers, (ii) complete collapse of markets as a result of hyperinflation or other catastrophes, and (iii) occurrence of persistent deviations from trend, which falls between the first two in terms of magnitude of effects. The chapter makes the basic point that there are relatively easy solutions to the first aspect of volatility (short-term fluctuations with quick reversion to the mean) but not to the second and third aspects, which present more daunting and persistent problems.

Managing Volatility

Without corrective measures, there can be very large fluctuations in replacement rates among retiring workers of different cohorts. Workers retiring in a year when equity and bond markets are booming would obtain a much higher pension than workers retiring when markets are stagnating. For instance, assuming an all domestic equity strategy, American workers who had invested their balances in a personal plan and retired in 1999 would have achieved a replacement rate more than 180 percent greater than workers who retired in 1995. This is because U.S. equities had a cumulative total return of over 180 percent between 1994 and 1998. In contrast, workers who retired in 1975 would have received a replacement rate that would have been nearly 50 percent lower than that obtainable in 1973, since the total real return on equities was negative 21 percent in 1973 and negative 34 percent in 1974. Similarly, Japanese workers that had invested in an all-domestic equity personal pension plan would have achieved a much lower replacement ratio in 1990 compared to 1989, since equity prices in Tokyo fell by 60 percent in 1990.

These would be very large fluctuations in replacement rates that could justify the concerns expressed by critics of personal pension plans. Because developing countries have shallower markets, the volatility of returns could be even higher, further weakening the case for systemic pension reform. However, various alternative strategies could be followed to mitigate the impact of high volatility in annual investment returns and, by extension, in the replacement rates of successive cohorts of retiring workers.[5] Some of these strategies are simple and can be implemented in any market environment, while others are more complex and require well-developed derivatives markets, the use of synthetic products, and highly sophisticated investment techniques. The simpler strategies, some of which are already practiced in a number of countries, include the following: balanced portfolios, gradual late shift to bonds, gradual purchase of fixed (nominal or real) annuities, use of phased withdrawals or purchase of variable annuities, and use of derivatives and synthetic products.

Balanced Portfolios

The first and most prominent strategy would be portfolio diversification. By investing in balanced portfolios of equities, bonds, and money market instruments, the volatility of returns during the accumulation period can be substantially reduced. This is common practice in most employer-sponsored private pension funds, especially in the United States where government regulations linked to the guarantee of pension benefits impose minimum funding requirements and force sponsoring employers to adopt conservative investment policies or to compensate for any shortfalls in pension reserves resulting from large fluctuations in asset prices. In several continental European countries, including Germany, the Netherlands, and Switzerland, government regulations impose quantitative limits on investment allocations that aim to reduce volatility (even though in most cases employers operate defined benefit plans and absorb the investment risk).[6] In Latin America, most countries have followed the example of Chile and have imposed upper limits on different classes of assets.

There is a trade-off between volatility (risk) and return. A less volatile portfolio would normally imply a lower return and a lower corresponding replacement rate and pension. The cost of lowering portfolio volatility can be quite significant if the equity premium is high, as has been the case in the United States and some European countries.[7] Volatility may also be reduced by investing in overseas assets, which diversifies country risk.

Gradual Late Shift to Bonds

A second strategy could involve switching gradually and progressively from an all-equity portfolio to a bond portfolio a few years before reaching retirement age. In this case the cost of lower volatility, measured in terms of lower average lifetime returns, can be minimized compared to the first option. This option could avoid exposure to serious equity market downturns at the end of the active life, when most of the pension fund has been accumulated and the worker does not have a great deal of time to make up any losses. The solution proposed here consists basically of having age-specific pension funds: those for younger workers investing mostly in equities and those for older workers investing a high proportion of their assets in government bonds. Both Chile and Mexico are contemplating the use of age-specific pension funds.[8]

Gradual Purchase of Fixed (Nominal or Real) Annuities

A third strategy could entail the gradual purchase over a number of years (say, five years before retirement) of several fixed (nominal or real) annuities. The annuities would start making payments as of the date of retirement. If five installments were used, four of the annuity contracts would be deferred annuities, starting to make payments not immediately after purchase but some time later. The United Kingdom already allows a gradual purchase of fixed annuities.[9]

Use of Phased Withdrawals or Purchase of Variable Annuities

A fourth solution could involve the use of phased withdrawals and/or purchase of variable annuities. Several countries, especially in the British Commonwealth, allow workers to withdraw the accumulated balances in their individual accounts in one lump sum. In contrast, the mandatory systems of Chile, Argentina, and other Latin American countries do not offer workers the option of withdrawing a lump sum (except for balances that exceed targeted pension levels). In these countries retiring workers can either purchase a fixed annuity (real in the case of Chile but nominal in the case of Argentina) from an insurance company or start a series of phased withdrawals from their pension fund accounts. Phased withdrawals take account of the life expectancy of retiring workers and their dependents but do not provide longevity insurance. Under the phased withdrawal option, workers obtain a market-related return on their declining balances. They are protected from low asset prices and low returns that might prevail at the time of their retirement and also benefit during their retirement from the higher returns offered by fund managers compared to providers of fixed annuities (perhaps because of a continuing equity premium). Variable annuities operate like phased withdrawals but they also provide longevity insurance.

Both phased withdrawals and variable annuities expose workers to the volatility of investment returns during their retirement years. Combining either of these approaches with the purchase of fixed annuities or investments in less risky assets would mitigate this risk. Combining them with purchase of a deferred fixed annuity that becomes effective at age 75 or 80 would probably provide a more economical solution with longevity insurance.

Use of Derivatives and Synthetic Products

In addition to these solutions that can be implemented without relying on sophisticated financial engineering, there are two other possibilities that involve the use of synthetic products and derivative financial contracts. Bodie and Crane (1998) and Bodie (1998) have analyzed the use of investment instruments that provide a floor on the value of a worker's assets over some period of time and also provide some share of the upside potential of the equity market as a means of protecting workers from the volatility of stock market returns.

An even more intriguing possibility is the use of portfolio insurance, such as that gained through the purchase of European put options, to protect the value of the balances of all workers who would be retiring within, say, a period of five years. The exercise price for these options could be equal to the current level of stock market prices or to a level that is 5 or even 10 percent lower. Thus a floor would be set on the impact of any market downturn.

The counterparts to the put options contracts could well be the very same pension fund management companies, although they would act on behalf of their younger cohorts. In other words, the put option contracts could be based on an intergenerational contract that would be similar in some respects to the contract that exists for social security systems, albeit with a very big difference. The put option contracts would be executed through the markets and their terms and conditions would be adjusted continuously in response to changing demand and supply factors. Such a solution would not be subject to the political pressures that cause a financial imbalance to arise, persist, and worsen before corrective action is taken, as has historically been the case with social security systems.[10]

It is of course unrealistic to suggest the use of put options and synthetic products in countries where capital markets are thin and underdeveloped. However, the growth of pension funds is likely to have a major positive impact on the development of capital markets. Thus, when the need to purchase portfolio insurance through put options is felt more strongly, which is likely to happen when pension funds reach a stage of maturity, the capital markets could have developed sufficient size and depth to be able to offer such sophisticated products.

Another way of providing a floor to the replacement rate is for the government to provide a minimum pension guarantee. This tends to be offered in countries, such as Chile, that have decided to close down the unfunded public pillar, but not in countries that continue to operate a first pillar, such as Argentina, since the public pension would provide a floor to the replacement rate. However, even in the former countries, the minimum pension guarantee is expressed either in absolute terms and adjusted on an ad hoc basis or in relation to average earnings. The minimum guaranteed replacement rate for high-income workers is much lower than for low-income ones.

The guarantee, which is provided free of charge, is financed from general revenue taxes and is available to workers with a minimum period of contributions (20 years in the case of Chile). These state guarantees protect low-income workers from the volatility of investment returns but offer limited protection to high-income workers. They are not, therefore, a substitute to the alternative approaches mentioned above. Like all state guarantees, they suffer serious problems of moral hazard.

Methodology

Despite the growing interest and attractiveness of defined contribution pension plans, there is not much empirical evidence to allow a systematic exploration of the impact of stock market volatility on replacement rates. The Chilean system has been in existence for some 18 years, which covers less than one-third of the 60-year span of the underlying pension contract and is still too short for drawing firm conclusions on the problems that might be caused by the volatility of investment returns.[11] Moreover, the number of old age pensioners is still very small. In the United States, defined contribution plans have grown at a dramatic rate over the past 15 years or so, a period, again. too short to allow empirical investigation.

Faced with a lack of directly relevant data, we use historical U.S. data to illustrate the effects of the solutions proposed in the previous section. First, we present simulations of what the performance of a defined contribution, fully funded pension scheme would have been over the past 126 years in the United States. The simulations assume that workers contribute 10 percent of their income for 40 years and live in retirement for 20 years. We calculate the capital accumulation ratios (the total accumulated capital divided by the final wage) and the replacement rates (the pension divided by the final wage) by using two basic types of annuities: real annuities in which the discount rate is equal to 2.5 percent,[12] and nominal annuities in which the discount rate is the 15-year bond yield prevailing at the time of retirement. In the case of nominal annuities, we report both the first-year and average replacement rates, since inflation erodes the real value of nominal annuity payouts. We abstract from all the complexities caused by differences in life expectancies, while for the sake of additional simplicity and because they are not the focus of the chapter, we do not take account of the operating fees and commissions charged by insurance companies and pension fund managers.[13]

Because the accumulation lasts for 40 years, we effectively have replacement rates for 86 cohorts. We compare the results with the hypothetical case (baseline) in which the return on pension fund investments is constant over time. The aim of this simulation is to analyze the deviations of actual

returns from the baseline case—their magnitude, frequency, and persis
tence. Then we evaluate the various solutions mentioned above using the
same approach.

In a defined contribution pension plan, three factors determine the value
of the accumulated capital of workers: the length of active life, the level of
contributions (which in turn depends on the contribution rate and the
wage level), and the net returns on pension fund investments. The capital
accumulation ratio is invariant to the use of real or nominal returns. The
annuity that retiring workers can purchase with their accumulated capital
depends on their life expectancy at retirement and the rate of interest that
is used to discount future payments. In the case of nominal annuities, the
annual replacement rate is eroded by inflation, and for this reason we
focus on the average replacement rate over a worker's retirement life.

Workers usually have some control over the first two factors (the length
of active life and level of contributions). The law establishes a normal
retirement age but does not preclude workers from working beyond that
age or from retiring early. There is also a minimum contribution rate to the
pension fund, but workers can contribute more or build up additional voluntary savings outside their pension account. By contrast, workers have no
control over the returns on financial assets or over interest rates. The solutions described in the previous section aim to mitigate the impact of the factors not controlled by workers but whose volatility can make an important
difference in the replacement rates that different workers obtain. The analysis assumes that workers adopt passive investment policies, investing in
indexed funds for the three main types of instruments and setting different asset allocation strategies for life with no opportunistic changes at different points in time. Nor does the analysis consider stock selection or market timing.

The simulations illustrate the replacement rate that workers would have
obtained from their individual retirement accounts had they regularly
saved a given percentage of their income during their active life, followed
the investment strategy, and purchased the annuity highlighted in each simulation. The simulations focus on the effects of the level and volatility of
asset returns on pension fund performance and on the replacement rates
that would be attainable under the specified terms. In order to isolate these
effects, we assume that participating workers from each cohort have earnings that increase over their active life at the average rate of wage growth,
obtained from historical series of earnings in the manufacturing sector.[14]
In order to allow for the upward sloping career-earning profiles of most
workers, we add 1 percentage point to each year's growth rate of wages.
The simulations also assume that the number of participating workers is
small enough to have no effect on the level and volatility of market returns.

The two baseline cases for the real and nominal annuities use the weighted average real and nominal returns on equities, bonds, and commercial paper with weights equal to 60 percent, 30 percent, and 10 percent, respectively. This is equal to 5.66 percent per annum in real terms and 7.69 percent in nominal terms.

Data

Sylla and Wilson provided the historical series of financial asset returns.[15] The database, which covers the period from 1871 to 1995, contains series for total nominal returns on Standard & Poor (S&P) stocks, 15-year U.S. bonds, and commercial paper. It also has series for the yield on U.S. bonds and commercial paper. To obtain the ex-post total real returns on these assets, we deflated the data with the Consumer Price Index.

The first three columns of tables 11.1 through 11.3 present some summary statistics of the inflation-adjusted Sylla-Wilson data for five, 25-year subperiods.[16] The final column represents the performance of an investment fund holding stocks, bonds, and commercial paper in proportions of 60 percent, 30 percent, and 10 percent, respectively.

The geometric average real return on equities for the whole period amounted to 6.87 percent against 2.81 percent for bonds and 3.11 percent for commercial paper. The balanced portfolio consisting of 60 percent equities, 30 percent bonds, and 10 percent commercial paper had an average return of 5.66 percent. Stocks were more volatile than the debt instruments or the balanced portfolio. The balanced portfolio had a lower return and

Table 11.1. Real Total Returns on Alternative Investments, Geometric Average, 1871–1995
(percentage)

Period	S&P stocks	15-year U.S. bonds	Commercial paper	Combination 60-30-10
1871–1895	6.84	6.89	7.69	7.15
1896–1920	3.78	−0.20	1.79	2.72
1921–1945	9.24	4.92	2.86	8.06
1946–1970	8.01	−1.25	0.45	4.79
1971–1995	6.55	3.93	2.90	5.67
Overall	6.87	2.81	3.11	5.66

Sources: Authors' calculations based on revised and updated data from Wilson and Jones (1987a, 1987b, 1997) and Sylla, Wilson, and Jones (1990, 1994). Data provided by R. Sylla and J. Wilson.

Table 11.2. Real Total Returns on Alternative Investments, Arithmetic Average, 1871–1995
(percentage)

Period	S&P stocks	15-year U.S. bonds	Commercial paper	Combination 60-30-10
1871–1895	7.72	6.93	7.73	7.48
1896–1920	5.60	0.01	1.95	3.56
1921–1945	12.15	5.28	3.10	9.18
1946–1970	9.33	−1.04	0.54	5.34
1971–1995	7.92	4.70	2.94	6.45
Overall	8.54	3.18	3.25	6.40

Sources: Authors' calculations based on revised and updated data from Wilson and Jones (1987a, 1987b , 1997) and Sylla, Wilson, and Jones (1990, 1994). Data provided by R. Sylla and J. Wilson.

Table 11.3. Real Total Returns on Alternative Investments, Standard Deviation, 1871–1995

Period	S&P stocks	15-year U.S. bonds	Commercial paper	Combination 60-30-10
1871–1895	0.1430	0.0311	0.0290	0.0875
1896–1920	0.1982	0.0640	0.0568	0.1337
1921–1945	0.2451	0.0904	0.0722	0.1539
1946–1970	0.1759	0.0658	0.0417	0.1096
1971–1995	0.1666	0.1328	0.0305	0.1289
Overall	0.1871	0.0883	0.0539	0.1242

Sources: Authors' calculations based on revised and updated data from Wilson and Jones (1987a, 1987b, 1997) and Sylla, Wilson, and Jones (1990, 1994). Data provided by R. Sylla and J. Wilson.

lower volatility than equities but a higher return and higher volatility than either of the debt instruments.

From an overall perspective commercial paper dominated bonds. For the whole period, the average return on commercial paper was higher, and the standard deviation lower, than for bonds. During the first subperiod 1871–1895, commercial paper also dominated stocks. This reflects the relative stage of development of U.S. financial markets at the end of the last century. Returns on commercial paper declined drastically in the subsequent periods. During the last subperiod, the variance of bond returns more than doubled compared to the earlier subperiod, reaching a level very close to the volatility of equity returns and more than four times the variance of commercial paper returns. These data suggest that for the whole period under review commercial paper was safer than government bonds. Allowing for the premium for inflation risk, which is higher for non-indexed, longer-term instruments, the risk-adjusted real return on commercial paper was even higher than the risk-adjusted real return on bonds.

For most of the period, there was a persistent premium of equity over bond returns. It was particularly high during the 25-year period from 1946 to 1970 (more than 9 percent) but fell to 2.6 percent in the subperiod 1971–95. Over the whole period the equity premium exceeded 4 percent.

The returns of the three classes of assets were positively correlated over the sample period (table 11.4). The correlation in the returns of equities and bonds was particularly high during the two subperiods when the equity premium was relatively low, suggesting that the benefits of diversification and holding bonds in order to hedge the risk of equities were rather limited.

Historical real equity returns fluctuated widely. Although over 25-year subperiods the fluctuation in the average return was not very high—ranging between a low of 3.78 percent for the 1896–1920 subperiod and a high of 9.24 percent during the 1921–1945 subperiod, there were shorter periods during which cumulative returns were either highly negative or highly positive. They were highly negative during 1915–1920, when they registered a cumulative fall of 44 percent; 1928–1931, when they fell by 57 percent; and 1972–1974, when they declined by 48 percent. Periods during which positive cumulative returns were very large include 1921–1922 (70 percent), 1924–1928 (234 percent), 1949–1952 (95 percent), 1954–1955 (90 percent), 1963–1965 (54 percent), and 1995–1998 (183 percent). These large cumulative fluctuations have important implications for replacement rates achieved by defined contribution personal pension plans.

Table 11.4. Real Total Returns on Alternative Investments, Correlations, 1871–1995

Period	Stocks – bonds	Stocks – commercial papers	Bonds – commercial papers
1871–1895	0.2106	–0.3512	0.5614
1896–1920	0.5964	0.2939	0.8886
1921–1945	0.1333	–0.0599	0.8501
1946–1970	0.0233	0.2949	0.6792
1971–1995	0.5848	0.3506	0.6076
Overall	0.3006	0.0862	0.6879

Sources: Authors' calculations based on revised and updated data from Wilson and Jones (1987a, 1987b, 1997) and Sylla, Wilson, and Jones (1990, 1994). Data provided by R. Sylla and J. Wilson.

The index of real wages is based on three historical series on remuneration in the manufacturing sector deflated by the Consumer Price Index. First, from 1891 to 1900 the series relies on average weekly hours and average hourly earnings in the manufacturing sector (identified as series 765 and 766 in U.S. Department of Commerce 1975) Secondly, from 1900 to 1948 the data correspond to the average annual earnings per full-time employee in the manufacturing sector (series 740 in U.S. Department of Commerce 1975). Finally, from 1949 to 1992 the data come from the National Income and Product Accounts, line manufacturing in tables 6.6b and 6.6c (U.S. Department of Commerce 1993).

The last two series, 1900–1948 and 1949–1992, are perfectly compatible, but the first one is not entirely compatible with the others and must be interpreted carefully. In order to have a series on real earnings covering the period 1871–1995, we extrapolated the overall average real growth rate of earnings (1.5 percent per annum) of the series 1891–1992 to the periods 1871–1890 and 1993–1995.

Table 11.5 presents some summary statistics on the growth rate of real earnings during 1871–1995 according to the index constructed with the data described above. This series is the one used in the simulations presented in this chapter. As already noted, in our simulations we add 1 percentage point in each year to reflect the age-related growth of wages.

Simulations with Real Annuities

To facilitate the discussion of our results, we first present our simulations using real annuities and then report the results of using nominal annuities. The real annuities are based on a 2.5 percent real rate of discount and make no allowance for differences in life expectancy.[17] For each case we report the capital accumulation ratio and the replacement rates. We show

Table 11.5. Real Earnings Growth Rate, 1871–1995

Period	Arithmetic average (percentage)	Geometric average (percentage)	Standard deviation
1871–1895	1.49	1.49	0.56
1896–1920	1.73	1.61	5.13
1921–1945	2.11	2.00	4.78
1946–1970	1.84	1.75	4.21
1971–1995	0.73	0.72	1.74
Overall	1.58	1.51	3.75

Source: Authors' calculations based on U.S. Department of Commerce (1975), series 765, 766, and 740.

the results for undiversified and balanced portfolios and then discuss the impact of undertaking three alternative strategies: a gradual late shift into bonds, a gradual purchase of annuities, and a purchase of variable annuities.

Undiversified and Balanced Funds

This section explores the performance of pension funds under four alternative portfolio strategies. Under each strategy the portfolio composition is the same every year. In the first two strategies there is no portfolio diversification among equities, bonds, and commercial paper—the individual accounts hold only equities (100-0-0) or only bonds (0-100-0). The last two strategies consist of accounts with balanced portfolios, holding combinations of equities, bonds, and commercial paper. The first combination is 60 percent, 30 percent, and 10 percent (60-30-10), respectively, and the second is 30 percent, 60 percent, and 10 percent (30-60-10). The last two strategies are part of the first type of corrective measures described in the introduction. In the United States private pension funds have a portfolio composition similar to the 60-30-10 strategy, while in Chile the portfolio composition is closer to 30-60-10.

In the baseline case, where the accounts obtain a fixed return of 5.66 percent every period, the average capital accumulation ratio amounts to 7.52, and the average replacement rate across all cohorts is 48.21 percent with a standard deviation of 5.65 percent. The volatility in the baseline case arises from fluctuations in real earnings. The cohorts that obtain the highest replacement rates are those retiring in the 1910s and in the 1990s, with replacement rates ranging from 50 to 58 percent. The cohort retiring in 1945 has the lowest replacement rate (39 percent). The max/min ratio (the ratio of the maximum to the minimum replacement rate) is only 1.46 in this case, while the coefficient of variation is 12 percent. These are the same for both the capital accumulation ratio and the replacement rates, since the same annuity rate is used throughout.

If the fixed rate of return is set equal to 6.87 percent—the geometric average for the return on equities—and the rate of earnings growth is set equal to 2.51 percent, the replacement rate for a 10 percent contribution rate, a 40/20 ratio of active to passive life, and a 2.5 percent real annuity, would amount to 65 percent. This compares with 48 percent for the baseline case and reflects the strong performance of the U.S. equity market over the past 120 years.

Tables 11.6 through 11.8 summarize the results, in terms of capital accumulation ratios and replacement rates, for the four portfolio strategies described above. The all-equity portfolio achieves the highest capital accumulation ratio (9.43) and highest average replacement (61 percent) but also has the highest volatility measured by the standard deviation, coefficient of

Table 11.6. Capital Accumulation Ratio for Alternative Portfolios, 2.5 Percent Real Annuities, Summary Statistics

Indicator	100-0-0	0-100-0	60-30-10	30-60-10	Baseline
Average (ratio to last wage)	9.43	3.53	6.55	4.85	7.52
Standard deviation	3.02	1.33	1.55	1.44	0.88
Maximum (ratio to last wage)	15.55	6.81	10.80	8.16	8.98
Minimum (ratio to last wage)	3.83	1.80	3.43	2.76	6.14
Coefficient of variation	0.32	0.38	0.24	0.30	0.12
Max/min ratio	4.06	3.78	3.15	2.96	1.46

Source: Authors' calculations.

Table 11.7. Replacement Rates for Alternative Portfolios, 2.5 Percent Real Annuities, Summary Statistics

Indicator	100-0-0	0-100-0	60-30-10	30-60-10	Baseline
Average (percent of last wage)	60.51	22.61	42.02	31.10	48.21
Standard deviation	19.34	8.56	9.93	9.21	5.65
Maximum (percent of last wage)	99.73	43.71	69.28	52.32	57.58
Minimum (percent of last wage)	24.59	11.57	21.99	17.68	39.36
Coefficient of variation	0.32	0.38	0.24	0.30	0.12
Max/min ratio	4.06	3.78	3.15	2.96	1.46

Source: Authors' calculations.

Table 11.8. Distribution of Replacement Rates, 2.5 Percent Real Annuities, Summary Statistics
(percentage)

Range	100-0-0	0-100-0	60-30-10	30-60-10	Baseline
0 to 30	1.1	73.6	11.5	56.3	0.0
30 to 60	56.3	26.4	85.1	43.7	100.0
Higher than 60	42.5	0.0	3.4	0.0	0.0

Source: Authors' calculations.

variation, or max/min ratio. In more than 40 percent of cohorts, the replacement rate exceeds 60 percent, while only 1 cohort (that retiring in 1921) obtains a replacement rate of less than 30 percent.

The all-equity and all-bond strategies show higher volatility, measured either by the coefficient of variation or the max/min ratio, than the balanced portfolio strategies. Perhaps because of the persistence of the equity premium, the all-equity strategy produces a higher replacement rate than the all-bond strategy for every single cohort. The maximum replacement rate for the all-equity strategy amounts to 100 percent (1966) but to only 44 percent (1996) for the all-bond strategy. The fact that the all-bond strategy always yields a lower replacement rate than any of the other three strategies underscores the historical weakness of the bond market relative to the equity market. The replacement rate of this strategy is also lower for all cohorts than in the baseline case. Investing only in government bonds, even those of the United States, would indeed have amounted to "reckless conservatism."

Among balanced portfolio strategies, the 60-30-10 strategy always results in a higher replacement rate than the 30-60-10 strategy. The 60-30-10 strategy performs better than holding an all-equity portfolio for only seven cohorts (1932, 1933, 1935, 1938, 1941, 1942, and 1943), but the difference is very small—less than 6 percentage points in the replacement rate.

The price for the much lower volatility of the balanced portfolio strategies, in terms of the coefficient of variation and the max/min ratio, is a much lower average capital accumulation ratio and replacement rate. For the 60-30-10 strategy these amount to 6.55 and 42 percent, respectively (against 9.43 and 61 percent for the all-equity strategy). The lower level of volatility of the balanced strategies is achieved by pulling down the high replacement rates of many cohorts in the all-equity portfolio rather than by raising the cohorts with low replacement rates. Under the 60-30-10 strategy, only 10 percent of the cohorts obtain a replacement rate above 60 percent. The performance of the balanced 60-30-10 strategy is close to that of the all-equity strategy for most of the period from 1920 to 1950 but is substantially below it in the period from 1950 to 1973, although it narrows again in the more recent period from 1974 to 1995.

Ranking the four strategies by average capital accumulation ratio or replacement rate gives the following results, in descending order: 100-0-0, 60-30-10, 30-60-10, and 0-100-0. The ranking according to volatility of outcomes is 60-30-10, 30-60-10, 0-100-0, and 100-0-0. If an investment strategy is defined as dominated if it yields a lower average level and a higher standard deviation of the replacement rate compared to another alternative strategy, then strategy 0-100-0 is dominated by both 60-30-10 and 30-60-10, while strategy 30-60-10 is dominated by 60-30-10.

In general, the lesson from the historical returns over the past 120 years is to avoid bonds, which have provided little hedging protection against the volatility of returns in the equity market. This is particularly the case in the subperiods when the equity premium is low but the correlation of returns between bonds and equities is quite high.

Gradual Late Shift To Bonds

The results of the first simulations, using U.S. data, suggest that the relevant investment strategies are those holding only stocks or a combination of 60 percent stocks, 30 percent bonds, and 10 percent commercial paper.

This section explores the effect of a gradual and progressive shift away from stocks toward bonds in the last five years of a person's working life (table 11.9). The objective of this strategy is to allow workers to benefit from the equity premium for most of their working lives but to gradually switch into the greater safety of bonds as they near retirement. If the equity market were to experience a major downturn close to their retirement, they would not have enough time to make up any large capital losses during their remaining working years. Tables 11.10 through 11.12 present the results of these simulations.

A gradual shift to bonds from an all-equity portfolio during the last five years of working life results in lower volatility, especially as measured by the max/min ratio but only a slight improvement in terms of the coefficient of variation. The gradual shift improves the replacement rates of 24 cohorts

Table 11.9. Portfolio Compositions for the Gradual and Progressive Shift to Bonds, Last Five Working Years
(portfolio allocations as a percentage of the total fund)

| | 100-0-0 | | | 60-30-10 | | |
| | Stocks | Bonds | Comm. paper. | Stocks | Bonds | Comm. paper. |
Year						
Ret – 6	100	0	0	60	30	10
Ret – 5	80	20	0	48	42	10
Ret – 4	60	40	0	36	54	10
Ret – 3	40	60	0	24	66	10
Ret – 2	20	80	0	12	78	10
Ret – 1	0	100	0	0	90	10

Note:Ret - i means i years before retirement age.
Source: Authors' assumptions.

Table 11.10. Capital Accumulation Ratios, Switching to Bonds, 2.5 Percent Real Annuities, Summary Statistics

| | All-equity case | | 60-30-10 case | |
Indicator	No switch	Switch	No switch	Switch
Average (ratio to last wage)	9.43	8.32	6.55	6.04
Standard deviation	3.02	2.42	1.55	1.55
Maximum (ratio to last wage)	15.55	12.73	10.80	9.48
Minimum (ratio to last wage)	3.83	4.14	3.43	3.42
Coefficient of variation	0.32	0.29	0.24	0.26
Max/min ratio	4.06	3.08	3.15	2.77

Source: Authors' calculations.

Table 11.11. Replacement Rates, Switching to Bonds, 2.5 Percent Real Annuities, Summary Statistics

Indicator	All-equity case		60-30-10 case	
	No switch	Switch	No switch	Switch
Average (percent of last wage)	60.51	53.37	42.02	38.71
Standard deviation	19.34	15.53	9.93	9.95
Maximum (percent of last wage)	99.73	81.66	69.28	60.79
Minimum (percent of last wage)	24.59	26.54	21.99	21.95
Coefficient of variation	0.32	0.29	0.24	0.26
Max/min ratio	4.06	3.08	3.15	2.77

Source: Authors' calculations.

Table 11.12. Distribution of Replacement Rates, Switching to Bonds, 2.5 Percent Real Annuities, Summary Statistics
(percentage)

Range	All-equity case		60-30-10 case	
	No switch	Switch	No switch	Switch
0 to 30	1.1	5.7	11.5	24.1
30 to 60	56.3	57.5	85.1	74.7
Higher than 60	42.5	36.8	3.4	1.1

Source: Authors' calculations.

and lowers those of all other cohorts. Cohorts retiring in the 1950s and 1960s obtain much lower replacement rates, while those retiring in the early 1930s obtain much higher replacement rates.

A similar approach from a 60-30-10 balanced portfolio would produce improved replacement rates for 22 cohorts and lower rates for all other cohorts. The positive or negative changes are, however, generally much smaller in magnitude. This is also reflected in the ambivalent improvement in overall measures of volatility. The max/min ratio falls from 3.15 to 2.77, but the coefficient of variation increases from 0.24 to 0.26.

The cost of the late switching to bonds from an all-equity portfolio in terms of a lower average replacement rate obtained by all the cohorts is 7 percentage points. This compares with 19 percentage points in the case of holding a balanced portfolio for the whole of a worker's active life. The replacement rate is above 60 percent in 37 percent of cohorts, while it is below 30 percent in only 6 percent of cohorts.

Because of the generally weak relative performance of bonds in the United States during the period under review, a gradual late shift into bonds does not produce significant benefits in lower volatility, even though its costs in terms of lower average replacement rates is also low. It appears to be superior than the strategy of always keeping a balanced portfolio in the sense that it achieves a higher average replacement rate with a lower max/min ratio and coefficient of variation. However, the "late balanced" strategy does not dominate the "always balanced" strategy because it reports a greater standard deviation (15 percent against 10 percent). For developing countries where the bond market may perform better relative to the equity market, or where the equity premium may be less persistent, the results of the gradual shift to bonds could be more promising.

Gradual Purchase of Annuities

The third solution mentioned in the introduction consists of allowing, encouraging, or even requiring workers to start buying several fixed annuities during the last years of their active life, instead of only one fixed annuity at retirement. Under this scheme workers would diversify two risks, one related to the profitability of the pension fund and the other related to changes in the annuity rate. The simulations assume a constant risk-free rate of interest of 2.5 percent and thus show only the effect of lowering the risk of changes in the profitability of the pension fund.

Because life in retirement is set at 20 years, the purchase of a fixed annuity is equivalent to investing in an asset that yields 2.5 percent.[18] Thus, the gradual purchase of annuities is equivalent to a gradual shift in this asset. Tables 11.13 and 11.14 present the simulations for the all-equity and 60-30-10 combination strategies. Five years before retirement workers start using 20 percent of their accumulated capital to buy an annuity every year.

The results are very close to those of a gradual late shift to bonds. The max/min ratio and coefficient of variation are a little lower but so is the

Table 11.13. Replacement Rates, Gradual Purchase of Annuities, 2.5 Percent Real Annuities, Summary Statistics

Indicator	All-equity case		60-30-10 case	
	One annuity	Five annuities	One annuity	Five annuities
Average (percent of last wage)	60.51	51.98	42.02	36.88
Standard deviation	19.34	14.30	9.93	7.49
Maximum (percent of last wage)	99.73	82.97	69.28	57.67
Minimum (percent of last wage)	24.59	27.80	21.99	24.40
Coefficient of variation	0.32	0.28	0.24	0.20
Max/min ratio	4.06	2.98	3.15	2.36

Source: Authors' calculations.

Table 11.14. Distribution of Replacement Rates, Gradual Purchase of Annuities, 2.5 Percent Real Annuities, Summary Statistics
(percentage)

Range	All-equity case		60-30-10 case	
	One annuity	Five annuities	One annuity	Five annuities
0 to 30	1.1	4.6	11.5	18.4
30 to 60	56.3	65.5	85.1	81.6
Higher than 60	42.5	29.9	3.4	0.0

Source: Authors' calculations.

average replacement rate.[19] Thirty percent of cohorts achieve a replacement rate above 60 percent, while only four cohorts (out of 86) have replacement rates below 30 percent.

Compared to the 60-30-10 strategy, there is significant improvement in terms of both a lower max/min ratio and a smaller coefficient of variation. Moreover, this is achieved at a small reduction of the average replacement rate from 42 percent to 37 percent. However, combining a balanced portfolio with a gradual purchase of annuities reduces the average replacement rate by 24 percentage points compared to the pure all-equity strategy. The price of lower volatility is thus quite high. Moreover, as already remarked, the reduction in the max/min ratio is achieved by lowering the maximum replacement rate without any increase in the minimum replacement rate.

Purchasing Variable Annuities

The results of the preceding simulations are based on the assumption that, at retirement, workers use the accumulated capital in their pension plan to buy a fixed real annuity (at a 2.5 percent real interest rate and a fixed life in retirement of 20 years). This section explores the possibility that workers use part or all of their accumulated capital to purchase a variable annuity. The part of the accumulated capital that is not used to purchase a fixed real annuity stays invested in the pension fund and earns the same return as the fund. Because in this chapter we assume that workers live in retirement for 20 years, use of variable annuities is equivalent to use of phased withdrawals. The balance kept in the pension fund is withdrawn gradually from the pension account during retirement. Each period retirees withdraw from their pension fund accounts a fraction of the remaining balance, which is equal to one divided by their remaining life. The amount withdrawn in each year varies in response to changes in investment returns.

In the simulations with phased withdrawals, the last 20 observations are lost since each simulation requires data until workers die, not just until they retire. Thus, instead of 87 cases (those cohorts retiring from 1910 until 1996), the simulations in this section cover only 67 cases (those cohorts retiring from 1910 until 1977). In the case with phased withdrawals, there is no unique replacement rate. It varies every year with the variations in asset returns. The results reported in tables 11.15 and 11.16 refer to the average replacement rate for individual cohorts. Again, because it is unaffected by the decision of how much, and how, to annuitize, no data on the capital accumulation ratios are reported.

The simulations in this section explore two cases: one in which all the accumulated capital is used for phased withdrawals (PW 100), and another in which only 50 percent of the capital is used to purchase a fixed real annuity and the other 50 percent is used for phased withdrawals (PW 50). We limit our analysis to the all-equity strategy.

Table 11.15 shows that under the all-equity strategy, the higher the proportion of the pension fund used for phased withdrawals, the higher the average replacement rate. Although the 50 percent phased withdrawal strategy has a smaller standard deviation, it is not a good strategy because for every single cohort it obtains a lower replacement. In fact, its average

Table 11.15. Average Replacement Rates for All-Equity and Phased Withdrawal Strategies, 2.5 Percent Real Annuities, Summary Statistics

Indicator	No PW	PW 50	PW 100
Average (percent of last wage)	61.85	72.36	113.79
Standard deviation	21.11	15.65	25.45
Maximum (percent of last wage)	99.73	104.10	165.13
Minimum (percent of last wage)	24.59	43.09	70.39
Coefficient of variation	0.34	0.22	0.22
Max/min ratio	4.06	2.42	2.35

Source: Authors' calculations.

Table 11.16. Distribution of Replacement Rates for All-Equity and Phased Withdrawal Strategies, 2.5 Percent Real Annuities, Summary Statistics
(percentage)

Indicator	No PW	PW 50	PW 100
0 to 30	1.5	0.0	0.0
30 to 60	52.2	1.5	0.0
Higher than 60	46.3	98.5	100.0

Source: Authors' calculations.

replacement rate is only marginally higher than the minimum replacement rate under the 100 percent phased withdrawal strategy. A comparison of the replacement rates for the cohort retiring in 1921 exemplifies the impact of continuing to invest in equities, even during a worker's retirement. Under the all-equity strategy that invests everything in a 2.5 percent real annuity on retirement, the replacement rate would be equal to 25 percent. But purchasing a variable annuity (100 percent phased withdrawal) would increase the replacement rate to 74 percent.[20]

Given the size and persistence of the equity premium over the past 120 years, it is not surprising that a strategy that focuses on holding equities, not only during the active life but also throughout the passive life of workers, would produce the best results in terms of replacement rates, even at the expense of a higher volatility. As shown in table 11.16, no cohort achieves a replacement rate of less than 60 percent, and the average is 114 percent, while the maximum is a staggering 165 percent. However, since it is not known if history will repeat itself, a more sanguine conclusion would, perhaps, be to advocate a 50 percent phased withdrawal strategy. Only one cohort obtains a replacement rate of less than 60 percent under this strategy, while the average replacement rate is 73 percent and the maximum reaches 104 percent.

Simulations with Nominal Annuities

This part of the chapter discusses replacement rates by using nominal rather than real annuities. Because we do not have historical data on annuity rates, we use the series of 15-year bond yields for calculating the annual payouts and comparing them to the final wage. We continue to abstract from operating fees and commissions as well as from the complexities caused by life expectancies.

As in the case of real annuities, we first present the results for strategies involving undiversified and balanced portfolios. But because the results of the simulations are broadly similar, we summarize the impact of undertaking the familiar three alternative strategies: a gradual late shift into bonds, a gradual purchase of annuities, and a purchase of variable annuities. Moreover, since the use of nominal annuities does not affect the capital accumulation ratios, we do not repeat them here. However, one complication that arises in the case of nominal annuities is that inflation erodes the real value of payouts. For this reason we report separately the first-year replacement rates and the average replacement rates. As in the case of variable annuities, we focus our analysis on the behavior of average replacement rates. But since we lose the last 19 observations, we report data for only 67 cohorts.

Before presenting the simulation results, we need to refer briefly to the behavior of nominal yields and inflation (table 11.17). Over the whole period under review, the 15-year bond yield averaged 4.72 percent. With inflation running at 2.03 percent, this implies a real rate of 2.64 percent, which is slightly higher than the 2.5 percent we used for real annuities in the preceding section. In the most recent period, nominal yields amounted on average to 8.72 percent against an inflation rate of 5.34 percent, giving a real rate of 3.21 percent. The real rate of interest was very high at the end of the last century and during the interwar period, but was very low from 1896 to 1920 and again in the period after World War II.

Undiversified and Balanced Portfolios

Because a different annuity rate is used for each cohort, there is greater variability in replacement rates than with the constant 2.5 percent real annuity of the preceding section. For the all-equity case, the max/min ratio is equal to 4.36 for first-year replacement rates and 4.79 for average replacement rates against 4.06 under real annuities (tables 11.18 and 11.19). The average replacement rate over the whole retirement life is slightly lower,

Table 11.17. Nominal Yields and Inflation, 1871–1995

Period	15-year bonds	Commercial paper	CPI inflation
1871–1895			
Average (percentage)	4.09	6.03	−1.61
Standard deviation	0.0069	0.0182	0.0151
1896–1920			
Average (percentage)	3.84	5.13	3.34
Standard deviation	0.0058	0.0128	0.0611
1921–1945			
Average (percentage)	3.10	2.40	0.02
Standard deviation	0.0080	0.0190	0.0539
1946–1970			
Average (percent)	3.86	3.57	3.08
Standard deviation	0.0147	0.0195	0.0390
1971–1995			
Average (percentage)	8.72	7.69	5.34
Standard deviation	0.0213	0.0297	0.0281
Overall			
Average (percentage)	4.72	4.96	2.03
Standard deviation	0.0239	0.0275	0.0490

Sources: Authors' calculations based on revised and updated data from Wilson and Jones (1987a, 1987b, 1997) and Sylla, Wilson, and Jones (1990, 1994). Data provided by R. Sylla and J. Wilson.

Table 11.18. First Replacement Rates for Alternative Portfolio Strategies, Nominal Annuities, Summary Statistics

Indicator	100-0-0	0-100-0	60-30-10	30-60-10	Baseline
Average (percent of last wage)	76.75	28.14	52.61	38.75	55.85
Standard deviation	27.32	10.99	13.82	11.97	15.16
Maximum (percent of last wage)	137.30	58.41	84.17	69.91	101.87
Minimum (percent of last wage)	31.47	15.66	28.45	23.98	40.87
Coefficient of variation	0.36	0.39	0.26	0.31	0.27
Max/min ratio	4.36	3.73	2.96	2.91	2.49

Note: In the calculation of the average replacement rate, 20 observations are lost and, therefore, the statistics cover only generations retiring between 1910 and 1976.
Source: Authors' calculations.

Table 11.19. Average Replacement Rates for Alternative Portfolio Strategies, Nominal Annuities, Summary Statistics

Indicator	100-0-0	0-100-0	60-30-10	30-60-10	Baseline
Average (percent of last wage)	55.03	19.67	37.80	27.60	45.40
Standard deviation	19.29	6.68	9.06	7.58	13.95
Maximum (percent of last wage)	107.62	29.60	66.56	43.51	71.69
Minimum (percent of last wage)	22.48	10.99	22.78	17.49	27.05
Coefficient of variation	0.35	0.34	0.24	0.27	0.31
Max/min ratio	4.79	2.69	2.92	2.49	2.65

Note: In the calculation of the average replacement rate, 20 observations are lost and, therefore, the statistics cover only generations retiring between 1910 and 1976.
Source: Authors' calculations.

amounting to 55 percent versus 61 percent. The maximum reaches 108 percent (1929), while the minimum is as low as 22 percent (1942).

The all-bond portfolio continues to perform very badly, with an overall average replacement rate of less than 20 percent, a maximum that is no higher than 30 percent, and a minimum that is as low as 11 percent. The 60-30-10 strategy achieves a substantial reduction in volatility (the max/min ratio declines from 4.79 to 2.92) but at a high cost in terms of a lower replacement rate of 17 percentage points (from 55 percent down to 38 percent).

The Three Alternative Strategies

The gradual late shift into bonds and the gradual purchase of annuities have very similar effects (tables 11.20 through 11.25). Volatility is reduced but at a considerable cost in terms of lower replacement rates. The use of nominal annuities causes greater variability across cohorts and the max/min ratios are generally higher than with real annuities.

Table 11.20. First Replacement Rates, Switching to Bonds, Nominal Annuities, Summary Statistics

Indicator	All-equity case		60-30-10 case	
	No switch	Switch	No switch	Switch
Average (percent of last wage)	76.75	68.18	52.61	48.70
Standard deviation	27.32	24.10	13.82	14.29
Maximum (percent of last wage)	137.30	113.08	84.17	79.46
Minimum (percent of last wage)	31.47	26.27	28.45	26.55
Coefficient of variation	0.36	0.35	0.26	0.29
Max/min ratio	4.36	4.30	2.96	2.99

Note: In the calculation of the average replacement rate, 20 observations are lost and, therefore, the statistics cover only generations retiring between 1910 and 1976.
Source: Authors' calculations.

Table 11.21. Average Replacement Rates, Switching to Bonds, Nominal Annuities, Summary Statistics

Indicator	All-equity case		60-30-10 case	
	No switch	Switch	No switch	Switch
Average (percent of last wage)	55.03	47.59	37.80	34.39
Standard deviation	19.29	13.66	9.06	8.02
Maximum (percent of last wage)	107.62	72.92	66.56	51.22
Minimum (percent of last wage)	22.48	18.47	22.78	18.66
Coefficient of variation	0.35	0.29	0.24	0.23
Max/min ratio	4.79	3.95	2.92	2.75

Note: In the calculation of the average replacement rate 20 observations are lost and, therefore, the statistics cover only generations retiring between 1910 and 1976.
Source: Authors' calculations.

Table 11.22. First Replacement Rates, Gradual Purchase of Annuities, Nominal Annuities, Summary Statistics

Indicator	All-equity case		60-30-10 case	
	One annuity	Five annuities	One annuity	Five annuities
Average (percent of last wage)	76.75	65.41	52.61	45.86
Standard deviation	27.32	22.14	13.82	12.62
Maximum (percent of last wage)	137.30	106.49	84.17	74.54
Minimum (percent of last wage)	31.47	26.83	28.45	26.01
Coefficient of variation	0.36	0.34	0.26	0.28
Max/min ratio	4.36	3.97	2.96	2.87

Note: In the calculation of the average replacement rate, 20 observations are lost and, therefore, the statistics cover only generations retiring between 1910 and 1976.
Source: Authors' calculations.

Table 11.23. Average Replacement Rates, Gradual Purchase of Annuities, Nominal Annuities, Summary Statistics

Indicator	All-equity case		60-30-10 case	
	One annuity	Five annuities	One annuity	Five annuities
Average (percent of last wage)	55.03	46.30	37.80	32.65
Standard deviation	19.29	13.41	9.06	7.23
Maximum (percent of last wage)	107.62	71.58	66.56	49.69
Minimum (percent of last wage)	22.48	18.91	22.78	18.28
Coefficient of variation	0.35	0.29	0.24	0.22
Max/min ratio	4.79	3.78	2.92	2.72

Note: In the calculation of the average replacement rate, 20 observations are lost and, therefore, the statistics cover only generations retiring between 1910 and 1976.
Source: Authors' calculations.

Table 11.24. First Replacement Rates for All-Equity and Phased Withdrawal Strategies, Nominal Annuities, Summary Statistics

Indicator	No PW	PW 50	PW 100
Average (percent of last wage)	61.85	96.71	157.75
Standard deviation	21.11	26.40	43.85
Maximum (percent of last wage)	99.73	140.77	214.01
Minimum (percent of last wage)	24.59	41.10	66.29
Coefficient of variation	0.34	0.27	0.28
Max/min ratio	4.06	3.43	3.23

Note: In the calculation of the average replacement rate, 20 observations are lost and, therefore, the statistics cover only generations retiring between 1910 and 1976.
Source: Authors' calculations.

Table 11.25. Average Replacement Rates for All-Equity and Phased Withdrawal Strategies, Nominal Annuities, Summary Statistics

Indicator	No PW	PW 50	PW 100
Average (percent of last wage)	55.03	70.08	112.64
Standard deviation	19.29	14.37	24.60
Maximum (percent of last wage)	107.62	100.51	165.29
Minimum (percent of last wage)	22.48	44.05	72.39
Coefficient of variation	0.35	0.21	0.22
Max/min ratio	4.79	2.28	2.28

Note: In the calculation of the average replacement rate, 20 observations are lost and, therefore, the statistics cover only generations retiring between 1910 and 1976.
Source: Authors' calculations.

The use of variable annuities seems to achieve the best results, lowering volatility but without sacrificing much in replacement rates. In this case more than two-thirds of the average replacement rates are between 90 percent and 120 percent, and only one-tenth of them are below 90 percent. This is clearly the result of the large and persistent equity premium of the past 100 years or so and the reduction in stock return volatility that can be achieved by participating for a longer period of time in the stock market. Table 11.26 presents volatility statistics for the average returns on stock held over different time spans. The longer a stock portfolio is held, the higher the average return and the lower the volatility of the returns (measured by the standard deviation and the max/min ratio). Again, an attractive compromise solution, given the great uncertainty about future returns, could well be the combination of variable and fixed annuities. In countries where social security offers real annuities, a combination of variable and nominal annuities would seem to make sense. But for workers for whom social security pensions are a small fraction of their income, a variable/real mix might be more appropriate.

Financial Engineering and Synthetic Products

As already noted, this chapter makes no attempt to assess the use of portfolio insurance and European put options to hedge the value of balances of workers who are near their retirement nor does it attempt to assess the use of synthetic products that provide a floor on the value of balances over some period of time while also allowing some sharing in the upside potential of the equity market. However, some evidence on such methods is available.

Bodie and Crane (1998) provide an interesting example of the potential use of financial engineering and synthetic products. They first establish that with a real rate of interest of 3 percent during both the accumulation and

Table 11.26. Average Returns on Stock over Different Time Spans
(percentage)

Indicator	20 years	40 years	60 years
Average	9.06	10.05	10.56
Standard deviation	2.14	1.87	1.46
Maximum	14.95	13.86	13.48
Minimum	5.88	6.66	7.30
Max/min ratio	2.54	2.08	1.85

Sources: Authors' calculations based on revised and updated data from Wilson and Jones (1987a, 1987b, 1997) and Sylla, Wilson, and Jones (1990, 1994). Data provided by R. Sylla and J. Wilson.

decumulation periods and a constant real wage, workers contributing for 40 years and living in retirement for 20 years would need a contribution rate of 11.84 percent to attain a targeted replacement rate of 60 percent (with a 10 percent contribution rate, this corresponds to a 51 percent replacement rate). They then assume that the S&P index has an average nominal return of 10 percent, a standard deviation of 20 percent, and a dividend yield of 3 percent and that inflation is also uncertain, with an average rate of 4 percent and a standard deviation of 0.5 percent. The simulated inflation reverts to the mean at a rate of 0.2, while there is positive correlation of 0.5 between the S&P index and inflation. On the basis of these assumptions, they run 100,000 simulations of an all-equity portfolio, producing an average replacement rate of 115 percent (implying an average real rate of return of 5 percent). However, in 34 percent of the cases the replacement rate is below the targeted 60 percent level. They also use a 60–40 allocation in equities and 3 percent inflation-indexed bonds (treasury inflation protected securities, or TIP) and find that the average replacement rate is then lower at 88 percent (implied average real return of 4.2 percent). In this case 29 percent of cases are below the targeted replacement rate. Additionally, they consider age-linked portfolios that invest a proportion equal to the age of the worker in TIPS and the rest in equities. This produces a lower average replacement rate of 83 percent (implied average rate of return of 4 percent), with 27 percent of cases below target. Finally, Bodie and Crane run two simulations with portfolio protection on an annual or five-year basis. They find that the annual protection is not efficient, but the five-year protection products achieve an average replacement rate of 128 percent with only 12 percent of cases below the target of 60 percent.

The simulations of Bodie and Crane show the potential benefits of financial engineering. However, they involve the purchase of indexed bonds and call options on equities. This would require a high level of sophistication in terms of using hedging products as well as regulating and supervising the financial institutions offering such products. This sophistication is not currently available, neither in developing countries nor the most advanced industrial countries. Moreover, use of these financial engineering techniques implies either that the government issues an immense amount of indexed bonds, which goes against the idea of containing government debts, or that other borrowers (corporations or mortgages for households) step up to fill the gap. The simpler approaches discussed in this chapter appear more feasible, although in the longer run the more sophisticated techniques discussed by Bodie and Crane could replace them, while the development of a true intergenerational marketable contract, as described in this chapter's introductory section, may also benefit from the growth of financial engineering.

Conclusion

This chapter explores simple financial strategies that can mitigate the impact of short-term volatility on personal pension plans. Sophisticated financial engineering promises more efficient solutions to this problem; however, its applicability in developing countries (and financial markets) may not be possible until important regulatory issues, among others, are resolved. Neither approach may be able to deal effectively with persistent deviations from the long-term trend. The use of a multipillar system may mitigate the impact of such deviations.

The preceding analysis has demonstrates that, on the basis of historical U.S. returns on equities, investing all workers' contributions in an all-equity index fund, and buying on retirement either a nominal annuity or a 2.5 percent real annuity, would have exposed workers of different cohorts to large fluctuations in replacement rates. While the average replacement rate would have amounted to around 60 percent, which is remarkably high with only a 10 percent contribution rate, the standard deviation would have been on the order of 20 percent, implying that one-fifth of workers would have a replacement rate either higher than 80 percent or lower than 40 percent. The maximum and minimum replacement rates would have ranged between 100 and 110 percent (depending on the type of annuity used) and 23 and 25 percent, respectively, resulting in a max/min ratio of between 4.0 and 4.8.

Investing everything in bonds, on the basis of their historical returns, would have produced much lower replacement rates while generating the same volatility and high max/min ratio. This would have been a consequence of the large and persistent equity premium that has characterized U.S. financial markets over the past 100 years or so.

Employing a more balanced portfolio—consisting of 60 percent in equities, 30 percent in bonds, and 10 percent in commercial paper—would have reduced the volatility of returns and the fluctuations in replacement rates. But the price of reduced volatility would have been a substantial reduction in the average replacement rate. Most of the improvement in the max/min ratio would have been obtained by reducing high replacement rates rather than by raising low ones.

Instead of using a balanced portfolio strategy throughout a worker's career, an alternative approach would use an all-equity portfolio for most of the active life and adopt either a gradual late shift into bonds or a gradual purchase of annuities. Both of these strategies would have achieved equivalent reductions in volatility and the max/min ratio at a significantly lower cost in terms of lower replacement rates.

However, in view of the persistence of the equity premium, the best approach would have been to buy a variable annuity either for the whole or for half of the accumulated capital. Using half the accumulated capital to purchase a fixed annuity (real or nominal) and the other half for phased withdrawals—which, under the assumptions used in this chapter, are equivalent to purchasing a variable annuity—would have achieved an average replacement rate of nearly 75 percent with a low max/min ratio of around 2.5. Of greater interest is that both the maximum and minimum replacement rates would have been much higher than under all the other strategies not using variable annuities.

The results would have been even better if all the capital were used for phased withdrawals, but this would have implied a huge exposure to the volatility of equity returns. Such an extreme approach would have been inadvisable, especially since the reported replacement rate for each cohort would have been an average of the variable annual replacement rates over a worker's retirement life.

Finally, use of synthetic products that provide portfolio protection would have achieved broadly similar results. In the long run, financial engineering and more sophisticated strategies may be more appropriate, but in developing countries the simpler solutions presented in this chapter would appear more feasible and probably equally effective.

Burtless (1998) reached similar conclusions. He suggested that workers could diversify their investment portfolios and place a portion of their retirement savings in bonds. He did not, however, recommend a late shift into bonds. He also proposed the use of installment annuities and even the use of 10 installments that would straddle the retirement year—five installment annuities before and five after they retire. Finally, he suggested that some of the accumulated capital could continue to be invested in equities, a proposal that is analogous to the use of variable annuities.

We have tried in this chapter to show that excessive concern about the impact of short-term volatility in stock markets may not be warranted. We are fully aware that annuity markets are very underdeveloped in most countries and that, once such markets develop, annuity prices are likely to fluctuate on a daily basis in response to changes in interest rates. We are also aware that the greater problem facing annuity markets is a sensible and realistic prediction of improvements in longevity. In fact, the biggest challenge facing annuity providers is the development of portable variable annuities along the lines suggested by Valdés-Prieto and Edwards (1997) and Valdés-Prieto (1998). Nevertheless, we believe that annuity markets will become more sophisticated in response to the greater demand for them generated by maturing pension systems based on individual accounts. The growth of financial engineering will also help in this process.

It is currently more difficult to see how to overcome the problems caused by persistent deviations from trend, when whole generations of workers may retire with either too high or too low pensions. The establishment of multipillar systems, comprising a public pillar based on the principles of redistribution and social insurance and a private pillar that has a symbiotic relationship with private capital and annuity markets, may provide an effective solution to this problem, although this remains to be proved.

Notes

1. The views expressed in this chapter are those of the authors and do not necessarily represent those of the World Bank or the International Monetary Fund. The authors are grateful to Estelle James for her insightful and extremely useful comments on an earlier version of the chapter. Thanks are also due to Gary Burtless, Salvador Valdés-Prieto, and Ajay Shah for their comments.

2. While the experience in the United States reflects the prevalence of a large equity premium over the past 120 years, it is not unique. Several other developed countries that have followed relatively stable and sound financial policies have also experienced large and persistent equity premia. The European Commission (1999) reports that since the 1920s equity premia in countries such as Australia, Canada, Denmark, Sweden, Switzerland, and the United Kingdom have been between 4.0 and 8.5 percent. Developing countries could benefit from similar equity premia in the future if they pursue policies that promote sound and stable financial systems.

3. Burtless (1998) also uses historical equity returns from the United States to discuss the impact of volatile equity returns on replacement rates and the internal rates of return earned by different cohorts. His objective is to critique proposals to privatize social security in the United States that overlook the impact of stock market volatility. Our objective is to discuss simple but feasible solutions to this problem.

4. For a review of the policy issues and likely causes of the underdevelopment of annuity markets, see James and Vittas (1999). There is a fast-growing literature on annuity markets in the United States led by academic researchers at the Massachusetts Institute of Technology and The Wharton School, while a research project sponsored by the World Bank focuses on annuity markets in a number of countries.

5. These alternative strategies do not address the problems caused by catastrophic collapses of markets or by persistent deviations from trend.

6. Notably, most of these quantitative limits have not been binding, although fund managers, especially in the Netherlands, have been pressing for their removal or relaxation.

7. Goetzmann and Jorion (1997) report data for equity returns in a large number of countries. These show that real equity returns were low in many countries that suffered from very high inflation or from interruptions

caused by war or financial crises. But a few European countries, such as the United Kingdom, Denmark, Sweden, and Switzerland, as well as the United States, reported uninterrupted real equity returns ranging from 5 to 8 percent (see Goetzmann and Jorion 1997, table 3).

8. Jagannathan and Kocherlakota (1996) and Bodie (1998) review the arguments for age-specific investment policies.

9. Burtless (1998) makes a similar proposal. He even goes further and suggests 10 installment annuities, starting five years before retirement and continuing for five years after retirement.

10. In private annuity markets, insurance companies try hard to forecast improvements in longevity and adjust their life tables and annuity prices accordingly. France lowered the normal retirement age in the social security system from 65 to 60 in the early 1980s, even though it was well known that, like the rest of Europe, French society was aging fast.

11. The Chilean experience has been characterized by high and volatile investment returns—the average rate of return amounted to more than 10 percent per year in real terms on pension fund assets, though less than 8 percent on average on individual account balances after the deduction of expenses.

12. Most countries do not offer real annuities and, as a result, workers have to assume the inflation risk during their life in retirement. Variable annuities as well as escalating annuities provide a partial (but complex) solution to this problem.

13. In the results the effect of these charges would be to proportionally scale down the level of replacement rates. We do not underestimate the impact of high fees on pensions. For a discussion of arrangements that would aim to lower fees by constraining choice, see James and others (1999).

14. We use earnings in the manufacturing sector to construct a real wage index due to the availability of data.

15. The data represent updated and revised estimates from previous research by Wilson and Jones (1987a, 1987b, 1997) and Sylla, Wilson, and Jones (1990, 1994).

16. All input and output data and charts are available from the authors.

17. In an earlier version of this chapter, we assumed a 4 percent real annuity and did not allow for the rising earnings profile of the average worker. Not surprisingly, we obtained very high replacement rates. At the suggestion of Estelle James, we lowered the real annuity to 2.5 percent and allowed for a 1 percent additional growth in wages. The combined effect of these changes in assumptions was to lower replacement rates considerably to more realistic levels.

18. As discussed in Brown (1999), annuity products benefit from the so-called mortality premium, although there is considerable debate about the

nature and size of this premium. However, any fixed annuity can be perceived as a bond paying a fixed nominal or real return in an ex-ante sense. This would be higher than the return of an ordinary bond by the amount of the mortality premium.

19. The results for the capital accumulation ratio are not shown since the final year's capital is already depleted by the purchase of a series of deferred annuities.

20. The implied strong conclusion needs to be mitigated by the realization that the replacement rates reported for the variable annuity cases are averages over the whole of the retirement life. There could be individual years when the value of the paid annuity could be very low and others when it could be very high.

References

Note: The word *processed* describes informally reproduced works that may not be commonly available through libraries.

Bodie, Zvi. 1998. "Financial Engineering and Social Security Reform." Boston University. Processed.

Bodie, Zvi, and Dwight B. Crane. 1998. "The Design and Production of New Retirement Savings Products." Harvard Business School Working Paper No. 98070. Cambridge, Mass.

Brown, Jeffrey. 1999. "Private Pensions, Mortality Risk, and the Decision to Annuitize." NBER Working Paper Series No. 7191. National Bureau of Economic Research. Cambridge, Mass.

Burtless, Gary. 1998. "Financial Market Risks of Individual Retirement Accounts: The Twentieth Century Record." The Brookings Institution. Washington, D.C. Processed.

European Commission. 1999. "Rebuilding Pensions: Security, Efficiency, Affordability." Brussels.

Goetzmann, William N., and Philippe Jorion. 1997. "A Century of Global Stock Markets." NBER Working Paper No. 5901. National Bureau of Economic Research. Cambridge, Mass.

Jagannathan, Ravi, and Narayana R. Kocherlakota. 1996. "Why Should Older People Invest Less in Stocks than Younger People?" *Quarterly Review—Federal Reserve Bank of Minneapolis* 20(3): 11–20.

James, Estelle, and Dimitri Vittas. 1999. "The Decumulation (Payout) Phase of Defined Contribution Pillars." World Bank Research Development Group. Processed.

James, Estelle, Gary Ferrier, James Smalhout, and Dimitri Vittas. 1999. "Mutual Funds and Institutional Investments—What Is the Most

Efficient Way to Set Up Individual Accounts in a Social Security System?" Policy Research Working Paper No. 2099. World Bank, Washington, D.C.

Sylla, Richard, Jack W. Wilson, and Charles P. Jones. 1990. "Financial Markets Panics and Volatility in the Long Run, 1830–1988." In Eugene W. White, ed., *Crashes and Panics: The Lessons from History.* New York: Dow Jones Irwin Press.

———. 1994. "U.S. Financial Markets and Long Term Economic Growth, 1790–1989." In Thomas Weiss and Donald Schaefer, eds., *Economic Development in Historical Perspective.* Stanford University Press.

U.S. Department of Commerce, Bureau of the Census. 1975. *Historical Statistics of the United States: Colonial Times to 1970.* Washington, D.C.

U.S. Department of Commerce, Bureau of Economic Analysis. 1993. *National Income and Product Accounts of the United States,* vols. 1 and 2. Washington, D.C.

Valdes-Priéto, Salvador. 1998. "Risks in Pensions and Annuities: Efficiency Designs." Social Protection Discussion Paper Series No. 9804. World Bank, Washington, D.C.

Valdes-Priéto, Salvador, and Gonzalo Edwards. 1998. "Jubilacion en los Sistemas Pensionales Privados." *El Trimestre Economico* 65 (January–March): 3–47.

Wilson, Jack W., and Charles P. Jones. 1987a. "Stocks, Bonds, Paper and Inflation: 1870–1985." *The Journal of Portfolio Management* 14(1): 20–24.

———. 1987b. "A Comparison of Annual Common Stock Returns: 1871–1925 with 1925–1985." *The Journal of Business* 60(2): 239–58.

———. 1997. "Long-term Returns and Risks for Bonds." *The Journal of Portfolio Management* 23(3): 15–28.

12

Gender Dimensions of Pension Reform in the Former Soviet Union

Paulette Castel and Louise Fox

THE ECONOMIC AND SOCIAL TRANSITION from communism has been extremely traumatic in the former Soviet Union (FSU),[1] both economically and socially. Poverty has increased as incomes and living standards have fallen sharply (Milanovic 1996). Fiscal systems have also collapsed, provoking major cuts in the cradle-to-grave cash transfers system. Consequently, pensions, the most important cash transfer system in both the Soviet and post-Soviet period, have had to bear a share of the cuts (Fox 1997). Pensions have historically been very important in preventing old age poverty among women (World Bank 1994). The FSU was no exception. As in Western Europe, pension systems were important in maintaining living standards of war widows in the post-World War II era. Even as the Soviet Union became wealthier, formal asset holding was uncommon, and this was true even in the rural sector because agriculture was collectivized. Pension systems provided the main income source for the last 15 years of women's lives (Fox 1994).

The Soviet pension system was particularly generous toward women. It allowed them to retire at age 55 (five years earlier than the normal retirement age for men) with 20 years of service; replaced 55 to 85 percent of previous wages; gave credit for years out of the labor force to have children; and provided for the retirement at age 50 of women with more than five children. While parts of the FSU were aging (such as the Baltics and the Ukraine) as a whole, the country was relatively young, and pension transfers were only about 6 percent of gross domestic product (GDP) in 1998.

Pension systems continued to be important in preventing the spread of poverty among the elderly during the transition in the FSU. Nonetheless, in most countries, as GDP and tax revenue fell, pension systems rapidly became unaffordable. In addition, transferring a large and increasing share of income through the public sector proved inconsistent with the market economy structures that countries were trying to establish. The pension system crowded out other important public expenditures. Consequently, countries throughout the FSU implemented painful pension reforms. While there are significant variations among countries, most followed the same basic model: (i) they increased retirement ages (reducing the real value of future obligations), and (ii) they adopted new formulas that tied pension rights more closely to contributions.

Pension reforms have important gender dimensions because the work histories of men and women tend to be different. Women normally have shorter and more disrupted working careers and are more likely to be low-income earners. Thus, changes in benefit formulas and eligibility rules designed to reduce future obligations can have different effects on the old age security of men and women, which would not be seen if other measures were taken to reduce future expenditures (for example, across the board cuts through reductions in indexation provisions).

In the FSU countries the legacy of apparent gender equality has meant that little attention has been given to the impact of the new reforms on women. The region's newly emerging feminization of poverty is challenging this situation (Larzeg 1999). As a result of high male mortality, women over 60 significantly outnumber men of this age. In addition, divorce and female-headed households are on the rise, implying an even greater dependence by women on pensions in their old age.

How will women fare compared to men under the new pension systems? This chapter considers that question by analyzing the differential impact of the pension reform on men and women in four FSU countries that have introduced four different types of pension systems: Kazakhstan, the Kyrgyz Republic, Latvia, and Moldova. In considering this question, the chapter is organized as follows. The first section presents each country and reviews the characteristics of the new pension systems. The second section explains the methodology used to compare the impact of the reforms on men and women. The third section presents and comments on the results of the level of benefits for women and men, the implicit financial returns obtained from the systems, and the net wealth changes resulting from the reforms. The final section discusses the policy implications.

Four Pension Reforms in the Former Soviet Union

Ten years ago, the four countries in this study were all part of the same nation-state. Despite differences in income levels and economic structure, they all had well-developed social service sectors, resulting in universal and high rates of educational attainment, low rates of infant mortality, declining fertility, and well-developed cash transfer systems (Fox 1994). Labor force participation was high, especially among women (given the income levels); wages and cash transfers were the main source of household income, even in rural areas, owing to the collectivization of agriculture. Nonetheless, despite Soviet efforts to homogenize the country, even before the transition, these four areas of the country were quite different. Today, the independent countries have very different economic characteristics.

Latvia (per capita income of US$2,430) is a small industrial country on the Baltic Sea, with strong links to Germany and the Nordic countries. Less than 10 percent of its population works in agriculture. After a burst of hyperinflation and a large income drop, it has recovered and realized positive wage growth for the past six years. Not only is privatization nearly complete, but an open trading regime is in place. With few natural resources, growth has come primarily from an expanding service sector (financial and high-technology services as well as more traditional re-export and port services) centered around Riga, the capital. It is demographically the most mature of the four countries, with the lowest fertility rate and nearly 14 percent of its population over age 65 in 1997.

Moldova (per capita income of US$540) is a much poorer and less developed country on the border between Romania and Russia. It is rural, with agriculture and agroprocessing remaining very important to GDP. Hurt by conflict along the Russian border in the early years (which caused a loss of about one-quarter of the population in the breakaway Dniester region), it has struggled to achieve positive growth rates. The recent Russian crisis (Russia is the main purchaser of Moldova's exports) has further damaged growth prospects. With nearly 10 percent of its population over 65, it is a surprisingly mature country given its income level.

The Kyrgyz Republic (per capita income of US$440) is a mountainous country in Central Asia, the poorest in the group. It is very rural, with 45 percent of GDP coming from agricultural production and 60 percent of its population living outside urban areas. Since independence in 1992, the country has successfully (albeit painfully) stabilized and privatized most economic activity. The Kyrgyz Republic realized an average of 8 percent GDP growth in 1996–97 (a figure strongly tied to the opening of a gold mine in the north), but growth has subsequently stalled on account of the Russian crisis. Moreover, it is the youngest country demographically, with the highest fertility rate and 5.6 percent of its population over 65.

Kazakhstan (per capita income of US$1,340) is a large, sparsely populated and mineral-rich country in Central Asia with a diverse economy. Sixty percent of the population is urban, and only 13 percent of the GDP comes from agriculture, while 30 percent of GDP comes from industry. At the time of independence, Kazakhstan inherited an economy deeply dependent on Soviet supply and trade networks and, therefore, suffered a large decline in output. Growth resumed in 1996, as privatization policies paid off, but declining commodity prices and the Russian crisis have caused growth to slow again. It is a young country, with 7 percent of the population over 65.

The Pension Reforms

In addition to being expensive, the inherited Soviet pension system was complex, combining elements of a European 1960's pay-as-you-go system with peculiar communist features. It was a system suited to a demographically young country, as retirement ages were low (55 for women and 60 for men). Pension benefits depended on final wage and years of service, not the amount of contributions (actually the difference did not matter since everyone worked for the state and there was full employment). Only 20 years of service were required for women, and 25 for men, to qualify for a full pension. In addition, the pension system was used to reward politically favored groups and to compensate for weaknesses of the Soviet system. For example, early retirement (up to 10 years earlier) for those who worked in heavy industry and the transportation sector compensated for a poor occupational health and safety system. Offering early pensions to ballet dancers, and wind instrument musicians, as well as the blind, compensated for the rigid labor markets and lack of occupational mobility. Finally, the overall income replacement was high. At the earliest retirement age, the rate was 55 percent of final wage, rising to 75–85 percent for more years of service or special service. These levels were much more generous than those found in Western European countries at a much higher level of income per capita (Fox 1997).

In addition to early retirement, women received several favorable advantages: pension credit for time spent out of the labor force raising children and early retirement for women who had raised five children or a disabled child up to at least the age of eight. Moreover, because of the compressed wage structure and small informal sector, women's generally lower earnings did not result in pensions that were considerably lower than men's.

Pension reform has taken a different turn in each country. Latvia implemented pension reform in several stages. The first stage took place in 1992, when the Soviet pension system was scaled back. Latvia adopted a simple formula basing pensions on years of service and the economywide average wage. Accrual rates were lowered as well. However, the low retirement age and all the special groups continued. By 1994 it was clear that even this system was too expensive and the retirement age would have to be increased, especially for women and special groups.

In 1995 a new law was submitted to Parliament that introduced a notional defined contribution scheme (NDC, see box 12.1), which bases pensions entirely on individual contributions and life expectancy at retirement.

Box 12.1. What Is a Notional Defined Contribution Pay-as-You-Go Scheme?

The scheme mimics a defined contribution funded scheme. Contributions are recorded in notional accounts that return notional interest until retirement. There are three main differences between a notional defined contribution (NDC) scheme and a fully funded scheme. First, worker's contributions are not invested in an NDC scheme but are only recorded as they are used to pay current pensioner benefits. Second, the "return" on contributions is not directly linked to the results on the financial market but set exogenously. The "interest rate" is most often related to the growth of the contributions. Third, at retirement benefits are calculated by dividing the amount accumulated in the notional account by the average number of months workers (with no gender differentiation) are expected to live at each specific age of retirement. Capital does not continue to earn notional interest during the payout phase. Indexation provisions are used to link the growth of benefits in payment to the performance of the economy.

Acquired rights under the old system were immediately converted in 1996 into notional capital in the new system.

Special groups were abolished and retirement ages for men and women are gradually being equalized. The state budget pays a contribution for up to 1.5 years for women on maternity leave. Pensions are no longer indexed to economywide average wage but to changes in the nominal price level. A second, funded tier will be introduced in July 2001 (Fox and Palmer 1999).

Kazakhstan was next to undertake a pension reform. It began slowly in 1996, with a gradual increase to 58 in the retirement age for women and 63 for men and the elimination of many early retirement provisions. The Chilean example inspired the more extensive reform in Kazakhstan, which took place in 1998. Fully funded individual accounts managed both privately and publicly are being developed, and the previous system is being gradually phased out.

Contributions are now split in two: 10 percent of gross wage is paid to a pension fund of the contributor's choice whereas another 15 percent is paid to the old State Pension Fund. The old State Pension Fund continues to pay existing benefits and provides new benefits based on the number of years worked under the old system. Contribution rates to this fund are expected to decline as the expenditures related to the old system decrease. This decline will occur gradually, for the reform did not reduce acquired rights. Disability and survivor's benefits have been converted to flat allowances unrelated to service or wage history and are financed by general revenues (Andrews 2000).

The government guarantees a minimum old age pension for those workers who complete 25 years of service if their combined pay-as-you-go and funded pension falls below the minimum amount. The minimum pension was equivalent to 25 percent of the nationwide average wage when the reform began, and was expected to be price indexed. Those who do not qualify for the minimum will receive an old age allowance close to the social assistance level, that is, approximately 7 percent of the nationwide average wage.

The Kyrgyz Republic took the first step toward pension reform in 1996 with the implementation of individual contribution record-keeping and the elimination of many early retirement provisions. In 1997 it introduced an NDC system (box 12.1). The reform was accompanied by a generous recalculation of all existing pensions and no increase in the retirement age (see Government of the Kyrgyz Republic 1997–1999). The system, however, was not sustainable in the short term, and the retirement age was at last gradually increased to 58 for women and 63 for men. There are no plans for a funded system.

Acquired rights in the old system were redefined and scaled down. Years of service accrued before 1996 qualify for a replacement rate of 1 percent of a worker's average wage. The latter is calculated on workers' five best consecutive years before 1996, although at 1997 prices. Workers' contributions in the new system earn an interest equivalent to 75 percent of the growth rate of the average wage. A particularity of the system is that there is no minimum pension but a flat base pension per year of service added to all workers' earning-related benefits. A minimum of five years of service is required to qualify for the base, and the full amount is paid to women and men who have completed 20 and 25 years of service, respectively. The total amount of the base cannot currently exceed 200 *Som*, which represented 25 percent of the average wage in 1998. The base will not be adjusted until it reaches 12 percent of the average wage (Castel 1998).

Moldova finally reformed its Soviet-era pension system in 1998 after an extremely difficult process. The old system clearly needed reform. Pension benefits were often paid months late and sometimes in the form of apples or onions that the government would accept in lieu of contributions. Nevertheless, the Parliament constantly rejected amendments to raise the retirement age or to scale back privileges. Parliament finally accepted a package that increased the retirement age, eliminated most of the early retirement provisions, and introduced a new defined benefit formula (Government of Moldova 1999). As in the Kyrgyz Republic, there are no plans to introduce a fully funded system.

Of the four countries, Moldova's new system is the closest to the old Soviet system. A minimum of 20 years of service is required to qualify for an old age pension. The first 35 years of service provide a replacement rate of 1.2 percent per year, and any additional years beyond this, as well as years worked after legal retirement age, provide 2 percent. The retirement age has been gradually increased until it has reached 60 for women and 65 for men. Periods of taking care of a child less than two year's old, a disabled child, or an elderly person (over 75 years)[2] still count as years of service. The reform introduced a minimum old age pension of 25 percent of the average wage (21.85 percent in the case of farmers). As with old age benefits, the latter is increased as per 2 percent for each additional year of service worked beyond 35 years or after the legal retirement age. Similarly, the minimum is proportionally reduced for those who do not have 35 years of service.

Years of service accrued before the reform qualify for a replacement rate of 0.4 percent of a worker's average wage and a flat amount of 57 Lei (approximately 16 percent of the average wage). Total benefits are a weighted average of the two components described above, according to the number of years of service realized in each system. Younger workers, who will work for 20 years or more after the reform, will lose all their acquired rights (Thompson and Yu 1997).

Main Changes for Women

Table 12.1 summarizes the key variables affecting women in the pension reforms. The trend has been to harmonize provisions across genders. All countries raised the minimum pension age for women (with a transition period). Only in Latvia will this age be equal to the men's minimum, albeit the lowest age for men among the four countries. Two countries eliminated the right to pension credit for time spent on maternity leave. Latvia maintained this provision, but it scaled back the entitlement and finances it from general revenues, not earmarked revenues.

Do these new systems reflect greater gender equality? Theoretically, they do, for the underlying philosophy of the reforms is to reduce intragenerational redistribution and improve labor market incentives. The pension systems were reformed to approximate market outcomes more closely, with the role of the state being to ensure intergenerational redistribution and efficient risk pooling. This implies that individuals bear direct responsibility for their choices about participation and exit from the labor force.

The social context in which these choices are made does, however, matter, particularly when it refers to women's traditional responsibility for raising children and grandchildren and the social value of this unpaid work. The Soviet system tried to compensate women directly for this time by (i) providing pension credit for time spent raising children and (ii) allowing women to retire five years earlier. The later provision, however, seems a rather inefficient approach. Although daughters frequently rely on their mothers to look after the children so they could work, by the time they are 55 most women are much healthier, on average, than men. Carrying this tradition forward into a market based, more individualistic system is

Table 12.1. Features of the New Pension System Affecting Women

	Latvia	Kazakhstan	Kyrgyz Republic	Moldova
Retirement age for women				
Old	55	55	55	55
New	60	58	58	60
Transition rate	6 months per year	6 months per year	4 months per year	6 months per year
Credit for time raising children	1.5 years for each child; maximum 2 children	n.a.	n.a.	2 years of service for each child
Memorandum				
Retirement age for men				
Old	60	60	60	60
New	65	63	63	65

n.a. Not applicable.
Source: Country legislation.

problematic. As shown in the next sections, disrupted careers and early retirements greatly affect women's old age security in the new systems.

This chapter does not consider survivor pensions in its analysis of the gender dimensions of pension systems principally because female labor force participation rates are so high in the FSU that survivor pensions are not a significant factor in women's old age security. Most women are already covered under the pension system based on their own participation. Because these systems do not permit having two public pensions, women usually receive survivor pensions in the period leading up to retirement if their spouse died before they retire. As a result, survivor pensions may be relevant primarily for preretirement income security for women.[3] Latvia eliminated survivor pensions for spouses an unnecessary expense at a time of cutbacks. The other three countries maintained them for spouses and for families with underage children (Latvia also maintains them for underage children), with a minimum equal to up to 100 percent of the minimum old age pension (in the Kyrgyz Republic). Kazakhstan has transferred them to general revenue financing.

Methodology

Definition of variables. In this chapter we are only concerned about the gender implications of the reforms; other features have been evaluated elsewhere. To do this we construct several variables to quantify gender differences in pension outcomes for women and men and follow well-established techniques of identifying the gender gap by comparing expected flows of income over time for the average woman and man in the country (Burkhauser and Warlick 1981). We construct three variables: the individual replacement rates, the implicit financial return on contributions, and the change in individual net wealth.

Replacement rates are calculated as the ratio (in percent) between a person's benefit and his or her average wage at retirement, as equation (1) shows:

(1)
$$RR_{i,a} = \frac{B_{i,a}}{W_i} \cdot 100.$$

In this formula, $RR_{i,a}$ is the replacement rate of the worker i retiring at age a; $B_{i,a}$, the level of his or her old age pension when at retirement; and W_i, his or her average wage. We assume a worker's average wage to be constant over the working life span. This measure ignores the time dimensions, both on the contribution side and the benefit side. A pension is a promise to pay a stream of benefits at a certain age or event (such as retirement) until death. It is usually paid through contributions over time. An easy way to compare both streams of cash is to calculate the implicit rate of return that would equalize them in formulas (2) and (2a):

(2)
$$B_{i,a} = PMT\left(r, K_{i,a}, -C_{i,a}\right)$$

(2a)
$$C_{i,a} = \sum_{t=0}^{t=a-1} \tau \cdot W_i \cdot (1+r)^t$$

In these formulas, r is the implicit rate of return; PMT is the financial function that provides the level of benefits (equal to $B_{i,a}$) that will exhaust a certain amount of accumulated contributions, $C_{i,a}$, over the expected number of retirement periods $K_{i,a}$. The expression (1) gives the level of benefits, $B_{i,a}$. The amount of accumulated contributions, $C_{i,a}$, is equal to the sum of the worker's wage multiplied by the contribution rate, , and the compounding interest earned on the contributions over the working life as if the latter had been invested at the interest rate or implicit rate of return, r.

The implicit rate of return is normally calculated in nominal terms. To avoid the difficulty of making assumptions about price and wage growth in each economy, we express this rate in relation to the wage growth. An implicit rate of return equal to zero is an implicit rate of return equal to wage growth.

If people work longer, they should realize a longer stream of wage income before retirement. This addition to income is not considered in the implicit rate of return analysis. This income stream should be higher than under the previous system, since the reforms reduce benefits and thus leave room for a cut in payroll taxes. These changes can be valued by

computing the net present value—at the time the reform is implemented—
of the flow of wages and pension incomes and comparing it to the present
value of such incomes in a no-reform case. We call this expression the
change in lifetime net wealth, and we use it to give a measure of the global result of these changes from the individual's perspective, as the set of formulas 3a to 3c shows:

(3a)
$$NZ = Z_{new} - Z_{old}$$

(3b)
$$Z_{old} = \left\{ \sum_{t=0}^{t=a-1} \frac{1-\tau}{(1-\beta)^t} \cdot W_i + \frac{1}{(1-\beta)^a} B_{i,a}^{old} \cdot \sum_{t=a}^{t=T} \frac{1}{(1-\beta)^t} \right\} \cdot \frac{100}{W_i}$$

(3c)
$$Z_{new} = \left\{ \sum_{t=0}^{t=b-1} \frac{1-\tau}{(1-\beta)^t} \cdot W_i + \frac{1}{(1-\beta)^b} \sum_{t=b}^{t=c-1} \frac{1-\mu}{(1-\beta)^t} W_i \right.$$
$$\left. + \frac{1}{(1-\beta)^c} B_{i,a}^{new} \cdot \sum_{t=c}^{t=T} \frac{1}{(1-\beta)^t} \right\} \cdot \frac{100}{W_i}$$

In these formulas, NZ is the lifetime wealth net change. Z_{old} and Z_{new} are
the flows of income under the old and new systems. They are expressed as
a percentage of a worker's wage. The contribution rate is assumed to be
changed at the period b, and τ and μ are the contribution rates before
and after this period. $B_{i,a}^{old}$ and $B_{i,a}^{new}$ are a worker's old age benefits before and after the reform. The starting period, 0, is the time the reform is
implemented.

In the calculation presented below, a discount rate β of 5 percent is
applied to the flow of future income. This rate should reflect households'
discount rate. Unfortunately, there is no available estimation of this parameter for any country in the Europe and Central Asia region. The discount
rate that the World Bank uses in economic evaluation of investment operations in the Europe and Central Asia region is currently about 10–12 percent in the case of industrial projects. Our estimate seems quite conservative if we consider that, evaluated as the opportunity cost for financial
resources, the discount rate should be higher than the real interest rate
because households often face borrowing constraints, especially at lower
income levels.

PROFILES OF WOMEN

Neither men nor women are homogeneous groups. We can, however, gen-
eralize about certain labor market characteristics, which tend to affect pension outcomes. Women tend to have interrupted labor force participation.

They take time out of the labor force to bear and raise children. They also have more periods of unemployment. Educational differences and experience, amount of hours worked, occupational segregation, and gender discrimination include reasons why women tend to have lower incomes than men. As transition economies move toward contribution-based systems, these tendencies should result in lower pensions for women, on average, as their total lifetime income will be lower than men's. Women also have higher life expectancy at retirement age than men, so they generally receive old age income over a longer period.

Table 12.2 shows the current differences in labor market characteristics in the countries in our study. While male and female labor force participation rates were high and very close during the previous regime, since the beginning of the transition women's rates have fallen in most of the former communist countries of Eastern Europe and Central Asia. In general, female rates fell even more than male rates, and the fall has been heavily concentrated in the younger and older categories (Barry and Reilly 1999). Recorded unemployment, however, is not significantly higher for women, which may reflect the lower participation rates at those ages most likely to suffer unemployment.

Comprehensive information is not available on how these differences translate in total years of contribution for men and women. For the purpose of our analysis, we generated average lengths of service based on each country's labor force participation by age and gender. Table 12.3 presents

Table 12.2. Labor Market Characteristics

	Kazakhstan	Kyrgyz Republic	Latvia	Moldova
Labor force participation, formal sector (percent of working-age population)				
Female	42.8	38.2	50.2	45.3
Male	52.5	45.6	59.0	52.6
Unemployment (percent of labor force)				
Female	6.4	7.5	16.3	n.a.
Male	5.7	7.0	15.4	n.a.
Wage gap (percent of male wage)				
Female	72.3	81.6	79.9	n.a.

n.a. Not available.
Sources: International Labor Organization; Kyrgyz Living Standards Measurement Survey; Organization for Economic Cooperation and Development-CEET 1997 database; E. Barry and M. Reilly (1999); World Bank data.

Table 12.3. Average Length of Service
(before pension)

Country	Year	Men	Women	Gender gap
Kazakhstan	1996	40	35	5.0
Kyrgyz Republic	1997	38.5	30.2	6.7
Latvia	1997	39.3	32.3	7.0
Moldova	1997	44	36.9	7.1
Bulgaria	1995	34.8	28.7	6.1
Poland	1998	36.9	32.0	4.9

Sources: Country data (Bulgaria and Poland); authors' calculations.

the results. As a reference, the table also reports figures in the case of Bulgaria and Poland, for which estimates are available. These numbers take into account that, in the prereform system, women were allowed to retire five years earlier. When we use them in the analysis, we make the assumption that women will not change their behavior. Thus far, this seems to be correct.

Women live significantly longer than men do in the FSU. Life expectancy and the expected length of the retirement period are central in valuing the pension. When unisex annuities are used (as they are in a pay-as-you-go system and in most defined contribution systems), women get a higher rate of return than men on contributions. Table 12.4 shows the gender gap difference in life expectancy in the four countries under consideration. The largest gap is observed in Kazakhstan.

Table 12.4. Life Expectancy

Country	Kazakhstan	Kyrgyz Republic	Latvia	Moldova
Year	1996	1997	1998	1997
At birth				
Female	70.4	71.4	74.9	70.3
Male	59.7	62.6	63.8	62.9
Age 60				
Female	20.4	19.1	19.9	18.8
Male	13.7	14.9	15.5	15.8
Age 65				
Female	17.4	15.6	16.0	15.3
Male	11.5	12.2	12.5	13.3

Sources: World Bank data; Kyrgyz Republic estimates.

Assumptions

Modeling the new pension system requires a series of assumptions. Many of the parameters are not known ex-ante, and some regulations still need to be issued. In our calculations we made the following general assumptions:

- *Characteristics of women and men.* The calculation of the level of benefits for men and women retiring under the new system requires projecting all the key values into the future: life expectancy, labor force participation, wage gap, unemployment gap, etc. This task is quite difficult in an Organization for Economic Cooperation and Development (OECD) country. In a transition economy—uncharted territory in economic history—this would be beyond heroic. Although the pension reform should also modify behavior, our analysis below simply assumes that the reported gender-specific characteristics will remain constant in the future.

- *Fully funded pillars.* The rate of return on contributions invested in the fully funded pillars created in Kazakhstan and Latvia is assumed to be 3 percentage points higher than the growth rate of the average wage in the economy, net of administrative costs. In Kazakhstan, with the reform, 10 percent of a worker's gross wage is invested in the funded pillar. In Latvia the second pillar will start functioning in 2002, receiving 2 percent of a worker's gross wage, which will increase by 1.25 percent every two years until it reaches 7 percent of a worker's gross wage in 2010.[4]

- *Overall contribution rates.* Our methodology requires an estimate of the contributions designated for future pensions. The official contribution rate assigned to the national pension fund (when a separate fund exists) or the second tier usually does not reflect the real cost of the public pension system. First, it does not take into account the long-term financial sustainability. The Kazakhstan reform, for example, implies an additional expenditure of about 1.7 percent of GDP over 20 years. Serving the additional public debt will imply additional taxes. Second, the contribution rate paid to the pension fund gives rights to other benefits: disability and survivors benefits as well as family allowance. The intertemporal cost of these benefits is impossible to evaluate at this point. Third, there are administrative costs in running a system, which may not be financed by contributions. If we ignored these issues, our comparisons across countries would be biased. Consequently, we decided that the best method of comparison would be to use the current cost of the old age system, and calculate what payroll tax would be required to cover these current expenditures. Table 12.5 presents these rates.

Table 12.5. Contribution Rate Estimates

(percentage of gross wage)[a]

	Kazakhstan	Kyrgyz Republic	Latvia	Moldova
Prereform situation				
Payroll tax earmarked for pensions	25.5	32.0	34.0	32.0
Payroll required to finance current old age benefits	33.2	37.5	27.5	29.7
Post-reform situation				
Projected payroll tax after 25 years	15	25	20	25

a. After payroll tax but before income tax.
Sources: Country legislation; authors' calculations.

PROBLEMS WITH THE METHODOLOGY

There are many weaknesses in the methodology, the most outstanding being the use of the old system as contrafactual. As discussed above, since the old systems were not affordable, it is unlikely that the benefits promised in the them would have been delivered to future generations. The analysis, however, does not focus on the absolute size of the changes but only on the differential impact of the reforms between men and women. The use of the old systems' legal benefits as a baseline clearly leads to overestimating the replacement rates and implicit financial returns in the old system, and to underestimating the changes in net wealth after the reform. It should not, however, affect the differential impact between men and women.

Finally, the calculation above does not include any estimation of the loss of welfare from the reduction of leisure (or time at home for unpaid work). The reason is that the value of leisure is difficult to estimate. If it is valued at the individual's wage rate, the increases in welfare related to work are simply offset by the loss of leisure. Retirement age increase would thus imply a welfare loss equal to the benefits not received due to later retirement. Under this assumption, if men receive higher wages, they suffer a greater loss of welfare, on average. The contrary might in fact be closer to the truth. A study in Ecuador (Rama and MacIsaac 1999) on the impact of downsizing on workers' earnings and welfare showed that women suffer higher income loss than men, but these difference did not appear when the questions was about welfare loss. In other words, women did not mind withdrawing from the labor force; they valued their time highly. A retirement age increase is just the opposite. As a result, our calculation of the net wealth changes, which does not take into account women's valuation of leisure, probably underestimates the overall negative impact of the pension reform on women.

Results

In this section we first use the three variables constructed above to estimate the gender differences nestled within the systems in each country. We follow a sequential approach to isolate the three gender-relevant aspects of the pension reforms. First we look at how the ratio of women's benefits to men's benefits would change with the reform, assuming both have a full work history and both earn the average wage. In this case any observed gender difference in replacement rates highlights the pure gender differences in benefit rules. Next we compute the gap in the implicit rate of return on contributions. Here the systems' subsidy to women based on longer life expectancy emerges. In a second stage we look at what happens to women if they continue to experience the labor market outcomes historically observed in these countries—lower wages and interrupted work histories. Again we first isolate the benefit gender gap, and then we use the implicit rate of return on contributions to see the combined impact of behavior, benefit rules, and life expectancy. We do a final analysis of the full relative impact of the reform using the net wealth variable.

Lastly, we check the sensitivity of the analysis to assumptions on the financial rate of return of the fully funded pillar. We look at how our results change for poorer workers, picking up the effect of the minimum benefit, which lowers the gender gap. We also analyze how the benefit gender gap changes through the transition by computing the ratio of replacement rates for several cohorts, and we look at the incentives for women to retire early.

Design Features: How Does the Design of the System Affect Gender Differences in Pension Outcomes?

Figure 12.1 shows the replacement rates for women as a ratio (in percentage) of those for men, using 60 and 65 as the retirement ages in the old and new systems, respectively, for both genders.[5] This ratio reflects the gender differentiation nestled within the system. In Latvia the old system had no gender gap in benefits. Accrual rates were the same for men and women. In the three other countries, however, women started accruing higher replacement rates at lower years of service under the old system. In Kazakhstan, these gender differences disappeared with a full working life under the old system as the maximum pension was reached. As a result, in figure 12.1 Kazakhstan looks just like Latvia. Only Moldova kept this feature within its new system, and it is the only one to show a benefit gender gap in the new system. Moldova even enlarged the gap because it doubled the benefit accrual rate for years of service completed after retirement age while maintaining a lower retirement age for women.

Figure 12.1. Ratios of Replacement Rates: Full Work History, Men and Women

In percentage of men benefit

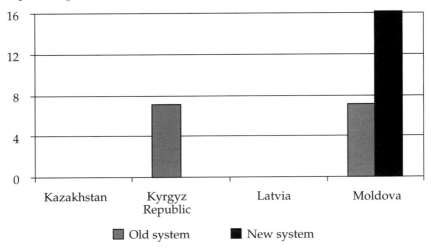

■ Old system   ■ New system

Source: Authors' calculations.

IMPLICIT RATE OF RETURN ON CONTRIBUTIONS

All countries show a gender gap in favor of women in rates of return under the old system. This gap decreases in all countries except Moldova in the reformed system (figure 12.2). It remains positive, however, as women at age 65 still have much higher life expectancy than men, so women's contributions still buy more benefits than do men's contributions. The highest gap overall is observed in Kazakhstan because this country shows the largest gender gap in life expectancy.[6]

How Does Incorporating Behavioral Differences and Labor Market Structures Change the Gender Gap?

This section analyses the gender gap once labor market outcomes for men and women are taken into account. As noted above, on average women earn less and have overall shorter working periods than men (tables 12.2 and 12.3). They also retire earlier. When we apply these characteristics (based on our country-specific profiles), on average women receive lower pension benefits than men in the new, as in the old, system (figure 12.3). The benefit gap widens (becomes more negative) after the reform because the new systems reward long service and early contributions and penalize early retirement.

Figure 12.2. Differences in Implicit Rates of Return: Full Work History, Men and Women

Relative to wage growth, women-men

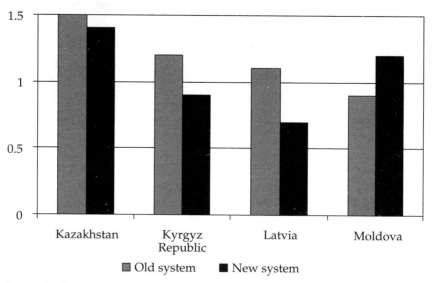

Source: Authors' calculations.

What factors drive the gender gap in each country under the new system? The gender gap widens in Kazakhstan, the Kyrgyz Republic, and Latvia because compound interest rates in defined contribution and notional account systems provide higher increments for the first years spent in the system (instead of the constant rate in the previous systems). In the Kyrgyz Republic, the base pension, which is not earnings related but linked to the number of years of service and capped at 20 years for women, moderates this effect. In Moldova the system strongly rewards length of service over 35 years. As average length of service for women is only 37 years, the shorter length of service (behavior effect) swamps the slight gender difference in accrual rates seen in figure 12.1. Finally, Kazakhstan and the Kyrgyz Republic permit but penalize retirement at younger ages since benefits are based on life expectancy at retirement, a key feature of defined contribution systems.

Role of maternity leave provisions

Figure 12.3 does not show the mitigating role of maternity leave provisions on the gender gap in Latvia and Moldova. In a defined contribution

**Figure 12.3. Ratios of Replacement Rates:
Observed Labor Market Outcomes**

In percent of men benefits

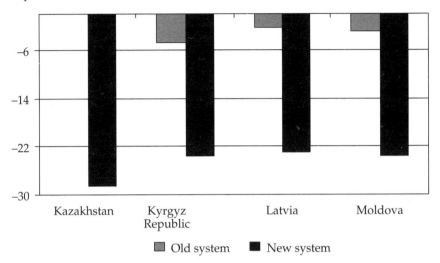

Source: Authors' calculations.

system, absences from the labor force have a larger effect on benefits if they occur early in the working career because of compounding effects. In Latvia the state budget pays contributions to the pension system during periods of maternity leave (1.5 years per child). This subsidy reduces the projected gender gap by as much as 23 percent. In Moldova maternity leave provisions reduce the benefit gender gap by one-half. A cross-subsidy from other contributors funds these provisions.

IMPLICIT RATE OF RETURN ON CONTRIBUTIONS

Women's longer life expectancy relative to men again generates higher rates of return on contributions but less in the new than in the old system (figure 12.4). The largest gap in the new systems is found in the Kyrgyz Republic because of the base pension. The base, added to the notional account component, represents a better financial return on contribution for women because on average women earn 25 percent less than men.

FULL IMPACT OF THE REFORM: CHANGES IN NET WEALTH

The decrease in pension obligations associated with reducing entitlements should bring about a surplus at current tax rates. This surplus could be saved, consumed by other branches of the government, or given back to the

**Figure 12.4. Differences in Rates of Return:
Observed Labor Market Outcomes**

Relative to wage growth, women minus men

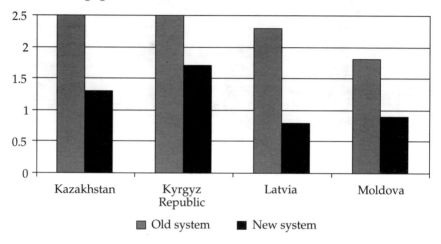

Source: Authors' calculations.

taxpayer in the form of reduced contributions. We assume that all of the decrease in contributions is passed on to the contributor in the form of higher wages. Table 12.5 shows our estimate of how much this reduction in contribution should be, based on fiscal projections of the systems.[7]

Under our financing assumptions, the present value of the expected flow of wages and benefits for new entrants is higher both for men and women after the reform, even if women continue to behave the same and the labor market generates the same outcomes (figure 12.5). Because men earn more than women over more years, the present value of men's projected income stream is always higher than the value for women, and the change is also more positive for them. But women do well, especially in Kazakhstan and Latvia. Three factors account for this result. First, the reduction of the contribution rate reduces the tax burden of the system, increasing take-home pay. This effect is projected to be high in Kazakhstan (even though it takes some time) and very low in Moldova. Second, the increase in the retirement age leads to increases in income during the working years. Third, our method calculates the present value of an expected stream of income (wages and pension benefits) at the beginning of the working life, so benefit reductions are heavily discounted (another factor favoring Kazakhstan). Because the benefit cut was large and the tax cut small in Moldova, the change in net wealth for women is near zero.

These effects are uncertain. The success of the reform in decreasing the tax burden will depend not only on the reform of the pension system, but also on the general economic environment and the capacity to collect the necessary level of contributions. Similarly, a retirement age increase will lead to an increase in working income only if there are jobs, and only if workers who must postpone retirement would not have become working pensioners under the previous regime. In Latvia and Kazakhstan the results also depend on how well the fully funded pillar functions.

Sensitivity Analysis

LOWER RATE OF RETURN ON FUNDING

The results presented in the above sections assume that in Latvia, as well as in Kazakhstan, workers' savings invested in the financial market show a rate of return 3 percent higher than wage growth. Actually, the rate could be higher or lower. Variations in the return on the financial market affect men more than women (table 12.6) because men accumulate over longer periods. The fall in benefits in both countries is limited by the minimum wage. On average, men's benefits fall relatively more than women's

Figure 12.5. Differences in Net Wealth: Observed Labor Market Outcomes

In number of annual wage, new - old system

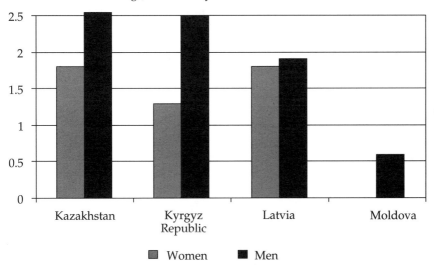

Source: Authors' calculations.

Table 12.6. Effects of Variations in Financial Rate of Return:[a]
Observed Labor Market Outcomes
(percentage of replacement rates obtained in baseline scenario)

	R = 0		R = 3		R = 6	
Country	Women	Men	Women	Men	Women	Men
Kazakhstan	80	43	100	100	229	248
Latvia	75	70	100	100	156	177

a. Expressed as the differential between the return of the financial market and wage growth.
Source: Authors' calculations.

in a downturn because women's expected benefit starts out lower and, therefore, the fall is broken earlier by the minimum. Pensioners in Kazakhstan are more vulnerable to a downturn because the fully funded pillar finances the total old age income.

LOWER INCOME

All four countries under study have introduced new provisions regarding old age minimum benefits. Table 12.7 summarizes their main characteristics. The minimum benefit in Kazakhstan plays two roles. As in the other countries, it serves to push up the level of benefit that low-income earners would earn if benefits were only earnings related, but it also provides a

Table 12.7. Old Age Pension Minimum Benefits Provisions

Country	Required service	Level when the new pension law was adopted	Added to benefits?	Indexing rules
Kazakhstan	25	25 percent of the average wage	No	Prices
Kyrgyz Republic	5	0.6 percent per year of service for women 0.5 percent per year of service for men up to a maximum of 12 percent of average wage	Yes	Wages
Latvia	10	28 percent of average wage	No	Ad hoc
Moldova	20	0.45 percent per year of service, up to a maximum of 16 percent of average wage, increased by 2 percent when service beyond 35 years and/or retirement age	No	Wages

Source: Country legislation.

guaranteed floor to all workers in case the financial market provides low returns. Indeed, without a minimum benefit, average women in Kazakhstan could receive old age income as low as 14 percent of the average wage if the returns in the financial market were not higher than the average wage growth.

In the four countries, low-income earners who contribute for many years will receive the minimum old age benefit. However, workers who are in agriculture or the informal sector for long periods of time may not qualify for the minimum in Kazakhstan or Moldova. The Kyrgyz Republic offers the broadest coverage and is the only country that still makes some gender differentiation when calculating the minimum old age benefit, making the Kyrgyz Republic the most beneficial country to women.

Women in Transition: What Is the Impact of the Reform on Different Age Cohorts of Women?

Since the new pension systems are introduced gradually, two types of transition issues must be considered. The first one, which usually attracts a great deal of attention, appears when funding is added. Some of workers' contributions are directed to the new scheme, thereby producing a shortfall in income in the public system. This transition cost associated with the creation of private pension funds has fiscal but not gender implications and, therefore, this chapter does not focus on it. The second type of transition issue, which does have a large gender dimension, relates to the gradual changes in eligibility criteria and pension formulas and their effects on different cohorts. In the previous sections we compared the old and new systems, as if workers have always been in one system or the other. In reality the new systems are introduced gradually. For at least the next 20 years, most pensioners will receive benefits that are a mix of rights acquired under the old and new systems. As a result, average replacement rates at retirement age will vary depending on a worker's age when the reform was implemented and the rate at which rights in the old system are phased out. This transition rate varies across the four countries depending on how the new systems recognize acquired rights under the old system, and, as a result, the evolution of the gender gap varies (figures 12.6 through 12.9).

Kazakhstan fully recognizes most existing rights, so the old system will survive for many years (figure 12.6). As a result, the transition period is long. The other three countries eliminated the old formulas. The Kyrgyz Republic and Moldova reduced acquired rights. In the Kyrgyz Republic, because of the introduction of the relatively high base pension of 30 percent of the average wage (figure 12.7), replacement rates only gradually started decreasing just after the reform.[8] This base will be allowed to fall gradually in real terms until it reaches the level of 12 percent of the average wage. The transition in Moldova (figure 12.8) is similar; the level of the base is, however,

**Figure 12.6. Kazakhstan:
Replacement Rates**

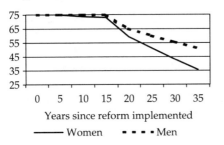

Years since reform implemented

———— Women   ▪ ▪ ▪ Men

Source: Authors' calculations.

**Figure 12.7. Kyrgyz Republic:
Replacement Rates**

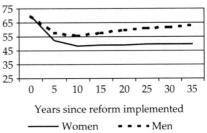

Years since reform implemented

———— Women   ▪ ▪ ▪ Men

Source: Authors' calculations.

**Figure 12.8. Moldova:
Replacement Rates**

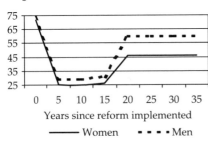

Years since reform implemented

———— Women   ▪ ▪ ▪ Men

Source: Authors' calculations.

**Figure 12.9. Latvia:
Replacement Rates**

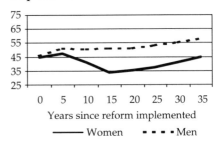

Years since reform implemented

———— Women   ▪ ▪ ▪ Men

Source: Authors' calculations.

much smaller and contrary to the Kyrgyz reform, and it will be eliminated at the end of the transition period.[9] Finally, in Latvia (figure 12.9) the reform shifted everyone into the new scheme, as if workers had always contributed 20 percent of their gross wage to their notional accounts.[10] The adjustment to the new system was thus almost immediate, and the calculation of all the benefit components began to be a function of life expectancy at retirement. As a result, women, who retire earlier than men under the transition rules, will initially experience a decrease in their replacement rate.

INCENTIVES TO WORK LONGER

Except for Kazakhstan, the adjustments in the pension systems introduced by the reforms have been swift for today's retiring women and will also be tough for future retiring women. Unless they begin to work past the minimum retirement age, their benefits will be cut by 30–50 percent. The minimum pension provides a floor on benefits, but this is quite low.

One of the main arguments in favor of defined contribution systems is that they can be structured to encourage longer working years. Will women respond to these incentives, change their behavior, and retire later? Certainly the incentives to work longer under defined contribution systems are strong, as Disney and Whitehouse (1999) show. However, experience in OECD countries suggests that other factors may be more important (Gruber and Wise 1999). In OECD countries the combined weight of other taxes and incentives discourage labor supply above pension age despite overall good health, and, as a result, workers exit from the labor force as soon as possible. It should be noted that this evidence comes from countries with weaker incentives to work longer and is mostly based on males. The working life for women in OECD countries is still increasing on average. However, in transition economies, the same factors encourage women to avail themselves of the early retirement provisions, as income tax rates are high, and total payroll taxes (including those needed to finance existing pensioners) remain steep. The pure defined contribution systems yield about the same rate of return on contributions for early or later retirement, while those with a base pension (Kyrgyz) or the defined benefit system (Moldova) encourage earlier retirement. If women have other income in the household or can work in the informal sector, the low pension may seem to provide enough income. If pensions represent the only income in cash in the household (such as in the agricultural sector), the decision to take a pension seems obvious. The brief evidence to date shows that despite reforms designed to reward increased contributions and a longer working life, most women in the FSU countries still take their pensions as early as possible and end up with a lower pension, on average, than men.

Conclusions

The transition from the Soviet period in the FSU involved a great deal of adjustment for almost everyone. Pension systems were not immune. The economic and ensuing fiscal collapse necessitated the reforms in the FSU. The transition goal of reducing the public sector was also an important element in the reforms. This element drove reforms towards reducing redistributions and basing pensions on actual contributions. Since women received relatively better treatment than did men in the Soviet system, it is not surprising that the introduction of reforms cut back these redistributions.

Considering that most benefits are not taxed but wages are, in pure replacement rate terms, postreform benefits will still be relatively high for women, if they participate in the workforce nearly all their working life. Time taken out to have children or a large portion of time spent in the informal sector will reduce benefits. Both Latvia and Moldova have tempered their systems with pension credit for women during the period after childbirth—1.5 years after the four months of maternity leave in Latvia and two years after maternity leave in Moldova. This helps to reduce the gender gap. It costs very little—less than 0.3 percent of GDP per year in Latvia. Note that in Latvia the cost is kept under control by financing it through a budget transfer to the pension fund. The Kyrgyz Republic and Moldova have reduced the gender gap by providing flat benefits per year of service. This makes these two systems more redistributive towards women than the pure defined contribution systems.

The principal issue in the four countries is the category of women who are 40 and above. They can take an early pension, and most will. But their pension will be low, especially if their wages were low. Will they be able to live on that pension at age 65, when they should have another 16 years to live, and at age 70, when their spouse has died and their children have moved away? This is a major social policy question, and a strong argument for raising minimum retirement ages.

Are women well served by these changes? Returning to our previous question, is this a step towards gender equality? On the whole, yes, as women and men face the same incentives in the labor market. Actually, women still benefit significantly more than men, for the unisex annuities provide a major redistribution toward women. At the same time, the new systems penalize women more for shifting their time and their human capital investments toward unpaid household work, despite both the private and social benefits of this work. And they may breed an increased poverty among lone elderly women, especially in Kazakhstan, where there is a high service requirement for the minimum pension and no compensation for time spent out of the labor force to have children.

A few policy changes could reduce this risk. First, reforming countries that do not offer some pension compensation for time spent having children should consider adding this feature. Second, defined contribution systems may wish to consider offering joint annuities. Higher levels of unpaid household work are usually found in middle- and upper-income households, as low-income households tend to need all the healthy earners working. In these households, there is usually a male earner who brings home the majority of the income. Public pay-as-you-go pension systems do a poor job of redistributing this lifetime household income over the pension period. The Soviet approach did not seem very appropriate, since it discouraged work and participation. Yet the individual annuities introduced in the new systems can leave women at their end of their lives with lower pensions, since they retire earlier and live longer. In the defined contribution schemes, a joint annuity purchase (as is required, for example, in Chile) could improve women's living standard after their husbands die.

This will, of course, be controversial because minimum vesting periods to avoid moral hazard necessarily involve some government intrusion into private relationship decisions such as marriage.

Third, FSU countries should move toward equal retirement ages for women and men at a higher age level. This would go a long way towards preventing old age poverty, since it would prevent women from making what could be in the long run a poor decision. Although women in the FSU have strongly opposed retirement age increases, the low pensions they will receive instead surely cannot be considered a victory.

Finally, countries should embark on a public information campaign to explain these changes to women and illuminate their choices and the costs of these choices in the new system. While we do not think the current incentives alone would be enough to get the majority of women to work longer, at least the choices could be made easier to understand. Given the importance attached to incentives and behavioral change in most pension reforms in the FSU, beginning this dialogue with this very large group of stakeholders is clearly important.

Notes

1. A preliminary version of this chapter was prepared for the World Bank conference entitled New Ideas about Old Age Security, held on September 14–15, 1999. The authors are grateful to the World Bank's Gender Board and the Social Protection Unit for funding for this research, and to Robert Holzmann, Peter Orszag, Karen O. Mason, Gert Wagnar, and seminar and conference participants for comments. The views expressed here are the authors' own and do not necessarily reflect those of the World Bank.

2. This also includes periods of study as a full-time student.

3. The high coverage of women in the formal pension system, even in low-income countries of the FSU, is one of the most striking features of the social protection system inherited from the Soviet period.

4. Legislation passed in January 2000 (after our analysis was complete) raised the upper limit on the second tier to 10 percentage points by 2010 in Latvia. We did not recalculate our figures, however, for the effect that far in the future would be very small.

5. This assumption is necessary to ensure comparability across countries but actually obscures gender differences in early retirement under the old system. For a description of these differences for Latvia, see Fox and Palmer (1999).

6. We assume that in Latvia and Kazakhstan annuity suppliers will not be able to discriminate by gender. If this were not the case, the gender gap on the implicit rate of return would shrink.

7. See citations in bibliography for our sources for projections. In Kazakhstan the reduction in the contribution rate is assumed to be very gradual because the transition period should be very long, since acquired rights were not scaled back. In Latvia the rate falls steadily until 2015. In the Kyrgyz Republic and Moldova, the contribution rate will be decreased between 2005 and 2010.

8. In the Kyrgyz system, each year of service completed before the reform earns approximately 1 percent replacement rate.

9. In Moldova each year of service realized in the previous system provides 0.4 percent of replacement rate, and a flat amount of 16 percent of the average wage.

10. For the workers retiring immediately, the calculation of the notional capital was based on the average wage recorded in the two years preceding the implementation of the reform. The number of years that enters in the calculation of the average wage will increase up to four for the workers retiring in 2000 and the years thereafter.

References

Note: The word *processed* describes informally reproduced works that may not be commonly available through libraries.

Andrews, Emily S. 2000. "Kazakhstan: An Ambitious Pension Reform." World Bank, Human Development Unit, Europe and Central Asia Region, World Bank, Washington, DC. Processed.

Barry D., and M. Reilly. 1999. "Female Labor Market Characteristics in Transitional Economies." UNICEF International Child Development Center. Processed.

Burkhauser, Richard V., and Jennifer L. Warlick. 1981. "Disentangling the Annuity from the Redistribution Aspect of Social Security in the United States." *Review of Income and Wealth* 27(4): 401–21.

Castel, Paulette. 1998. "The Kyrgyz Republic: Fiscal Implications of the Pension Reform." Poverty Reduction and Economic Management, Europe and Central Asia Region, World Bank, Washington, DC. Processed.

Disney, Richard, and Edward Whitehouse. 1999. "Pension Plans and Retirement Incentives." Social Protection Discussion Paper No. 9924. World Bank, Washington, D.C.

Fox, Louise. 1994. "Old Age Security in Transitional Economies." Policy Research Working Paper No. 1257. World Bank, Washington, D.C.

————. 1997. "Pension Reform in the Post-Communist Transition Economies." In National Research Council, eds., *Transforming Post-Communist Political Economies*. Washington, D.C.: National Academic Press.

Fox, Louise, and Edward Palmer. 1999. "Latvian Pension Reform." World Bank Social Protection Discussion Paper No. 9922. World Bank, Washington, D.C.

Government of Latvia. 1998. "The Law on State Pension." Latvian-English version. Consensus Programme Phase.

Government of Moldova. 1999. "Law on the State Social Security." English version. World Bank, Washington, D.C.

Government of the Kyrgyz Republic. 1997–1999 (legislation). "Pension Law," "Amendments to the Pension Law," and "Governmental Decree on the Pension Law." English version. World Bank, Washington, D.C.

Gruber, Jonathon, and David Wise. 1999. *Social Security and Retirement Around the World*. National Bureau of Economic Research Conference Report. Chicago and London: University of Chicago Press.

Larzeg, Mania. 1999. "Making the Transition Work for Women in Europe and Central Asia." World Bank Discussion Paper No. 411. Poverty Reduction and Economic Management Unit, Europe and Central Asia Region, World Bank, Washington, D.C.

Milanovic, Branko. 1996. "Income, Inequality and Poverty during the Transition: A Survey of the Evidence." *Moct-Most: Economic Policy in Transitional Economies* 6(1): 131–47.

Rama, Martin, and Dona MacIsaac. 1999. "Earnings and Welfare after Downsizing: Central Bank Employees in Ecuador." *World Bank Economic Review* 13: 1.

Thompson, Alan A., and Xiaoqing Yu. 1997. "Program of the Social Protection Reform of the Republic of Moldova." Human Development Unit, Europe and Central Asia Region, World Bank, Washington, D.C. Processed.

World Bank. 1994. *Averting the Old Age Crisis: Policies to Protect the Old and Promote Growth*. New York: Oxford University Press.

13

Extending Coverage in Multipillar Pension Systems: Constraints and Hypotheses, Preliminary Evidence, and Future Research Agenda

Robert Holzmann, Truman Packard, and Jose Cuesta

OF THE WORLD'S SIX BILLION PEOPLE IN 1999, only 15 percent or less have access to a formal system of retirement income support.[1] To the extent that households can rely on traditional arrangements and alternative investments in retirement security, there may be little cause for worry. However, with the aging of populations, urbanization, and globalization, the elderly will have reduced access to informal, traditional safety nets in the family or community. Economic development may not be fast and comprehensive enough for individuals to accumulate sufficient real and financial assets over their working lives, rendering them increasingly vulnerable to the risk of poverty in old age. This danger ties the concern with low rates of coverage closely to the World Bank's mission of eradicating poverty. For this reason the Bank has proposed a multipillar pension system to provide adequate pensions for the working population and to cushion against economic, demographic, and political risks to income support in retirement. Many countries in the world have started or are contemplating a move toward a multipillar pension system, but evidence so far suggests that such a move has done little to increase coverage of the workforce and may perhaps contribute to a decline in coverage in some countries.

The alternatives to a contributory, mandated scheme of old age income support are noncontributory schemes in the form of demogrants, social pensions, and universal or specially targeted social assistance. While universal and non-means-tested benefits are effective in addressing old age poverty, they are often expensive and inefficient. Means-tested benefits are potentially efficient but difficult to administer to be effective. Working through community support and nongovernment organizations presents a potential alternative to reach the elderly poor, but there is little evidence of the effectiveness and long-term sustainability of relying on organized civil society. The viability of noncontributory systems of income support for the elderly poor in an environment of scarce public resources and low administrative capacity is the subject of separate research.[2]

The limited coverage of contributory, multipillar pension systems and the difficulties of providing effective and efficient income support for the elderly through noncontributory schemes calls for an investigation of the relative merits and economic trade-offs of each. The investigation requires a better understanding of the constraints to broader coverage under a multipillar scheme. Such a scheme ideally consists of (i) a publicly managed, unfunded, and defined benefit pillar, which is tax or contribution financed and should take care of poverty and redistributive concerns; (ii) a privately managed, fully funded, and defined contribution pillar, which takes care of income replacement and is financed by earnings-related contributions—both of these are mandatory—and (iii) voluntary saving for old age in the form of assets, insurance contracts, housing, and so forth. Because pension reforms mostly start from the existing systems and are constrained by national preferences, the economic environment, and the costs of transition, however, the resulting pillars are of varying size and structure (Holzmann 2000; Schwarz 1999). Yet even an ideal multipillar structure may not be able to attract all individuals in the labor force. International evidence hints at a strong correlation between the level of coverage under a formal pension system and the income level of an economy (see figure 13.1). This correlation suggests that administrative and other efforts to achieve complete coverage may come at a price for individuals and the economy.

This chapter discusses the governmental, institutional, and market-oriented failures that deter rational individuals and households from participating in reformed multipillar pension systems. To this end, the structure of the chapter is as follows: the second section outlines briefly why coverage extension may be beneficial beyond providing old age income support, identifies the main barriers impeding it, and highlights drawbacks of aggressively expanding coverage in contributory pension systems. The third section reviews the coverage experience in reformed schemes, focusing on Chile, which, since its reform in 1981, has the longest experience with a funded pillar of individual accounts, and Argentina, whose adoption of a "mixed" model in 1994 presents its own set of implications for coverage. In the fourth section the main hypotheses on the barriers to coverage and

Figure 13.1. Relation between Coverage and Income Per Capita in 1990s

Contributors/labor force (percent)

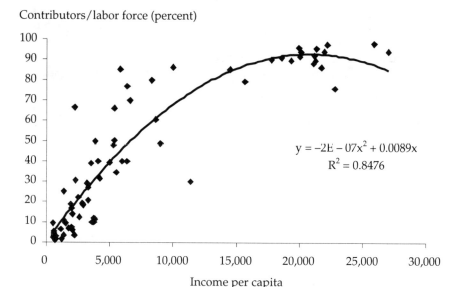

$$y = -2E - 07x^2 + 0.0089x$$
$$R^2 = 0.8476$$

Income per capita

Source: World Bank staff.

obstacles to extending access to the multipillar pension system are organized into five groups: (i) the case of the poor, (ii) the case of the self-
employed, (iii) transactions costs, (iv) system design issues, and (v) system
credibility. The fifth section presents very preliminary econometric evidence
on some of the hypotheses based on existing data from Chile and Argentina;
the sixth section concludes.

The Broader Benefits, Barriers and Drawbacks to Extending Coverage

The benefits and barriers to increased coverage extend beyond the pension
system itself and income security concerns in old age. The benefits are largely attributed to the expected formalization of the work relationship in a
world of increasing risk and waning reliance on strained traditional systems of social security brought on by aging, urbanization, and globalization. A wide range of failures by government and market institutions presents barriers to greater coverage. For this reason an improvement in the
benefit-contribution link alone will have only a marginal, if any, impact on

coverage, and as a result, increased coverage may come at a cost. The arguments in favor of increasing coverage as well as some of the principal drawbacks are addressed below.

- The main benefits from increased coverage under a multipillar pension scheme arise in the following ways:
- Coverage implies formalized work relations that promote better labor conditions, enforceable labor rights, and access to formal social risk management instruments besides pensions, such as health, accident, sickness or unemployment protection (Holzmann and Jorgensen 1999).
- Moving from the informal to the formal sector, which often entails mandatory participation in a pension system, may effect economic growth. If the informal sector uses less productive technology with higher transaction costs, labor force movement to the formal sector will enhance overall productivity and, in an endogenous growth model, can lead to a higher growth path (Corsetti and Schmidt-Hebbel 1994).
- Expanded coverage and formal labor force participation will further strengthen the overall revenue position of the government, which, in turn, may allow for additional growth-supporting and poverty-reducing expenditures.
- Partial presaving under a multipillar scheme should also better secure the provision of future benefits. Reliance on the multipillar system allows households to diversify income risk through foreign investments of pension fund resources.
- Expanded coverage under a multipillar scheme strengthens the secondary effects of the move from an unfunded pay-as-you-go (PAYG) system to one of funded pillars, including a contribution to national savings and financial market development (Holzmann 1997).
- Additional secondary benefits presented in the literature include an institutional shift toward less reciprocal market arrangements that broadens household choice (Barr 1998); greater productivity from lifting institutional constraints that confine households to unproductive liquid investments (Alderman and Paxson 1992); and economic growth from increasing access to savings and the efficiency of investment through greater participation in the formal capital market (Serrano 1999).

The main barriers to increasing coverage are linked with market imperfections and the regime switch that a move from the informal to the formal sector implies (see figure 13.2). Design improvements in the multipillar over the single-pillar PAYG systems may have some, but perhaps only limited, effects. Section four describes the main barriers in detail, which include the following:

Figure 13.2. Informal Sector in Latin America:
Percentage of Economically Active Population

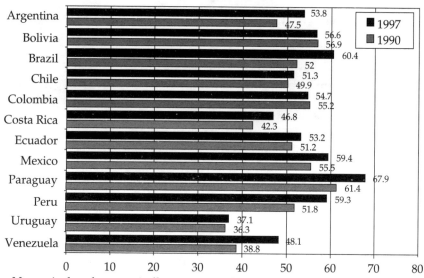

Nonagricultural economically active population informally employed (percent)

Source: ILO (1998); excludes agricultural employment.

- *Imperfections in the output market.* In many countries access to the formal output market is linked with strict licensing regulation for the producer of goods and services. While strict regulation may be motivated by consumer protection, insiders and administrative incapacity restrict license access in many cases.
- *Imperfection and regulations on the factor markets.* Heavy regulation of the labor market provides ample incentives for entrepreneurs to keep workers off the official payroll. Limited access to credits for consumers and producers in the financial market creates another set of conditions that make it rational to pursue informal activities and avoid participation in the mandated pension scheme.
- *The regime switch implied by a move to the formal sector.* While workers may gain access to a broader range of benefits, these typically imply high contribution rates for the whole bundle of services and payment, in principle, of all direct and indirect taxes, related and unrelated to social security.
- *Bad system design and/or administrative weaknesses.* The example most often cited is a weak link between contributions and benefits that renders contributions akin to a wage tax that individuals seek to avoid.

An expansion of coverage, however, is not free of cost. As mentioned above, even an actuarially fair system provides a strong rationale for individuals to avoid from formal social security. Hence, attempts to force increased coverage under a multipillar system through administrative and other means probably implies drawbacks:

- Disregarding the argument of myopia to motivate mandated participation, forcing individuals to participate in a (broadly actuarially fair) pension system implies the imposition of a savings path they may not have chosen on their own. In a world of perfect capital markets, individuals could offset the forced saving through borrowing ("dis-saving"). In an imperfect world, forced savings lead to individual welfare losses.
- If individuals consider the net costs of forced participation to be too high, they will try to avoid and evade the mandated contribution, typically achieving the latter by moving into informal-sector activities. While they choose this move to enhance their individual welfare, it is likely to have negative effects on the economy, including the choice of lower production technology and higher transaction costs, including corruption.
- The strategies for avoiding contributions can be manifold. Employees in sectors with strong union representation will attempt to shift the burden to the employer, to the detriment of the outsiders and employment. In the case of low competition output markets, the employer will try to shift the burden to the consumer. If the self-employed are not required to participate in the system or can more easily avoid the burden, employees will notionally change to self-employed status, which may weaken their bargaining power and overall access to social programs.
- Forced participation at high individual costs may weaken an existing informal safety net. Workers that care for their parents (and children) in an informal manner will have fewer resources to share with them, possibly increasing poverty among the current elderly not covered under formal provisions.

Pension Reform and Coverage: Illustrations from Chile and Argentina

Much of the literature on pension reform presents the single-pillar PAYG model as a manifestation of government failure. Where the objective of governments has been to achieve greater equity through a redistribution of income within and between generations, the state has often established

mechanisms that not only fail to bring about greater equity but also introduce distortions into the labor market that retard job creation in the formal
sector and lead to a loss of productivity. The increase in coverage expected after the transition from an unfunded PAYG system to a multipillar
system with funded individual accounts is attributed to the correction of
these distortions through reform. The labor market benefits of transition-
ing from PAYG to multipillar are widely held to include the following
(World Bank 1994):

- The creation of a stronger link between contributions and retirement
  benefits that reduces the motivation to evade by eliminating a perceived unrecoverable *tax* on income
- A reduction in payroll taxes and in the cost of hiring incurred by
  formal-sector employers
- Greater flexibility and cross-sector mobility in the labor market
  enabled by portable pension benefits
- Reduction in incentives for early retirement and nonretention of
  experienced labor

The simulations of transition from PAYG to multipillar on which the
incentive-driven coverage expansion is predicted are typically performed
using overlapping generations (OLG) models with perfect foresight (see
Auerbach and Kotlikoff 1987), raising the question of why participation in
formal pension systems should be mandated. Publicly mandated pension
systems are typically motivated by considerations of myopia (the failure
of individuals to perceive future utility); insufficient or lacking financial
market instruments; and protection of public resources against moral hazard and opportunistic behavior. The first two arguments imply that a mandated pension system should replicate the savings behavior rational individuals would manifest if they had full access to perfect market instruments.
Since it is difficult to design a collective system that accommodates the preferences of all individuals, however, it follows that any mandated scheme
creates distortions and any contribution has a tax element, no matter how
tightly the contribution rate is linked with benefits. This suggests that, all
things being equal, moving to a multipillar scheme may reduce the tax element, but the effect is likely to be small and, hence, have limited positive
incentive effects on coverage. If other obstacles and institutional barriers
remain unchanged, lower coverage may even result. The case of the
reformed systems in Latin America seems to validate these considerations,
as illustrated by the experience of Chile and Argentina (see table 13.1).

Of the countries in Latin America that have reformed their public PAYG
plans and established systems of defined contributions into individual
accounts, only in the case of Chile, where payroll taxes fell from 19 percent
to 13 percent (including commissions and the premium paid for disability coverage), has sufficient time elapsed to provide relevant empirical

Table 13.1. Features of Reformed Pension Systems that May Influence the Decision to Participate

Feature	Chile's AFP system, 1981	Argentina's integrated system, 1994
Nature of reform	Public defined benefit (PAYG) changed to private defined contribution (all workers)	Separate regimes Public split consolidated. into public PAYG and private defined contribution
What happens to the old system?	Phased out	Continues with changes
Is second-pillar mandatory for new choice of labor force entrants?	Yes	No. Workers have a one-off participating in PAYG or AFJP system
Treatment of self-employed	Voluntary	Obligatory
Structure of public pillar	Minimum Pension Guarantee (MPG) Social assistance	Flat and minimum pension
Financing acquired rights under old PAYG	Recognition bonds financed with future general taxation	Compensatory pensions financed partially through current payroll taxes
Total contribution rate for new system:		
- for old age annuity	10	8
- disability/survivors/commissions	3	3
- public pillar and social assistance	General revenues	16
Total contribution rate:		
–before reform	19	27
–after reform	13	27
–employer/worker	0/13	16/11 employer contribution is pure PAYG taxation, for the universal flat benefit
Collection of contributions	Decentralized: employers pay to fund managers, with follow-up enforcement by regulator	Centralized: employers/workers pay contributions, along with taxes on income and other tribute, to single tax authority (DGI)
Second-pillar commission structure	*Fixed:* although variable on contributions, on combination, no discounts	*Variable:* on contributions, discounts for length of period affiliated/ contributing to AFJP
Maximum percentage of portfolio allowed in:		
–Domestic equities	30	63
–Foreign securities	12	17
–Government securities (in 1994)	50	65
Second-pillar contributors as portion of affiliates (percentage)	57	48

Source: Country legislation, information compiled by authors.

evidence of such an adjustment. Figure 13.3 shows a disaggregated picture
of how nonagricultural employment in Chile has evolved by sector from
1980 to 1997.

In Chile, where the Administradoras de Fondos de Pensiones (AFP) system of funded individual accounts has been in full operation for nearly 19
years, the portion of the workforce that is informally employed has
increased from 49.9 percent in 1990 to 51.3 percent in 1997. This relatively
static picture of the trends in sector choice supports the assertion that the
tighter link between contributions and benefits and the lower cost of formal-sector hiring brought about by pension reform may be a necessary, but
insufficient, condition either for formalization of the factors of production
or to attract widespread participation in the new multipillar systems. This
argument is further supported by studies of the Chilean labor market that
conclude that the new pension system has not caused significant changes
in the number of workers, as a portion of total employment, who contribute
regularly to social security (Cortazar 1997).

**Figure 13.3. Chile: Sector Allocation of Economically Active
Population, 1980–97**

Nonagricultural economically active population (percent)

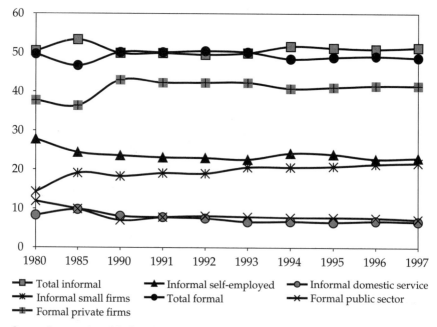

Source: International Labor Organization (ILO) (1998)

On the other hand, the data in figure 13.3 demonstrate that while informal-sector participation has risen dramatically in other Latin American countries, sector participation trends in Chile have remained relatively stable since the introduction of the AFP system. Although there is insufficient empirical evidence to support the claim that a fully funded pension system of individual accounts will lead to a formalization of the workforce, pension reform in Chile may have played an important part in slowing the growth of the informal sector (Schmidt-Hebbel 1998), although probably in concert with high rates of economic growth and employment creation in the formal sector.

While International Labor Organization (ILO) data on sector participation are only a second-best indicator of coverage of formal pension systems, the size of the informal sector is likely to be highly correlated with the portion of the labor force that does not regularly contribute to a retirement account. Unlike the national PAYG schemes that they replace, retirement benefits in defined contribution systems are based on accumulated contributions and the returns they earn from investment. Under the reformed systems, regular contribution is critical to adequate income replacement in retirement, making "coverage" a more active, intentional concept than under the defined benefit framework and creating a group of "partially covered" workers (James 1999).

While worker affiliation to the AFP system in Chile may have increased since the reform, the portion of affiliated workers who regularly contribute to their individual accounts has actually fallen (Arenas de Mesa 1999; Mastragelo 1998; see figure 13.4). A similar, if more accelerated, fall in the number of contributing affiliates has occurred in Argentina since the introduction of its private Administradoras de Fondos de Jubilaciones y Pensiones (AFJP) pension pillar.[3] Thus, while the percentage of economically active workers considered "informal" may not exactly indicate the size of the *uncovered* population, a large and dynamic informal sector facilitates irregular contribution patterns by providing ample opportunity for unregulated/uncovered employment and easy exit and reentry to formal-sector jobs (World Bank 1999). In effect, a large informal economy transforms first- and second-pillar forced savings into third-pillar (voluntary) investment choices. Each individual and household is then faced with the decision of whether or not to participate in the formal pension system, depending on the set of viable alternatives to which they have access and the efficiency of each investment in terms of reliability and returns.

Barriers to Participation: A Set of Hypotheses

This section presents a number of hypotheses as to why rational workers/households choose to avoid participating in multipillar pension

Figure 13.4. Affiliates and Contributors in Chile and Argentina

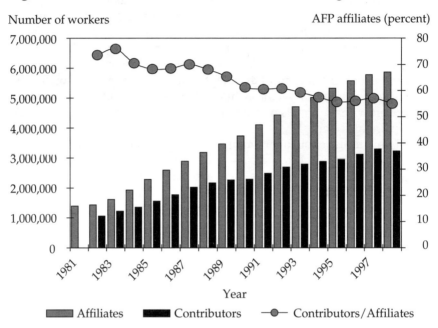

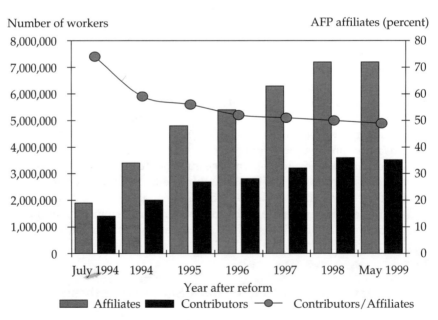

Source: SAFP (1998); SAFJP (1999).

systems. The hypotheses are grouped into five broad categories relating to (i) the poor, (ii) the self-employed, (iii) transactions costs, (iv) system design issues, and (v) system credibility. A short discussion and suggestions for further research follow each hypothesis.

The Poor

Pension systems funded through mandatory contributions can lead to welfare losses for households for which rates of discount are high and credit constraints are binding. In most developing countries a large segment of the population may simply be too poor to participate in contributory pension systems. While household income may be just enough to meet immediate, basic needs for survival, saving for old age may not be rational. The rate of discount on future consumption in poorer households is higher than that of wealthier households. Poorer households will put much greater value on consumption today than on consumption tomorrow or far into the future. If the time preference rate is higher than the market rate of interest and credit is expensive or rationed, the shadow discount rate is even greater.[4] Thus, for lower income households, mandatory contributions can lead to major welfare losses, and participation in a formal pension system in which savings are illiquid may place an intolerable constraint on household efforts to smooth consumption. Household data from Chile and Argentina show a sharp rise in rates of participation in the formal pension system as income decile rises from the poorest to the richest (figures 13.5 and 13.6).

In a related argument, income security in old age may not be the primary risk concern of poor households. The profile of risks faced by the poor may more prominently feature less predictable shocks to income, such as disability and sudden illness. The link between income (nutrition/health) and mortality strengthens this line of argument, that is, poorer people would rather consume income today than save and consume in the future when, because of their relatively higher mortality, they may not be around to savor deferred consumption in retirement. Myopia, the failure to recognize future utility, also explains the greater priority for immediate consumption.[5]

These factors combine to augment the implicit tax component of mandated retirement savings for poorer households. To illustrate, assuming a market rate of return of 5 percent in real terms and a subjective discount rate as typically estimated in the range of 18 to 20 percent, then simple compounding of contributions and discounting of actuarially fair benefits lead to some 20 cents per dollar of contribution. Put differently, the implicit tax share can be as high as 80 percent.

Traditional systems of old age security may still provide better risk management for poorer households in developing economies. There is ample evidence that poorer, economically active agents (as individuals, as households, and

Figure 13.5. Chile: Participation Increases with Income Contribution by Income Decile, 1997

Workers in decile (percent)

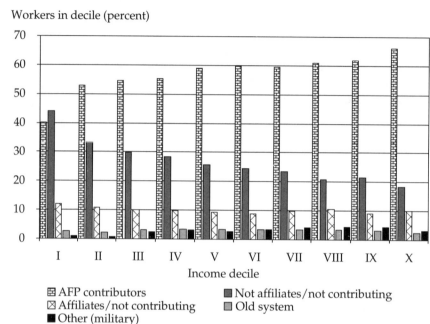

Income decile

☒ AFP contributors   ■ Not affiliates/not contributing
☒ Affiliates/not contributing   □ Old system
■ Other (military)

Source: CASEN survey, 1996.

within households) engage in consumption-smoothing and exhibit risk management in view of fluctuating income. Where formal insurance markets have failed to coalesce or may have broken down due to moral hazard and adverse selection stemming from information asymmetries, the extended family and community have been able to partially fill the gap.

The majority of the world's old people rely solely on informal and traditional arrangements for income security (World Bank 1994). These traditional strategies can take the form of larger families or preferences for male offspring in rural agricultural economies and in labor markets that wage-discriminate against women (Hoddinott 1992). Households may still depend heavily on reciprocal relationships within tribe or extended family; remittances arising from rural-to-urban and international migration of household members (Hoddinott 1992; Lucas and Stark 1985); strategic marriage arrangements (Stark 1995); intrahousehold arrangements; the establishment of a portfolio of assets with uncorrelated risks (Stark 1990); the purchase of livestock or jewelry; the forward sale of agricultural crops; and community-based credit schemes.

The portfolio of strategies taken by risk-averse households will necessarily depend on the relative costs and benefits of each and their efficiency in balancing returns with risk (Holzmann and Jorgensen 1999). A portfolio of informal assets may have higher returns (education of oneself or education of a child) and lower risks (beholden children) than those afforded by formal pensions. Formal pension systems based on compulsory savings may impose liquidity constraints on households pursuing informal/traditional arrangements for retirement security, thereby crowding out such arrangements. Furthermore, "coverage" offered under the formal pension system may not substitute for investment in informal arrangements that are often multifunctional (covering risks other than old age poverty) and flexible to a worker's (the household's) particular need.

The transition costs of moving from informal to formal regimes of retirement security are too high. Just as the transition from an unfunded PAYG system to a funded multipillar can impose a double burden on a "transition generation" of workers, the move out of a regime of informal strategies into a formal pension system may also impose high costs. Upon moving into

Figure 13.6. Argentina: Participation Increases with Income Contribution by Income Decile, 1997

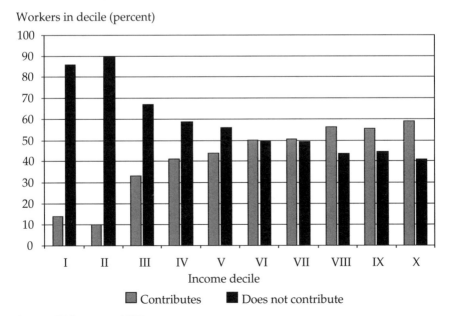

Workers in decile (percent)

Income decile

■ Contributes   ■ Does not contribute

Source: EDS survey, 1997.

a formal system, workers informally supporting an elderly parent—workers who have credible expectations that their own children will provide similar support when grown—would be expected to continue their support in addition to funding their own retirement. Similarly, opting for the formal system may brand a worker/household as untrusting or disdainful of "traditional ways." Once branded untrustworthy, the worker/household may be locked out of reciprocal systems of risk management, heightening vulnerability to shocks other than the inability to work in old age.

The Self-Employed

Contributory pension systems impose constraints on productive investments of the informally self-employed. The constraints imposed by formal pension systems on the self-employed (especially the poor self-employed) are more binding on their investments in productive inputs than on their ability to smooth consumption. The rate of interest on borrowing for investment in small enterprise can be very high—even infinite—while the net marginal returns to a unit of capital invested in small enterprise may be considerably higher than the returns from investing the same unit of capital in an AFP account. Avoidance of the formal pension system may be optimal, given capital and credit constraints on productive investment choices of the self-employed and the opportunity costs of vesting scarce capital in an illiquid retirement account.

Where formal retirement security is bundled with unrelated government regulations and taxes, the costs of compliance may be too high. Coverage under a formal pension system is often nested deeply within the broader regulatory framework of the formal economy. Participation may require compliance with regulations and labor standards unrelated to the provision of income security in old age.

How retirement contributions are collected can also impose secondary costs. While recognized efficiency gains exist from the collection of contributions together with other taxes, where collection is centralized, the self-employed (and employers in small firms) will find it difficult to divorce their participation in the pension system from overall compliance with a tax code they may continue to perceive as unjust (Schwarz 1998). Pension contributions, even if perfectly linked to benefits, are then perceived, by association, as another tax to evade. Participation in the pension system can, therefore, invite constraints on the rational, individually utility-maximizing behavior of informal economic agents (De Soto 1989; Tokman 1992). There is a likely trade-off between fiscal efficiency from linking contribution collection to collection of taxes and the incentives to participate. The more the state relies on pension systems to increase collection of unrelated taxes and enforce labor regulations, the deeper it will cut into incentives to participate.

Moreover, a fixed contribution rate and the inability to draw on their saved funds in times of hardship may place unacceptable constraints on the self-employed, whose income may be episodic and financial needs less predictable. This is especially true of farmers and the rural, nonfarm self-employed whose wealth resides in illiquid forms (accruals in farming capital and "on the hoof," but little cash) and whose income is largely seasonal. An AFP account might be more attractive to agents with irregular incomes if they were allowed to use their retirement balances as collateral to borrow and/or withdraw a limited amount in case of emergencies, with penalties for failure to replace the withdrawn amount after a specified period.

Self-employment may attract individuals who prefer to bear a greater share of old age income risk than to rely on government-mandated pension systems. There may be a high degree of self-selection in informal self-employment. The self-employed may prefer to bear a larger share of retirement income risk and take a more active role in managing their long-term savings and investments. They may even be relatively less myopic than wage or salaried workers. Research should examine whether the self-employed as a group take greater precautions for retirement security by analyzing the past labor market status/sector choice (salaried or self-employment) among the current elderly not receiving pension benefits (past evaders).

A casual poll of taxi drivers in Santiago and Buenos Aires revealed that at least some self-employed pursue alternative market strategies for retirement security, investing in financial sector instruments other than the second-pillar retirement accounts. In Chile term life insurance policies (*seguro de vida con ahorro*), available since 1995, seem to offer a competitive alternative investment.[6] Private insurance companies in Chile report that, while it is likely that the policies are prohibitive for poorer households, considerable demand exists for these life insurance/savings facilities among middle- and lower-income groups, especially younger age cohorts for whom premiums are low.

System Transactions Costs

The cost of pension fund administration cuts into account balances, lowers returns, and increases the implicit tax on participation. There is a mutually reinforcing vicious cycle between low rates of participation in the new multipillar pension systems and their high administrative costs. The fewer the workers who affiliate and regularly contribute to the system, the harder it is for the fund managers to lower costs by exploiting economies of scale. If costs to the workers remain high, the returns from the system will be low relative to the returns that can be earned from other formal and informal retirement investments, making the opportunity costs of participation prohibitive for poorer households.

There is a large body of literature on the commissions and fees charged by second-pillar fund managers and whether these commissions are high relative to the fees charged by similar agents—banks and mutual fund managers—in developing capital markets. These costs are especially high for poorer households and workers who frequently enter and exit the formal labor force (Srinivas and Yermo 1999). The prices exacted by the AFP mangers in Chile's second pillar have been blamed for increasing the perceived tax component of retirement contributions (Torche and Wagner 1997) and encouraging evasion.

Valdes-Priéto (1998) finds that in Chile, while AFP commissions are lower than those charged by mutual funds, the charges on an AFP retirement savings accounts are 60 percent greater than those on a regular savings deposit in a private bank. Other researchers contend that charging commissions as a percentage of wages is cheaper over the course of the workers' contributing life than commissions as a percentage of earnings or accumulated balance. A branch of this research suggests that AFP commissions are competitive, especially when considering the additional educational services that the pension fund managers provide to their affiliates. The level of commissions and fees may be justified when the value of the "financial education" received by the average affiliate—who may have no other contact with the formal financial sector—is fully taken into account. This claim requires further investigation.

The transaction costs of providing financial services to the working poor are too high to attract the interest of fund managers, eliminating incentives to affiliate rural and urban informal-sector workers. Where a market for private management of pension savings has developed, the high costs of providing financial services to contributors with lower and more irregular incomes may deter fund managers from affiliating informal-sector workers. The costs of collecting contributions from frequently mobile workers and of reporting individual account balances to informal affiliates may be high when compared to the low commissions (as a percentage of wages) fund managers can earn. Furthermore, providing savings facilities to workers with lower surplus incomes involves diseconomies of scale. Disincentives to the AFPs are compounded in the case of informal workers in rural areas where transaction costs are even greater due to population dispersion and information asymmetries.

However, much has been learned in the last 20 years from the practical experience of community-based organizations and microfinance institutions (MFIs) that have developed methodologies to dramatically reduce the costs of providing financial services to the working poor. MFIs have experimented with different ways of structuring financial contracts and with developing supervision mechanisms that reduce information asymmetries and consequent costs. Emerging evidence reveals a demand among the working poor for formal savings facilities (Alderman and Paxson 1992; CGAP 1997a). In Bolivia, organizations like BancoSol (formerly PRODEM) already offer medium- and long-term savings accounts to their clients as well as positive returns to shareholders (CGAP 1997b).

While most MFIs lack the capacity to invest workers' savings, they can still play an important role. The greatest costs to AFPs from affiliating the urban and rural poor arise from contribution collection and disclosure of account information. These are services for which the MFIs hold an institutional comparative advantage. There should be room for trade in financial services between AFPs and MFIs.

System Design Issues

The benefit structure of minimum pension guarantees introduces deterrents to the participation of poorer households as well as perverse incentives and moral hazard. Minimum pensions guaranteed by the government are often blamed for being both deterrents to participation and the source of moral hazard. A poverty trap may be created when poorer households that do not expect to qualify for the formal minimum pension guarantee decide not to participate. The minimum guarantee can also create incentives for workers to participate only until they have complied with vesting requirements, and to evade thereafter.

In the Chilean AFP system the government guarantees a minimum pension to affiliates who have contributed for at least 20 years. In Argentina, workers must contribute to the system for 30 years before qualifying for the state-guaranteed minimum pension. Evidence exists in both Chile and Argentina of strategic underreporting of wages by workers—especially the self-employed—who may be seeking only the government-guaranteed minimum. The barrier to participation posed by discrete vesting requirements could be removed by applying both vesting and the guaranteed benefit continuously. For example, a worker that contributes to Argentina's reformed system for only 25 and not the required 30 years would receive some benefit proportional to his or her years of contribution instead of not receiving any benefit.

The strongest motivation to regularly contribute to a second-pillar retirement account is not income security in old age but access to health insurance and better health care. Surveys of the informally employed reveal a greater demand for formal health insurance above all other forms of insurance, including retirement insurance (ILO 1997). The greater demand for health coverage is not surprising since the returns from a worker's investment in health insurance are usually enjoyed over his or her lifetime, while those from formal social security and pensions are only enjoyed in old age. All other things being equal, the tighter that access to health coverage (or disability) is bundled together with the pension system, the more attractive regular participation will seem.

Although the self-employed in Chile are excused from participation in the pension system, many informally self-employed who are otherwise neither regulated nor directly taxed contribute to an AFP in order to gain access to health insurance (both to FONASA, Chile's state health insurance scheme, and to the ISAPRES, the country's private providers). There are even reports of workers contributing to an AFP for a determined period in order to secure access to health care when they need it most, such as during pregnancy. In Argentina health insurance was separated from the privately managed pension system, and is still financed through payroll taxes to union-organized group policies called *obras sociales*; however, access to health insurance and care is just as tightly linked to participation in the reformed pension system as it is in Chile.

Where employers are required to pay a larger payroll contribution relative to workers, the employer will have more to lose (gain) from participation (evasion) than the worker will have to gain (lose). With the introduction of the multipillar model, employer contributions are often retained to finance government liabilities from the old regime, and/or first-pillar benefits, while workers' contributions are left to accumulate in a second-pillar account. While the worker's contribution to the second pillar may no longer be perceived as a pure tax, the employer's contribution to the first pillar on the worker's behalf may be.

The ratio of employer-to-worker contributions can influence the decision to participate or to evade. High employer contributions relative to the contributions of workers provide the employer with a greater incentive to evade and to informalize his or her workers. Even if the worker fully perceives future utility (is "clairvoyant") and would like to benefit from participating in the formal system, the decision to contribute may not be his or hers to make.

A shift in the employer/worker split can correspond to a shift in the bargaining position (and threat points) of each in negotiating terms of employment, including whether the contract will be formal or informal. The extent to which the employer/worker contribution split will affect the decision to participate (to comply) will be determined by the elasticity of labor supply (affected by range of informal employment opportunities) and the existence (and importance) of institutions (such as unions and with labor codes) that prevent employers from shifting the entire burden of payroll taxes onto the worker by reducing net wages.[7] If the employer does not coerce evasion outright, the employer may collude with the worker to avoid the costs of participating by adding a portion of would-be retirement contributions to the workers' take-home pay (Schwarz 1998). All other things being equal, a higher ratio of employer/worker contributions is expected to lead to lower participation in the formal system.

The establishment of a specialized private pension fund industry to manage mandated worker savings can discourage competition and slow a downward adjustment in commissions. Observers suggest that the regulatory framework for the new second pillars, while designed to protect affiliates, often creates biases against competition, efficiency, and specialization. The PAYG fully funded reforms in Latin America often "confer a collective monopoly of managing mandated savings" to the new fund management industry, excluding other financial intermediaries from competition for affiliates and limiting market forces that would in time lower second-pillar costs[8] (Shah 1997). In Argentina there is growing concern that recent market consolidation will further hurt competition, and as the AFJPs increase their efficiency and cut their costs, these savings are not being passed on to affiliates.[9]

Current regulation of pension fund investment causes distortions, limits returns, and restricts workers' choices, making participation less attractive relative to market alternatives. The regulation of the market structure and investment decisions of second-pillar fund managers has been described as draconian (Vittas 1996). Although strict regulations may be justified to safeguard workers' retirement savings from the risks of developing capital markets in the first few years after a pension reform, they impose significant costs over time. Analysis of pension fund investment performance in Chile, Argentina, and Peru has shown that restrictions on investments (especially on investment in equity and foreign issues) create distortions in asset management, limit opportunities for diversification, and constrain workers' choices, since the funds in these countries are earning almost the same rates of return (Srinivas and Yermo 1999).

The limit of one pension fund per fund administrator further constrains the investment choices of account holders. In most countries that have adopted the multipillar pension model, the investment of a worker's savings is restricted to a single fund that is invested mostly in government bonds.[10] This restriction makes it impossible for workers to shift the risk/return profile of their investment in the second-pillar account from a more aggressive holding when they are still young and risk-tolerant/return-hungry to more conservative fare as they become older and more risk-averse (Shah 1997).

The financing of the transition toward multipillar and/or the new benefit structure make participation for some participants less attractive. Moving from single-pillar PAYG to a multipillar system imposes a double burden on transition generations if the implicit debt made explicit is repaid and the reform does not create sufficient externalities (such as lower labor market distortions or growth effects from financial market development) that can be used to repay this debt (Holzmann 1998). Since these externalities take time to materialize, transitory budgetary financing will lead to an increased tax burden for the working population, with the size and effects depending on the form of taxation (labor, income, or consumption tax). However, in many cases the additional taxation will lead to incentives to avoid or evade formal labor market participation.

The negative participation (and decreased coverage) among certain groups of the working population, particularly the poor, will worsen if the new benefit structure provides a lower rate of return. Not everybody under the old PAYG system received a low (implicit) rate of return—the rate was sometimes high for the poor due to high minimum pensions and low eligibility requirements, and individuals with very steep earnings profiles and pensions calculated on the last year's earnings only.

Credibility of Reformed Systems

Households may put little stock in the promises of government. Reformed pension systems may be suffering from an inherited lack of credibility associated with formal pension institutions. Individual preference/tolerance for risk may to an extent determine workers' or households' idiosyncratic rates of time preference. Under a public PAYG system, risk to the worker is defined by his or her failure to receive the promised pension. Even if workers were fully aware of the implicit guarantees in the benefits defined by social security legislation, they might have perceived a high political risk to their promised pension stemming directly from a government's lack of credibility. If the government had a track record of frequently changing the "rules of the game" (vesting requirements, the benefit formula, or minimum pension guarantees), if the inflation tax was high, and if funds earmarked to pay retirement benefits were mismanaged or depleted, workers might have considered the risk of not receiving a PAYG pension to be too high and, thus, may have heavily discounted the returns to being covered. The high risk of not receiving the defined benefit, coupled with high transaction costs of compliance or costs (in other taxes) of participating in the formal economy, may have fully eliminated returns to participation in the system.

Both real and perceived political risk is a difficult and enduring legacy that may inevitably color workers' perceptions of any government mandated retirement security program. Postreform, the political risk to the new system perceived by workers may still be high, even if reforming governments have attempted to start with a clean slate by establishing new private pensions institutions and new public authorities to regulate them. Workers may not put stock in the reform of a government that has frequently changed vesting and benefit rules in the past.

Households may find the burden of financial risk in the postreform systems to be too high. Exposure to capital market investment may (positively or negatively) influence the decision to participate or to evade. A criticism of defined contribution systems is that they require workers to assume too much risk to their income security in retirement. While under public PAYG regimes government assumed a hefty share of risk (longevity and financial risk), under the reformed systems workers are often burdened with the full weight of risk.[11] Although these risks stem from many sources (systemic, demographic, and financial) and can be minimized in a variety of ways, we are concerned with how workers will behave—whether or not they will choose to participate in the new system—when suddenly confronted by a new set of financial risks shortly after a reform.

Under a fully funded system of individual accounts, risk is defined by greater certainty of receiving some pension but uncertainty as to the level of the pension or of an accumulated balance sufficient to guarantee adequate income in retirement. However, the premise that systemic or financial risks (real or perceived) somehow affect workers' decision to participate rests on the assumption that workers have information on the workings of the financial sector or have had the opportunity to build expectations of these workings, either through participation in the form of self-investments or through the participation of a close friend or family member (learning by observing). To the extent that workers have previously (i) held financial assets, including a bank account with time-deposits and/or (ii) have relatives who have held financial assets, the premise is stronger.[12]

If, on the other hand, workers have had no previous contact with the financial sector and no experience of the earnings and losses that can be made on the capital market—if, as is often the case, workers are paid in cash and do not even have a bank account—they may not even have a benchmark perception of the risks and returns from participating in the new system. Systemic and financial risks would not enter into the rational worker's perceptions and decisionmaking. These workers may even fail to perceive the elimination of the pure tax component of mandatory retirement contributions.

Workers may be uncomfortable with the "privatization of social security" and have little faith in the profit motives of the private sector. While the credibility of the government and that of the publicly managed pension system may not have been high in the past, the credibility of the new private fund managers in the funded pillar may not be much higher. This may reflect a simple lack of information or familiarity with the financial sector; mistrust in the profit motives of the capitalist system and its visible representatives—the financial market institutions; or a negative past experience with a unregulated or government-related financial system, that is, "crony capitalism."

Increased disclosure and education can partially overcome the fist two obstacles to greater credibility, while structural and political changes in the pension system as well as the financial sector are required to overcome the last obstacle. In Eastern Europe and Central Asia where disclosure is minimal, information about financial markets is scarce, and the impact of recent economic shocks has been widely felt, governments have established publicly administered "accumulation funds" alongside the new privately managed pension funds to ease the transition. Any measure aimed at increasing the credibility of a privately managed system, however, requires time for its impact to be felt.

The list of hypotheses presented in this section is by no means exhaustive. Rather than providing a single explanation as to why workers/households choose to evade participation in multipillar pension systems, the discussion suggests that the roots of the coverage problem are multiple and intertwined.

Preliminary Econometric Evidence from Chile and Argentina

In this section we discuss the results of exploratory econometric tests performed on data from the 1996 CASEN in Chile and the 1997 EDS in Argentina. In order to substantiate the prior section, we have attempted to test as many of the hypotheses as the available data will permit. The annex provides the tabulated results of our analysis as well as a fuller discussion of the data employed and its limitations. Readers are cautioned from the onset that the surveys chosen are not uniform in breadth or depth and, thus, the results presented in this section cannot be compared. Furthermore, the results are preliminary and are intended primarily to illustrate the need for sharply focused data collection and further research.

Methodology and Choice of Variables

We have chosen a simple methodology to test several of the hypotheses outlined in section four—the estimation of probits on participation in the formal pension system. This method evaluates the significance, positive or negative impact, that a number of explanatory variables have on the probability that a working-age individual will contribute to the formal (AFP or any) pension system.

The variables included in the probits were selected with an eye to the hypotheses in section 5 and the richness of each database. We do not claim that our selection is either exclusive or exhaustive. A number of alternative variables to those chosen could have been used to test the hypotheses—whether, for example, traditional social security strategies substitute for the formal system (gender rather than simply number of children, or contribution to the household of resident elderly rather than their number). In several instances we were obliged to construct imperfect, proxy variables to test our hypotheses; to illustrate, we used a targeted housing benefit to measure liquidity constraint.

We grouped the variables into sets according to the hypotheses being tested. The first set of variables reports on the impact of the individual characteristics (gender, marital status, age category, and educational attainment). This last variable has the additional benefit of acting as an instrument for income.[13] A second set of variables test whether the demographic and geographic characteristics of the household (number of children and number of elderly residing in the household and dummy variables accounting for region and urban/rural location) affect the probability of contributing toward a pension. The third set, welfare variables, includes both individual and household characteristics: the former refers to the contribution to health systems, while the latter refer to the existence of students receiving private education in the household.

For the probits on data from Chile, the set of variables capturing labor characteristics includes a composite index of labor status: this index starts at zero, for those out of the labor market, and rises with the unemployed, and increasing degrees of formality. *Formality* is defined over two main parameters: the existence of a contract and the time tenure of the job (permanent versus temporary/occasional). Our definition of formality does not include contribution to the pension system, although we would expect the probability of regularly contributing to an AFP account to increase with both the existence of a contract and tenure. In addition, we include dummy variables isolating the self-employed in three key sectors: agriculture, manufacturing, and services. The inclusion of these dummies simultaneously tests whether self-employment is in itself a decisive variable on contributions to AFPs *and* how that impact varies across sectors. Finally, we explore the role of incomes accruing from sources other than labor and access to credit using two dummies.

To the extent possible, we used variables in our estimates for Argentina equivalent to those for Chile. We included individual and household characteristics, constructed a similar informality index, and used a housing-finance subsidy to proxy for credit constraint. To accommodate asymmetries in the chosen surveys, we used a single variable for contribution to the health system. Furthermore, we placed greater emphasis on reported secondary jobs in order to capture the influence of secondary employment—particularly secondary self-employment—on a worker's decision to contribute to a pension system in Argentina.

The Determinants of Pension Participation in Chile

The results from the probits for Chile show few surprises (see table A13.1 in annex). As education rises so does the probability of contributing to an AFP account (or to any pension regime). Hence, not only are larger stocks of human capital a determinant of participation, but ultimately higher income level increases the probability of regular contribution. Women are less likely to contribute than men, and even less so if they are married. However, in general, married individuals tend to participate more. We attribute these phenomena to differentials in labor participation: women, particularly married women, participate much less in the labor market than do men.[14] Consequently, they are less exposed to the government's mandate to contribute to the pension system.

As anticipated, the relationship between age and likelihood of contribution does not follow a linear trend. However, our results suggest that as individuals age over 40, the probability that they will contribute to an AFP decreases with respect to the control group (those 15–29 in 1996).[15] Although this is understandable for age groups near or beyond the retirement age, it is counterintuitive for the 40–49 age group. Note that the counterintuitive result disappears when we consider contributions to *any* pension system.

As expected, household demographics affect the probability of contribution both to AFP and other systems. Each additional child a family has lowers the likelihood that individuals in that household will contribute. However, the reverse holds for the number of elderly in the household. This result may indicate that more children reduce time supplied to the labor market as a result of childcare responsibilities, while the presence of elderly relatives, who may fulfill this function, increases the number hours working-age household members will sell. Note that the test on the specification of the number of children indicates a linear specification: it might be that older siblings are not given the responsibility of caring for younger siblings or, more likely, that even if they are, this does *not* significantly effect the labor supply decision.

Living in Greater Santiago increases the likelihood of contributing to AFP but not to other pension schemes, while living in rural areas decreases that probability. This result supports the hypothesis that the transaction costs that usually accompany the provision of financial services in rural areas may be dissuading the AFP supply and worker demand alike. There also appears to be a clear link between AFP participation and contribution to the health system. The likelihood of contributing to the pension system increases as we move from the indigent and the poor up the income ladder to the less poor. Enrollment in an ISAPRE increases the probability of AFP contribution (and pension contribution generally) the most. Interestingly, those who purchase more exclusive health insurance are *less* likely to contribute.

The most significant variable in our exercise is a worker's degree of formality (as defined previously). As formality increases, it is more likely that the individual participates in the AFP system. Typically informal occupations such as the self-employed exhibit decreasing probability to contribute to an AFP, this being especially true in the agricultural and manufacturing sectors. The critical factor that is most likely driving this result in Chile is that the self-employed are *not* required to participate in the pension system. The result reflects the lower rates of contribution shown in earlier descriptive statistics. However, that the only group of workers that are not forced to participate largely chooses to participate less than salaried workers could be used as evidence to support a number of hypotheses: that agents *are* myopic,; that superior, alternative strategies of minimizing income risk in retirement prevail; or that the self-employed are less myopic and pursue alternative strategies more suitable to their needs.

The Determinants of Pension Participation in Argentina

Once again, readers must use caution in interpreting the results of our estimates (see table A13.2 in annex). The construction of the key variable, *contribution to the pension system*, in the EDS introduces a structural bias into the model. Since only private sector wage employees are asked whether they contribute to the pension system, all other occupational categories are *automatically* classified as noncontributors. Furthermore, some of the data used to construct the variables included in the Chilean estimate are unavailable in the EDS database. A further bias in the results arises from the urban sample frame employed in the EDS. As demonstrated from the estimates using data from Chile, the determinants of participation in the pension system have a significant rural/urban dimension.

These caveats notwithstanding, the results in Argentina, as in Chile, show few surprises. Education has a positive and significant sign. Individual characteristics all have the predicted signs and are significant, except for gender. As age increases, we observe increases in the probability of contribution, except, of course, for those of retirement age, 65 and older. Household demographic variables also behave as predicted. The linear specification of the number of children in the household is preferable to nonlinear specifications: the sign on the variable is both negative and significant. In Argentina, as well as Chile, a large number of children may be substituting for formal social security, while the number of elderly in the household raises the probability of contribution.

Geographically, living in the province of Buenos Aires, as opposed to other regions, has no noticeable impact on contribution. This is interesting as, to a large extent, Argentina and Chile are geographically comparable with a big metropolis for the capital and extremely distant regions. However, the metropolitan region in Chile was found significant even for the all-pension regime probit estimation. Whether information or infrastructure costs play an important role is difficult to gauge, since we have no information on rural areas in Argentina.

As in the Chilean estimate, degree of formality is the most significant determinant in our estimates, even when, due to the limitations of the EDS questionnaire, the formality index in Argentina leaves out a critical variable, the "nature of labor contract." As explained earlier, self-employment dramatically decreases the probability of observing pensions contributions, reflecting the bias in the EDS questionnaire. More interestingly, having a second occupation in addition to salaried employment (secondary self-employment) does *not* reduce but increases the probability of contribution. This result contradicts the fundamental assumption implicit in the construction of the EDS questionnaire, namely, individuals in activities other than salaried employment do not contribute to formal social security.

Finally, contributions for health are again strongly associated with contribution toward pensions, probably reflecting the tight link between Argentina's *obras sociales* and the Integrated Prestación Adicional por Permanencia (PAP)/AFJP system. The educational welfare variables and access to credit variables (the latter also a proxy: subsidized housing finance, as in Chile) were found not to be significant.

The exploratory econometric exercise has many (data) limitations, and this strongly supports the call for development of a specialized data set to permit better discrimination between alternative and complementary hypotheses for nonparticipation in a multipillar pension system. Still, despite its limitations, the exercise heavily supports the conjecture that individual/family circumstances matter for participation in a formal pension scheme, and most parameter estimates are consistent with the underlying hypotheses, particularly the following:

- The lower participation of the poor/less educated in a mandated pension scheme.
- The special situation of the self-employed—although the currently available data do not allow us to distinguish between the effects of credit constraints or differences in risk-taking behavior.
- The effect of household composition on participation and the potential influence of informal/traditional retirement strategies.
- The interaction between the pension system and access to other social programs, most importantly health coverage.

To confirm these results, to distinguish between competing explanations and, equally important, to test other hypotheses such as the impact of transaction costs and system design, more and different data are required.

Conclusion

This chapter provides a set of preliminary hypotheses to explain low rates of participation in reformed social security systems, with special emphasis on reforms in two Latin American countries and their implications. The hypotheses claim that the working poor and self-employed continue to have a specific and strong rationale for avoiding participation in the multipillar pension system and that high transactions costs, systemic and design issues, and problems of credibility negatively influence the decision to participate on the part of all members in the labor force.

Some of the established hypotheses have been subjected to exploratory econometric testing using available household survey data for Chile and Argentina. While the available data preclude testing of all the hypotheses that have been discussed, or an empirical discrimination among them, they support the conjecture that socioeconomic characteristics matter for (non) participation and that the poor, the uneducated, and the self-employed pose a special challenge to the extension of pension coverage. In addition to a more social security focused survey, comparative analysis is required to confirm the results presented in this chapter and to test those hypotheses related to the different pension institutions reforming governments have chosen to put in place. Work in this vein has already begun.

An important underlying implication of the hypotheses presented in this chapter is that rather than any fundamental flaw in the multipillar pension framework, reforms have not gone far enough toward making formal retirement security portable, flexible, and inexpensive. While these reforms may not lead to full coverage of the labor force, they should ease the problem of inadequate retirement income for an important share of the population, reduce the scope and need for noncontributory assistance, and provide important social and economic benefits beyond income security in old age.

Notes

1. The chapter has profited from many useful comments and suggestions during its preparation and from the discussion at the research conference. Special thanks go to Indermit Gill, Anita Schwarz, Charles Griffin, Estelle James, Louise Fox, Juan Yermo, P. S. Srinivas, Miguel Navarro, Olivia Mitchell, Rafael Rofman, Salvador Valdés-Prieto, John Hoddinott, and

Abigail Barr for their insights and comments. All errors are, of course, the responsibility of the authors.

2. Poverty and the Elderly: Investigations into the Effectiveness and Efficiency of Noncontributory Schemes for Old Age, World Bank project, under preparation.

3. Readers should note that a deep recession brought on by the Tequila Crisis out of Mexico shortly followed the introduction of the AFJP pillar in Argentina in 1994. The steep fall in regular contributors is likely explained by a rapid rise in unemployment, which reached 18 percent in 1995.

4. The shadow discount rate for the poor can reach 10 or more percent in real terms per annum even if the rate of time preference is merely 4 percent and the interest rate 2 percent. For a framework of distributive considerations and numeric simulations under market imperfections, see Holzmann (1984, 1990).

5. Much of the literature on time preference assumes that the rate of discount is exogenous. New theories of endogenous discount rates suggest that not only will rates of time preference fall as agents gain in optimism for the future but also that agents play an active part in increasing optimism by pursuing strategies that will increase the likelihood of higher future utility—investing *in future oriented capital* (Becker and Mulligan 1997). In a related point, households are more likely to make investments in such future-oriented capital if they have better information about what they will need to maintain (or increase) welfare when they can no longer work. Recent research shows that giving workers an estimate of their income needs in retirement can decrease myopia (Mitchell 1999).

6. Similar to policies offered in the United States, the *seguro de vida con ahorro* in Chile offers an attractive insurance/savings option. Santander's policy, Super Futuro, guarantees a market rate of return on the savings portion that will not fall below UF + 4 percent. Policyholders can insure up to a certain amount in benefits in case of death without having to undergo medical examination. Partial withdrawals can be made from the savings account after three years of paying premiums. At the legal age of retirement, the policyholder can withdraw the full balance in his or her savings. Although premiums are taxed, the returns to the savings account and withdrawals are tax-exempt (conventionally, tax-exempt-exempt, or TEE). A close study of the profile of policy buyers in Chile should be considered, since the features of the life insurance with savings policies resemble funded defined benefit/deferred annuity plans. The self-employed may be demonstrating a preference for pension plans with an absolute return guarantee over the relative return guarantee offered by the AFP system. Alternatively, they may simply value the access, however limited, to a portion of their savings. Allowing workers to withdraw a portion of their savings could imply very low balances at the time of retirement. Evidence from

Singapore suggests that workers are likely to exhaust their retirement savings if access is permitted.

7. Recent findings from labor market analysis in Brazil would complement the "contribution split/bargaining position" hypothesis. Gill and Neri (1998) find that since labor market institutions favor workers and strengthen their bargaining position in negotiating the terms of the contract, workers in the formal and the informal sector are able to take employers to court to demand coverage under any of Brazil's social security and unemployment insurance programs.

8. While the creation of a special pension-fund industry might be justified in the first few years after a reform—and it is certainly prudent to build fire walls between workers' savings and fragile financial institutions—over time these precautions should not be allowed protect an entrenched AFP market from outside competition.

9. Since the inception of the system in 1994, the Superintendencia de Administradoras de Fondos de Jubilaciones y Pensiones has noted that as the price of disability and survivors insurance premiums has fallen, AFJP commissions have remained steady.

10. In Mexico a second fund, primarily of equity holdings, is contemplated in the 1995 reform legislation but has yet to be implemented. A second fund with lower risk investments was included in the Chilean AFP system in November 1999, and a third fund of riskier, higher return investments aimed at younger affiliates and the self-employed has been proposed.

11. How risk to retirement income security is diversified post reform varies from country to country. In Chile, El Salvador, Mexico, and Peru the worker bears a greater share of financial risk. In Argentina, Uruguay, Colombia, and Bolivia, the tax-financed pillar retains a large portion of risk.

12. The "learning by observing/by doing" hypothesis presents additional motivation for an investigation of workers' economic and financial awareness.

13. In fact, while education is highly correlated with individuals' incomes, it has lower correlation with other variables.

14. This is true in Chile and across Latin America.

15. Note that individuals in the 15–29 group in 1996 are the only group that was not yet in the labor market at the time of the 1981 reform. These are the only workers who did not choose between the old PAYG and the new AFP system.

References

Note: The word *processed* describes informally reproduced works that may not be commonly available through libraries.

Alderman, H., and C. Paxson. 1992. "Do the Poor Ensure? A Synthesis of the Literature on Risk and Consumption in Developing Countries." World Bank Policy Research Paper No. 1008. Washington, D.C.

Arenas de Mesa. 1999. "Fiscal Effects of Social Security Reform in Chile: The Case of the Minimum Pension." Paper presented at the APEC Second Regional Forum on Pension Fund Reforms, Viña del Mar, Chile, April 26–27, 1999.

Auerbach, Alan, and Lawrence J. Kotlikoff. 1987. *Dynamic Fiscal Policy*. New York: Cambridge University Press.

Barr, A. M. 1998. "Enterprise Performance and the Functional Diversity of Social Capital." WPS/98-1, Center for the Study of African Economies, University of Oxford.

Becker, G., and Casey Mulligan. 1997. "The Endogenous Determination of Time Preference." *The Quarterly Journal of Economics*, August.

Cerda, Luis, and Gloria Grandolini. 1998. "The 1997 Pension Reform in Mexico." Policy Research Working Paper. World Bank, Latin America and the Caribbean Regional Office, Finance, Private Sector, and Infrastructure Unit. Washington, D.C.

CGAP (Consultative Group to Assist the Poorest). 1997a. "Introducing Savings in Microcredit Institutions: When and How?" CGAP Focus Note No. 8. CGAP. World Bank, Washington, D.C.

———. 1997b. "The Challenge of Growth for Micro-Finance Institutions: The BancoSol Experience." CGAP Focus Note No. 6. CGAP. World Bank, Washington, D.C.

Corsetti, G., and K. Schmidt-Hebbel. 1994. "An Endogenous Growth Model of Social Security and the Size of the Informal Sector." World Bank, Policy Research Department, Macroeconomic and Growth Division. Washington, D.C.

Cortazar, R. 1997. "Chile: The Evolution and Reform of the Labor Market." In S. Edwards and N. Lustig, *Labor Markets in Latin America: Combining Social Protection with Market Flexibility*. Washington, D.C.: Brookings Institute Press.

De Soto, H. 1989. *The Other Path: The Invisible Revolution in the Third World*. I. B. Tauris & Co. Ltd.

Gill, Indermit, and Marcelo Neri. 1998. "Do Labor Laws Matter? The Pressure Points in Brazilian Labor Legislation." Draft World Bank-IPEA Study.

Hoddinott, J. 1992. "Rotten Kids or Manipulative Parents: Are Children Old-Age Security in Western Kenya?" *Economic Development and Cultural Change* 40(3): 545–66.

Holzmann, Robert. 1984. "Lebenseinkommen und Verteilungsanalyse—Ein Methodischer Rahmen fuer eine Neuorientierung der Verteilung-spolitik." In Berlin and others, ed., *Studies in Contemporary Economics*. Springer.

_____. 1990. "The Welfare Effects of Public Expenditure Programs Reconsidered." International Monetary Fund (IMF) Staff Papers 37, No. 2. Washington, D.C.

_____. 1997. "Pension Reform, Financial Market Development and Economic Growth: Preliminary Evidence from Chile." *IMF Staff Papers* 44(2).

_____. 1998. "Financing the Transition to Multi-Pillar." Social Protection Discussion Paper No. 9809. World Bank, Washington, D.C.

_____. 2000. "The World Bank Approach to Pension Reform." *International Social Security Review* 53(1): 11–34.

Holzmann, Robert, and Steen Jorgensen. 1999. "Social Protection as Social Risk Management: Conceptual Underpinnings for the Social Protection Sector Strategy Paper." Social Protection Discussion Paper No. 9904. World Bank, Washington, D.C.

International Labor Organization (ILO). 1997. "Social Security for the Informal Sector: Investigating the Feasibility of Pilot Projects in Benin, India, El Salvador and Tanzania." Issues in Social Protection Discussion Paper No. 5.

_____. 1998. "Panorama Laboral: America Latina y el Caribe." Oficina Internacional del Trabajo (OIT), Ginebra.

James, E. 1999. "Coverage Under Old Age Security Systems and Protection for the Uninsured: What Are the Issues?" Presentation given at IDB conference on Social Protection. Processed.

Lucas, E .B., and O. Stark. 1985. "Motivations to Remit: Evidence from Botswana." *Journal of Political Economy* 93(5): 901–18.

Mastragelo. 1998. "La Experiencia Chilena en Materia de Cobertura." In Adolfo Rodriguez Herrera, ed., *America Latina: Seguridad Social y Exclusion.*

Mitchell, Olivia. 1999. "Building an Environment for Pension Reform in Developing Countries." Social Protection Discussion Paper No. 9803. World Bank, Washington, D.C.

Queisser, M. 1998. "The Second Generation Pension Reforms in Latin America." OECD, Development Center Studies.

SAFP (Superintendencia de Administradoras de Fondos de Pensiones). 1998. *Evolucion del Sistema Chileno de Pensiones,* No. 3 (1981–1997).

SAFJP. (Superintendencia de Administradoras de Fondos de Jubilaciones y Pensiones). 1999. El Régimen de Capitalización a Cínco Años de la Reforma Provisional. Buenos Aires.

Schmidt-Hebbel, K. 1998. "Chile's Takeoff: Facts, Challenges, Lessons." Economic Development Institute, World Bank, Washington, D.C. Processed.

Schwarz, A. 1998. "Comment to 'The Shift to a Funded Social Security System in Argentina.'" In Martin Feldstein, ed., *Privatizing Social Security.* University of Chicago Press.

———. 1999. "Taking Stock of Pension Reforms Around the World." Social Protection Discussion Paper No. 9917. World Bank, Washington, D.C.

Serrano, Carlos. 1999. "Social Security Reform, Income Distribution, Fiscal Policy and Capital Accumulation." Policy Research Working Paper No. 2055. World Bank, Latin America and Caribbean Region, Finance, Private Sector and Infrastructure Unit. Washington, D.C.

Shah, Hemant. 1997 "Towards Better Regulation of Private Pension Funds." Policy Research Working Paper No. 1791. World Bank, Latin America and the Caribbean Regional Office, Technical Dept., Advisory Group. Washington, D.C.

Srinivas, P. S., and Juan Yermo. 1999. *Do Investment Regulations Compromise Pension Fund Performance? Evidence from Latin America.* World Bank, Washington, D.C.

Stark, O. 1990. *The Migration of Labor.* Basil Blackwell.

———. 1995. *Altruism and Beyond: An Economic Analysis of Transfers and Exchanges within Families and Groups.* Cambridge University Press.

Tokman, V., ed. 1992. *Beyond Regulation: The Informal Economy in Latin America.* World Employment Program, ILO.

Torche, Aristide, and Gert Wagner. 1997. "Prevision Social: Valoracion Individual de un Beneficio Mandatado." *Cuadernos de Economia,* No. 103, PUCC.

Valdés-Prieto, S. 1998. "Las Comisiones de las AFPs: Caras o Baratas?" World Bank, Washington, D.C. Processed.

Vittas, D. 1996. "Pension Funds and Capital Markets." FSD Note No. 71, February. World Bank, Washington D.C.

World Bank. 1994. *Averting the Old Age Crisis: Policies to Protect the Old and Promote Growth.* World Bank Policy Research Report No. 13584. New York: Oxford University Press.

———. 1999. "Costa Rica: Strategy for Pension Reform." Latin America and the Caribbean Department, Country Operations Division, Washington, D.C.

Annex

Empirical Analysis of Available Household Data from Chile and Argentina and Ongoing and Future Research

This annex describes (i) the selected survey data from Chile and Argentina and discusses the limitations in the data, (ii) presents the results of tests of as many of the hypotheses outlined in section 4 as the available data will permit, and (iii) reviews ongoing and future research efforts.

Data Description and Data Limitations

From the array of household and labor surveys conducted in Chile and Argentina, we selected the 1996 CASEN and the 1997 EDS for our analysis.1 These two surveys provide for each country the latest available information required for our investigation, namely (i) data on participation in the government-mandated pension system and (ii) data on socioeconomic characteristics of individuals and households (education, occupation, and incomes) necessary to identify the factors that determine participation in formal social security.

Limitations in the data seriously constrained our empirical work. First, neither of the surveys chosen have pensions or social insurance as their primary or secondary focus. Rather, the surveys are intended to assess the accessibility, coverage, and targeting of social assistance programs. Second, and more importantly, the surveys are not uniform in breadth or depth and, thus, the results cannot be compared. While the Chilean survey—the CASEN—reports on the affiliation and contribution to social security of all individuals in the active labor force regardless of sector (private or public) and occupation status (employees, employer, self-employed), the survey for Argentina, the EDS, asks *only* private sector employees whether or not they contribute to a pension system (that is, whether contributions are deducted from their salaries for retirement schemes). Furthermore, the CASEN survey specifies to which regime (AFP, SSS, CAPREDENA, etc.) within the social security system a worker is affiliated and regularly contributes, while the EDS survey does not specify the particular plan (AFJP, PAP) to which a worker in Argentina contributes.

While the responses of the self-employed in Chile reveal important information on the demand for public pensions and the motivations to contribute, the failure of the EDS, as well as of Argentina's *Encuesta Permanente de Hogares* (EPH), to question the self-employed on their participation in government-mandated social security is particularly surprising since the self-employed are required to contribute in Argentina. This omission in the data from Argentina not only ignores a critical and frequently unprotected sector of the economy but also introduces to our results a serious structural bias.

Methodology and Results

We propose a simple methodology to test the hypotheses outlined in section four—the estimation of probits on participation in the formal pension system (defined via regular contribution). This method evaluates the significance, positive or negative influence, and impact that a number of explanatory variables have on the probability that a specific event will be observed. For our purposes, the event is specified as contribution to the (AFP or any) pension system by individuals of working age. While the available data allow differentiation between analysis of participation in the funded versus the PAYG systems in Chile for which two probits are estimated, the dependent variable for our probit on Argentina is "contribution to a pension system."

The main results are presented in table A13.1 (Chile) and table A13.2 (Argentina).

Ongoing and Future Research

This section describes ongoing research on the barriers to participation in reformed pension systems. These efforts include a comparative study linking coverage under the reformed pension systems of Chile and Argentina and social risk management and an evaluation of coverage expansion policies in other Latin American countries that have reformed social security.

Table A13.1. Chile: Results from Probits on CASEN 1996 Data

Dependent variable	Contribution to AFP			Contribution toward any pension system			mean (x)
	Coefficient	z-value	Elasticity	Coefficient	z-value	Elasticity	
Individual characteristics							
Years of school	0.0031	2.25[a]	0.039	0.0069	4.88	0.076	7.35
Female dummy	-0.05	-2.67	-0.043	-0.064	-3.37	-0.051	0.512
Marital status reference							
Single							
Married	0.221	11.01	0.214	0.276	13.72	0.239	0.568
Married female dummy	-0.561	-20.63	-0.271	-0.665	-23.85	-0.291	0.28
Age groups:							
15–29	reference						
30–39	0.109	6.44	0.04	0.15	8.6	0.049	0.218
40–49	-0.109	-5.37	-0.026	0.092	4.5	0.022	0.156
50–59	-0.384	-15.02	-0.073	-0.004	-0.17[b]	-0.0007	0.112
60–65	-0.781	-16.58	-0.074	-0.241	-5.78	-0.021	0.056
65–plus	-1.189	-17.32	-0.196	-0.602	-12.22	-0.09	0.097
Household characteristics							
Number of children	-0.012	-2.1[a]	-0.024	-0.03	-5.21	-0.056	1.2
Number of aged	0.05	4.12	0.04	0.028	2.36[a]	0.021	0.48
Santiago dummy	0.039	2.57	0.015	0.036	2.26[a]	0.012	0.233
Rural dummy	-0.056	-3.43	-0.025	-0.092	-5.48	-0.037	0.263
Welfare variables							
Contributions to health system							
Public system							
Fonasa categories A, B	reference						
Fonasa categories C, D	0.587	35.18	0.18	0.548	32.61	0.151	0.179
Private Systems:							
ISAPRES	0.808	45.83	0.232	0.655	36.39	0.17	0.169
Other private systems	-0.48	-17.81	-0.098	-0.694	-24.62	-0.129	0.121
Private education household	-0.038	-1.69[b]	-0.005	-0.017	-0.443[b]	-0.0013	0.081
Dummy:							
Labor characteristics							
Labor status (formality index)	0.443	123.55	1.719	0.484	114.15	1.711	2.29
Agricultural self-employed dummy	-0.193	-4.99	-0.012	-0.074	-2.26[a]	-0.004	0.038
Manufacture self-employed dummy	-0.763	-6.832	-0.013	-0.661	-6.39	-0.011	0.01
Service self-employed dummy	0.216	2.01[a]		0.0008	0.95[b]	0.105	0.002

(Table continues on next page)

Table A13.1 continued

Dependent variable	Contribution to AFP			Contribution toward any pension system			mean (x)
	Coefficient	z-value	Elasticity	Coefficient	z-value	Elasticity	
Financial variables							
Financial income household dummy	−0.063	−4.27	−0.013	−0.034	−2.282[a]	−0.004	0.532
Public housing credit access dummy	0.011	0.02[b]	0.001	0.097	3.71	0.01	0.07
Constant	−2.136	−89.53		−2.15	−85.51		
Number of observations	95337 (23)	26845.9		95337 (23)	24364.1		
Wald Chi2 (n–d · freedom)							
Log likelihood	−23521.1			−22244.1			
Test on linearity of number of children:							
Chi2(1)	0.67				1.62		
Prob > Chi	20.412				0.203		

Note: Wald statistic tests the significance of the model. The null hypothesis on the test for linearity of "number of children" is the linear specification.
a. Indicates variable is not significant at the 99 percent confidence level, but is significant up to 95 percent.
b. Indicates variable is significant at confidence levels lower than 95 percent.
Source: Authors' calculations.

Table A13.2. Argentina: Results from Probits on EDS 1997 Data

Dependent variable	Contributions to a pension system			Mean (x)
	Coefficient	z–value	elasticity	
Individual characteristics				
Years of school	0.021	2.51	0.467	10.22
Female dummy	−0.098	−1.23[b]	−0.107	0.492
Marital status				
Single	reference			
Married	0.974	8.62	0.309	0.141
Married female dummy	−1.019	−6.86	−0.018	0.081
Age groups:				
15–29	reference			
30–39	0.648	3.95	0.042	0.029
40–49	1.239	8.54	0.061	0.022
50–59	0.861	6.1	0.058	0.03
60–65	0.633	3.04	0.011	0.009
65–plus	−1.302	−4.66	−0.035	0.012

(Table continued on next page)

Table A13.2 continued

| | Contributions to a pension system | | | |
Dependent variable	Coefficient	z–value	elasticity	Mean (x)
Household characteristics				
Number of children	–0.139	–4.21	–0.291	0.93
Number of aged	0.136	2.24[a]	0.061	0.201
Buenos Aires dummy	0.061	0.99[b]	0.063	0.46
Welfare variables				
Contributions to health system dummy	0.478	6.9	0.198	0.187
Private education household dummy	–0.034	–0.391[b]	–0.020	0.256
Labor characteristics				
Labor status (formality index)	0.365	25.59	0.892	1.115
Workers with secondary occupations other than waged, dummy	0.703	2.08	0.002	0.001
Self–employed dummy	–3.002	–10.07	–0.262	0.039
Financial variables				
Financial income household dummy	n.a.	–0.126	–0.029	0.105
Public housing credit access dummy	–1.33[a]			
Constant	–2.371	–22.34		
Number of observations	14045			
Wald Chi2(n–d.freedom)	1276.7 (18)			
Log likelihood	–2645.7			
Pseudo–R2	0.438			
Test on linearity of number of children:				
Chi2(1)	0.61			
Prob > Chi2	0.435			

n.a. Not applicable.
a. Indicates variable is not significant at the 99 percent confidence level, but is significant up to 95 percent.
b. Indicates variable is significant at confidence levels lower than 95 percent.
Source: Authors' calculations.

Comparison of Coverage and Household Social Risk Management in Chile and Argentina

Although this chapter makes a first attempt at explicative analysis for low rates of participation in reformed pension systems in Chile and Argentina, limitations of the data currently available severely constrain the depth of investigation. However, the contrasting political and economic environments under which social security reform was undertaken, the varying depth of reforms, and the differences in the formal pensions institutions that were adopted in Chile and Argentina provide an excellent opportunity for rich, comparative analysis. A comparative approach to the study of coverage and household social risk management will allow for the isolation of the impact of important structural differences between the two reformed pension systems on the decision to participate (as hypothesized above).

Of particular importance to the examination of household participation and coverage will be (i) contrasts in the role of government in each of the reformed systems, (ii) the structure of government guarantees, (iii) the finance of transition costs, (iv) centralized versus decentralized collection systems, and (v) treatment of the self-employed under the two regimes— voluntary versus compulsory participation in the reformed systems—and the effect, if any, mandated participation has had on the extent of coverage.[2] A *Social Risk Management Survey* (SRMS)—focused on risks to income in old age and combining elements of labor, household, consumption, and expenditure surveys—will be conducted in Chile and Argentina to gather data on household awareness of the reformed systems, preferences for alternative retirement security investments, financial literacy, access to credit, perceptions of mortality, and contingent risk-coping strategies.

The Effectiveness of Government Interventions to Increase Coverage

Several governments that have adopted the multipillar pension framework have included special features and mechanisms in their reforms to "graduate" workers into regularly contributing to a second-pillar account. The efficiency of these programs has yet to be formally assessed or their impact on coverage to be measured. Some of the programs that should be evaluated include the following:

- *The social quota in Mexico.* Private sector workers in Mexico began to affiliate with pension fund managers in February 1997. By December 1997, most privately employed formal-sector workers (96 percent) formerly covered under the public PAYG system had elected a private fund manager to invest their retirement savings. Partly as an incentive for workers to affiliate with the new system, the government deposits pesos of US$1 per day into the retirement accounts of contributors, indexed to the consumer price index and estimated to be between 1 and 5.5 percent of worker salary, depending on the workers' incomes. On average, the social quota will be equivalent to 2.2 percent of wages (Cerda and Grandolini 1998). The pension authorities have yet to report on the impact the social quota has had in terms of new affiliates to the formal pension system.
- *Second-pillar account subsidies in Colombia.* Colombia introduced a new pension system of privately managed accounts in 1994. The government

has experimented with a targeted program that subsidizes contributions into the second-pillar retirement accounts for informal-sector workers. The subsidy is meant to integrate the informally employed into the formal system. Formal-sector workers earning more than four minimum wages contribute an additional 1 percent of their income that, along with matching transfers from the government, makes up a publicly managed Solidarity Fund. Revenue from this fund is used to subsidize the participation of lower-income workers. Because the subsidy is targeted to certain areas, however, it not universal to poorer workers (Queisser 1998).

- *Subsidized second-pillar participation in Uruguay.* In Uruguay, participation in each pillar of the reformed pension system is determined by a worker's level of income. Authorities have reported a rise in participation in the national pension system since the government undertook a structural reform of social security in 1996. The Uruguayan government attributes this rise not only to the correction of perverse incentives that prevailed under the old PAYG scheme, but also to the option afforded to workers whose income falls below a certain threshold[3] to split their pension contributions between the remaining PAYG pillar and their individual retirement accounts. To encourage the participation of lower-income workers, reform legislation allows workers earning less than 5,000 pesos per month to contribute up to half of their mandatory 7.5 percent PAYG contribution (3.75 percent) into an individual retirement account. The government absorbs this loss of revenue to the first pillar as an explicit subsidy.

An evaluation of each specific intervention, along with an overview of policies applied to increase social security coverage in developed economies, would form a core of "best practice" that currently does not exist.

Overview of SRMS/PRIESO Questionnaire—Chile

This section provides an overall description of the Social Risk Management Survey, or SRMS (*Encuesta de Prevision de Riesgos Sociales – PRIESO*), piloted in Santiago, Chile, in the fall of 1999. The SRMS combines elements of labor, household, consumption, and expenditure surveys and will additionally gather data on household awareness of the reformed pension system, preferences for alternative retirement security investments, financial literacy, access to credit, perceptions of mortality, and contingent risk-coping strategies. The survey is intended to overcome the limitations of currently available household data.

The SRMS is structured to identify and evaluate the strategies taken by individuals—and by groups of individuals in the household—in the face of a series of risks to income. The survey emphasizes those risks that affect the individual and, by extension, his or her household. The questionnaire explores both institutional strategies as well as informal or traditional strategies taken by households in the face of income risks arising from the inability to work in old age, disability, work accident, and the death of an income-earning spouse.

The survey focuses principally on the Chilean pension system, specifically the motivations of working-age individuals when they decide to contribute or not to contribute to an individual retirement account. Following a set of introductory questions in Module I meant to identify characteristics of individuals and the composition of the household to which they belong, Module II of the SRMS, Risk Recall and Perception, constructs a history of past and present shocks to income and measures the expectation of future risks that can influence the decision to undertake risk-minimizing strategies. Module III, Evaluation of the Pension System, examines the knowledge and attitudes of both covered (contributing) and noncovered workers toward the pension system.

The remaining three modules seek to map the set of alternative strategies to participation in the formal social security system. These alternative strategies have been divided into three broad categories: Financial Strategies (Module IV), strategies that rely on Intra- and Interhousehold relationships (Module V), and, finally, strategies related to the Labor Market (Module VI). The survey seeks to identify, evaluate, and quantify (i) the relevance of inter- and intrahousehold transfers to the decision to participate in the formal pension system, (ii) access to credit and personal savings—either complementary to or substitute for an AFP account, and (iii) variations in the household's supply of labor as a countercyclical risk-coping mechanism. At the end of Module V, a series of questions are asked to measure respondents' economic and financial awareness. These questions cover knowledge of basic economic indicators like the inflation rate and the rate of unemployment, as well as more sophisticated indicators such as the level of the stock market index. The data arising from these questions will allow researchers to test the extent to which economic and financial awareness differs between contributing and noncontributing workers.

The SRMS will be conducted on a sample of 2,500 respondents of working age (14 years and older) from the Santiago metropolitan area (including peripheral rural areas), drawn from the sample frame of the 1998 CASEN survey. Relative weights will be assigned to maintain statistical representation by labor market status (employed/unemployed), occupation (dependent worker/employer/self-employed), gender (male/female), and location (urban/rural). The selection of the respondent in each household will be random and unrelated to that individual's relation to the household head.

The full questionnaire is available on the World Wide Web at *http://www.worldbank.org/sp*, and readers are encouraged to review the survey, in English or Spanish, and to provide comments to the authors.

Notes

1. Social Development Survey (Encuesta de Desarrollo Social, or EDS), 1997, and the National Socioeconomic Characterization Survey (Encuesta de Caracterizacion Socieconomica Nacional, or CASEN), 1996.

2. To illustrate, to the extent to which the self-employed voluntarily affiliate with a Chilean AFP, the significance of income level, occupation, and a number of household factors on the decision to participate can be examined.

3. Workers earning the average wage in Uruguay can qualify for the contribution split.